Botulinum Toxin for Facial Harmony

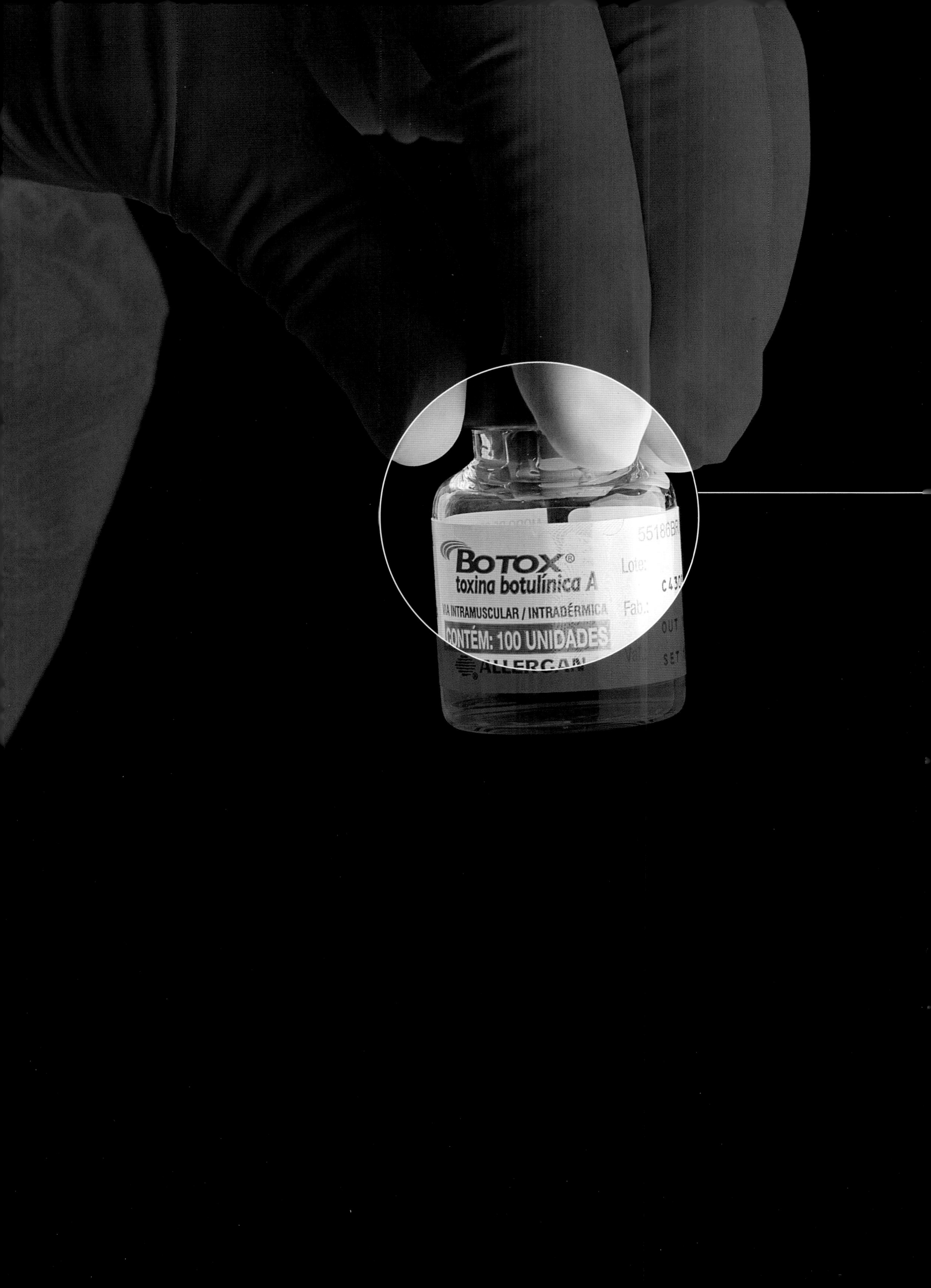
55186BR
BOTOX®
toxina botulínica A
VIA INTRAMUSCULAR / INTRADÉRMICA
CONTÉM: 100 UNIDADES
ALLERGAN
Lote:
Fab.:

Acknowledgments

I would like to express my gratitude to Dr Paulo Vinícius Soares for the idea and encouragement to write this book. It is an honor to be trusted by this great professional. I am also grateful and have great respect for Bill Hartman, Leah Huffman, Bryn Grisham, Sue Robinson, Sue Zubek, and the entire Quintessence crew involved in giving life to this book. You amaze me with your work. My special thanks to Dr Rubelisa Cândido Gomes de Oliveira for assisting us with the scientific format of this book. Your organization is deeply appreciated. My dear Denise Riley, I am so grateful for the uncountable hours spent on finding the right terms for my books. You are like a sister to me. I wish to thank my secretary, Carina Morais, for her perfectionism and unselfish friendship. I also would like to thank my friends at the Miami Anatomical Research Center—Allan Weinstein, Eduardo Sadao, Heloise Peixoto, Justin Fraioli, Jorge Carrasco, and Maylin Perez Carrasco—for their effort in keeping up with our courses that help educate so many professionals. I wish to acknowledge my first supporter, Dr Francisco Leite Pinto, as well as my friend Dr Newton Fahl Jr, who taught me the meaning of "possessing the knowledge." To my friend Dr Fernando Saad, thanks for your true friendship and for the "true vertical line." Dr Francisco Célio Dantas, thank you so much for all those years as a partner in our mission to educate. Dr Maria Geovânia Ferreira, even after 20 years of partnership your competence still surprises me. Dear anatomists Márcia Viotti and Rogério Zambonato, you amaze all students with your skillful dissections. Congratulations! Thank you, Alberto Van Lima, for spending so many nights working hard to produce such beautiful images all these years. I also would like to express my gratitude to Professor Luis Fernando Naldi for our discussions about esthetic facial references. My grateful thanks to Professor Paula Cardoso and Rafael Decurcio for their noble work at ABO in Goiás. I would like to sincerely thank Rafael Araújo Câmara for his support. Thanks also go to my colleagues from SBOE and SBTI for all the knowledge I have received from you. I greatly respect these two associations. My greatest respect and gratitude goes to all those who have selflessly given their precious bodies to science. To my dear patients who allowed me to use their photos and clinical history to improve the knowledge of so many health professionals through this book, I cannot thank you enough. I would also like to acknowledge the important role of so many teachers I have had throughout my lifetime. I will always carry with me your teachings. Finally, my eternal gratitude to the greatest teacher of all, Jesus, for the daily blessings.

contents

Extra content
Extra content is available online. QR codes throughout the book link to PDFs, PowerPoint presentations, and videos that can be used by the professional to facilitate better treatment planning and delivery of care. Scan the QR code here to access this supplementary information. The full list of links may also be found at www.quintpub.com/BTX.

Foreword

Esthetics should be considered part of dentistry as a whole instead of just a specialty. Regardless of our expertise, a common goal in dentistry will always be to integrate, preserve, or recreate function, biology, structure, and esthetics. Therefore, there is no dentistry without esthetics and no facial esthetics without dentistry.

As the well-known plastic surgeon Ivo Pitanguy once said, "Before performing facial plastic surgeries, we should first take care of the smile." A smile works as a postcard of ourselves, a universal expression unique to human beings. Consequently, esthetics has an essential role as a means to generate self-esteem, confidence, well-being, and joy.

In order to be able to produce esthetic smiles, we first should understand the face itself. All professionals who work with smile rehabilitation should be experts on the face. We have noticed a lack of facial knowledge by dentists as well as a lack of knowledge of smiles by plastic surgeons. This gap should not exist. The integration of these two worlds will transform the way we impact people's lives by modifying their facial expressions.

Patients who need or want more confident smiles deserve a complete orofacial analysis that should be made by a team of professionals with extensive knowledge in areas that include orthognathics, orthodontics, orthopedics, total prosthesis, cephalometry, dentogingival esthetics, airways, occlusion, perioral procedures, dermatology, and plastic surgery procedures. Instead of elaborating esthetically perfect projects, it is essential to obtain harmonious results that will meet the morphopsychologic desires of our patients.

Being an orofacial expert involves more art than math—an art that produces predictable results through the detailed study of facial anatomy and clinical practice of the procedures. This explains why I became a fan of Altamiro, a pioneer and artist of orofacial esthetics. In my point of view, this book will become a reference on this topic due to the great skill of the author in organizing and expressing his ideas, his vast clinical experience, his wonderful results achieved, and his educational method used to gather all of his knowledge. Without a doubt, this masterpiece will help all dentists who wish to go beyond their current scope. For all these reasons, it is a great honor to introduce this book. Best wishes and good luck in this journey.

Christian Coachman, DDS, CDT
Founder of Digital Smile Design

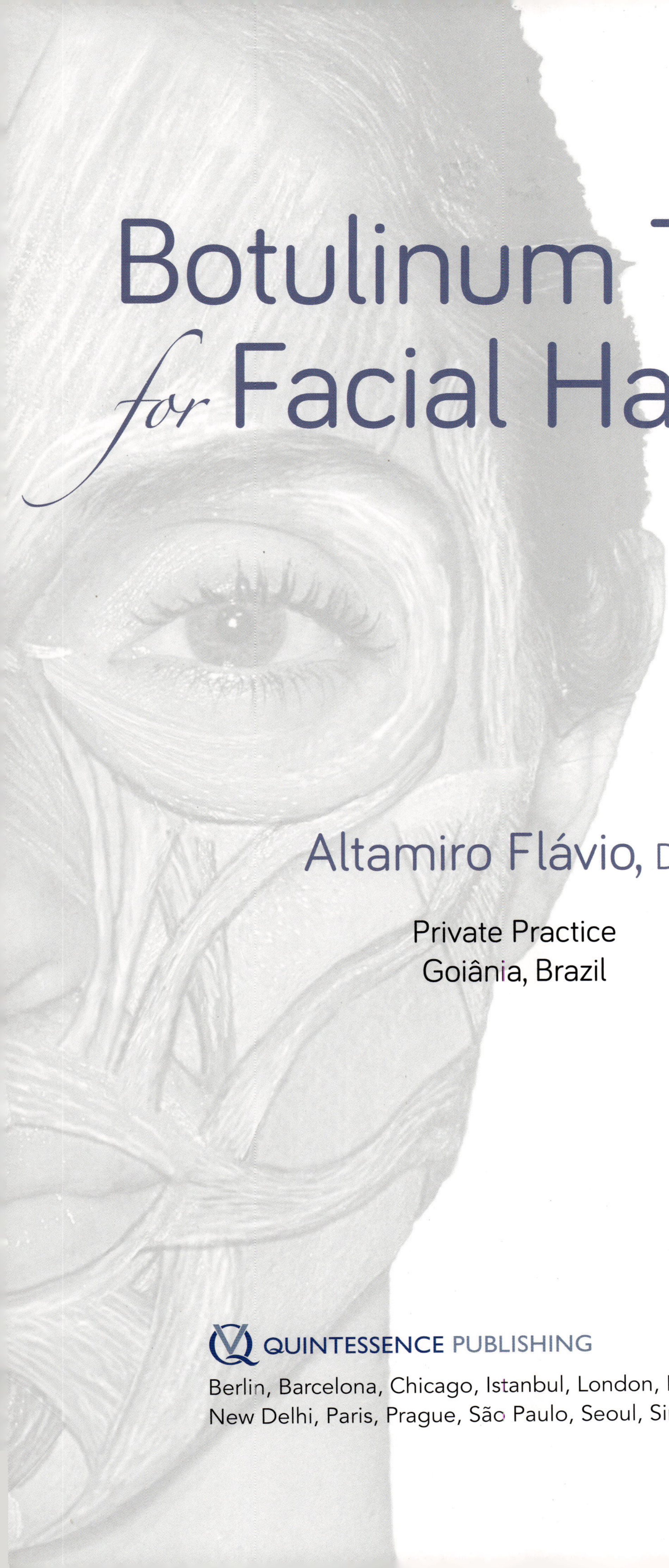

Botulinum Toxin *for* Facial Harmony

Altamiro Flávio, DDS

Private Practice
Goiânia, Brazil

QUINTESSENCE PUBLISHING

Berlin, Barcelona, Chicago, Istanbul, London, Milan, Moscow,
New Delhi, Paris, Prague, São Paulo, Seoul, Singapore, Tokyo, Warsaw

Dedication

This book is dedicated to my parents, who with their example of life and love showed me the path that I now teach my children. I would have loved to be able to show you this book. To my brother, Antônio Eugênio Pacheco, a nature lover and the master of overcoming life's difficulties. To my sister, Marya Olimpia Pacheco, who has found the balance between strength and tenderness and is the most ethical person I have ever met. To my beloved wife, Cláudia Bittar, for her hard work and dedication that keeps our family united. To my beloved children—Gabriel Pacheco, my best friend, and Ana Sofia Pacheco, my turning point for happiness—for all the joy they have given me.

Library of Congress Cataloging-in-Publication Data

Names: Flávio, Altamiro, author.
Title: Botulinum toxin for facial harmony / Altamiro Flávio.
Description: Hanover Park, IL : Quintessence Publishing Co Inc, [2018] | Includes bibliographical references and index.
Identifiers: LCCN 2018011314 | ISBN 9780867157871 (hardcover)
Subjects: | MESH: Botulinum Toxins, Type A--therapeutic use | Cosmetic Techniques | Facial Muscles--drug effects | Case Reports
Classification: LCC RL120.B66 | NLM QV 140 | DDC 615.7/78--dc23
LC record available at https://lccn.loc.gov/2018011314

QUINTESSENCE PUBLISHING USA

Quintessence Publishing Co, Inc
411 N Raddant Road
Batavia, IL 60510
www.quintpub.com

5 4 3 2 1

Editor: Leah Huffman
Design: Sue Zubek
Production: Sue Robinson

Printed in China

preface

Throughout these 25 years working as a teacher, sometimes I catch myself rereading old educational materials, and I find that the only knowledge we keep is that which we use in our daily practice. This book was based on this concept. All information provided has clinical applicability. When you are 50 years old, it is only natural to start evaluating what is really worthwhile in life. My goal was to write an objective book that could effectively guide professionals who want to provide the different benefits of botulinum toxin to their patients. Even before thinking about treating a patient, we as professionals must concentrate on not causing any injury, so I chose to describe the limits and risks of the most delicate procedures. Science has several theories, some feasible and others not so much. This fact has always confused readers of scientific works. Therefore, I was cautious enough to prove several of the contents in the book through numerous clinical cases, carefully retreated and described in an objective way.

My students often complain that botulinum toxin treatments only last 5 months. When they do this, I ask them to name one type of antibiotic, anti-inflammatory, anesthetic, or antidepressant that has an effect that lasts as long. In fact, the duration time is one of the greatest advantages of the toxin. I see these complaints as an acknowledgment of the toxin's benefits and a subconscious desire for the effect to last longer.

Other students ask themselves why God in his infinite perfection did not allow all human beings to be beautiful. I posit that perhaps this was on purpose so we as humans can develop the skill to love others regardless of their outward appearance. Nonetheless, it is the professional's responsibility to study hard to offer health and esthetics to his or her patients.

I get excited when I see the final results of treatment in my daily practice. This professional accomplishment is a great reward. I rarely have patients who are not secure enough to accept the esthetic procedures. While they understand that aging is a natural part of life, they do not want changes to their face, so these esthetic procedures allow them to maintain their appearance a little longer.

Finally, during the course of reading this book, the reader will find a lot of numbers; these numbers help us to find the correct dimensions and proportions. Because each face has different measurements, we need numbers and proportions to provide specific treatments. It is part of my philosophy to create "one smile for each face."

God bless you all. And please enjoy the reading.

Foreword

The challenge of our generation is to look young and youthful for the longest time possible. Botulinum toxin (BTX) is useful in the treatment of many diseases. Dental clinicians are experts on the head and neck area and have a deep comprehension of the anatomy and physiology of the muscles of the face. BTX has been applied in conjunction with hyaluronic acids for the treatment of facial asymmetry, temporomandibular disorders and facial pain, bruxism and clenching, and age-related or other esthetic concerns. The clinical application of BTX can help to control parafunctional habits, improve facial esthetics, and altogether change patients' quality of life.

It is my pleasure to introduce this book written by my mentor on this subject, Dr Altamiro Flávio. The book is divided between the fundamental concepts of BTX application and protocols to use in various clinical situations. This handbook is designed to be a practical introductory and reference guide for students, clinicians, and researchers. The author has gathered the necessary knowledge, clinical fundamentals, scientific evidence, and technical skills and protocols to write the constituent chapters.

I hope you enjoy this book and can achieve success with BTX application in your patients.

Paulo V. Soares, DDS, MS, PhD
School of Dentistry
Federal University of Uberlândia, Brazil

CHAPTER 01

Basic Principles of Botulinum Toxin

Box 1-1 Serotypes of BTX

A, B, C1, C2, D, E, F, G, H, and I
A and B have different clinical uses.
C, E, and F are used experimentally.

Box 1-2 Characteristics of BTX-A and BTX-B

A	B
Broad range of indications	Shorter duration of effect
Used in different countries	Therapeutic use
Well-described in the literature	Increased pain when injected
Marketed as Botox (onabotulinumtoxinA, Allergan), Dysport (abobotulinumtoxinA, Ipsen), and Xeomin (incobotulinumtoxinA, Merz)	Marketed as Myobloc (rimabotulinumtoxinB, Solstice Neurosciences) and NeuroBloc (no FDA license, Eisai)

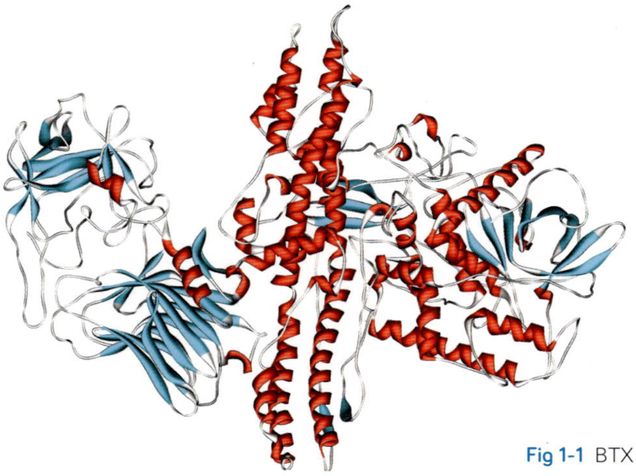

Fig 1-1 BTX neurotoxic protein.

Botulinum toxin (BTX) is a biologic agent manufactured in a laboratory in the form of a crystalline stable substance, freeze-dried in human albumin, and supplied in a sterile, vacuum-dried vial to be reconstituted in a saline solution. It is naturally produced by *Clostridium botulinum*, a gram-positive anaerobic bacterium that produces several distinct serotypes of BTX (Box 1-1).[1–3] In terms of cosmeceutical therapy, type A is the only one that shows a clinically important biologic activity, and hence it is the most often studied and used serotype of BTX.[4] Type B is also commercially available to treat cervical dystonia and for patients resistant to BTX-A,[5–8] but it is generally associated with a higher incidence of pain when injected and a short-lasting effect, although it has a faster onset than type A[9–13] (Box 1-2).

BTX is an organic macromolecule made up of amino acids linked together by peptide bonds (polypeptide chains). Biochemically it consists of a 50-kDa light chain and a 100-kDa heavy chain (Fig 1-1) connected by protease-sensitive disulfide bridges; the bond of these chains results in a

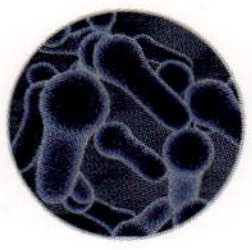

Fig 1-2 Timeline of BTX discovery.

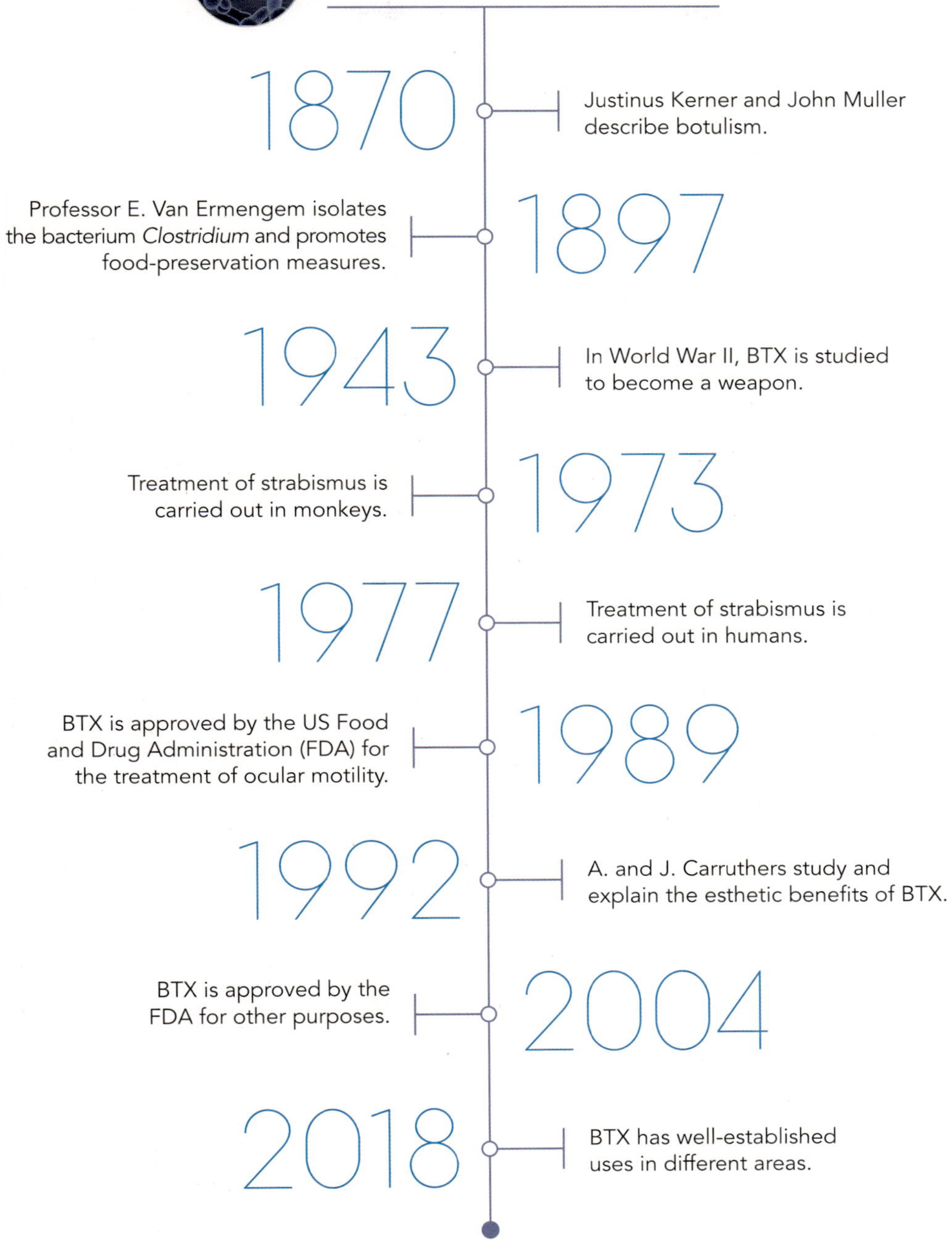

150-kDa protein.[14,15] This toxin is protected by larger nontoxic proteins and by hemagglutinin. The final weight of these multimeric complexes varies from 700 kDa for BTX-B to 900 kDa for BTX-A, reflecting the weight of the surface proteins that form such protection.[1,2,16,17]

Figure 1-2 illustrates a brief history of the discovery and scientific developments surrounding BTX.

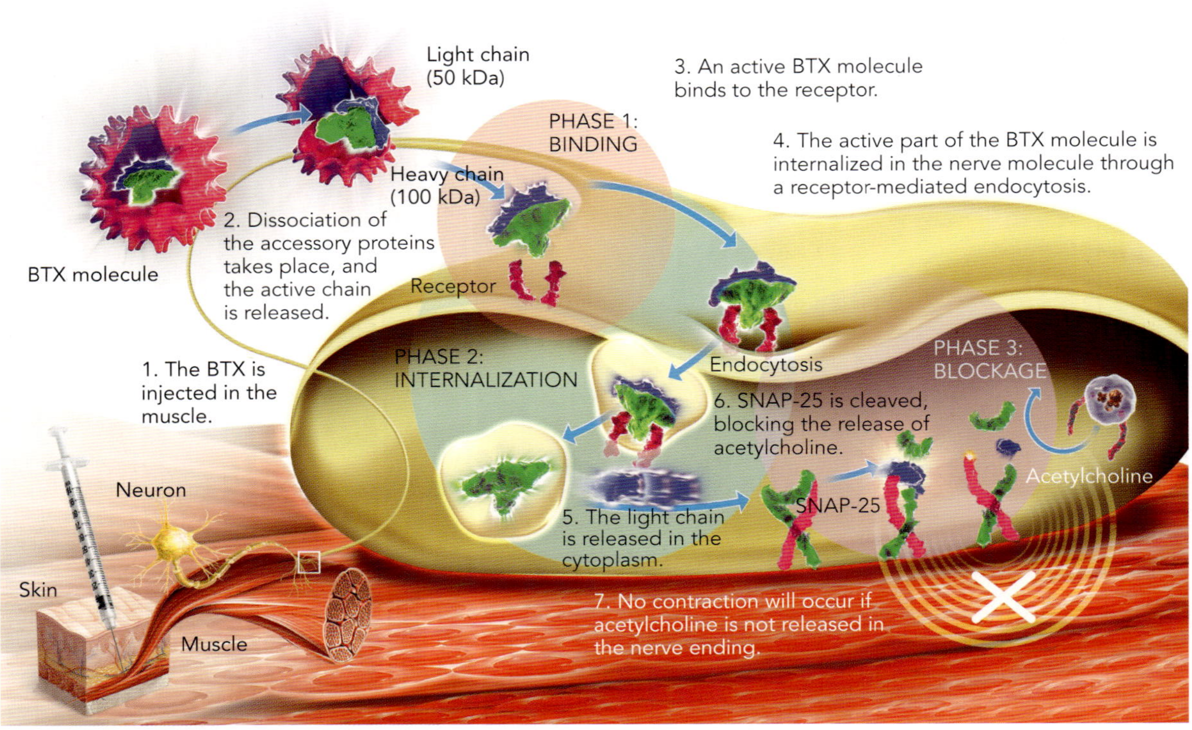

Fig 1-3 Mechanism of action of BTX.

Mechanism of Action of BTX

BTX-A should be injected in the muscle so that it disperses and diffuses to cholinergic nerve endings, where its mechanism of action takes place. BTX essentially breaks down fusion proteins (synaptosomal-associated protein 25 [SNAP-25]) responsible for the release of the neurotransmitter acetylcholine (ACh), thereby inhibiting muscle contraction in the fibers that receive the BTX injection.[16–20] Figure 1-3 shows a detailed illustration of this process, as outlined below.

Once injected, BTX dissociates from the accessory proteins through the action of proteases. Immediately afterward, it is irreversibly bound to high-affinity specific receptors in the neuromuscular junction (NMJ). This is phase 1: binding.

Once the BTX molecule is bound to the receptor at the nerve cell membrane surface, the heavy chain allows the toxin to enter the cell through a membrane invagination, resulting in the formation of a vesicle that will surround the two chains of BTX. This process takes 20 minutes and is called *receptor-mediated endocytosis*. This is phase 2: internalization.

The light chain is then separated from the heavy chain by the dissociation of disulfide bridges through the action of proteases. Under an acidification condition, it is released from the vesicle to the neuronal cytoplasm. Once at the cytosol, the light chain performs its metalloproteinase activity at the intracellular targets that regulate the exocytosis of ACh vesicles. Such targets are part of the SNARE complex (soluble N-ethylmaleimide-sensitive factor attachment receptor) responsible for the binding and coupling of ACh vesicles. This complex is formed by the fusion of three proteins: SNAP-25, VAMP (vesicle-associated membrane protein), and syntaxin 1a.

The light chain of BTX-A, through a zinc-dependent endopeptidase and under an acidic pH, cleaves SNAP-25. (VAMP is cleaved by BTX-B, -D, and -F, and syntaxin 1a is cleaved by BTX-C.) This cleavage prevents the release of the neurotransmitter ACh. This is phase 3: blockage or proteolytic cleavage.

By inhibiting release of ACh from synaptic vesicles, BTX chemically denervates muscles and glands; this process is known as *chemodenervation*. This mechanism is specific to BTX-A and has wide clinical applications, including the modulation of muscle contraction, whose effect is clinically observed for 3 to 4 months. It may also be used to reduce hyperhidrosis for up to 12 months and excessive salivation for up to 6 months.

Box 1-3 **Onset and duration of action of BTX**

Onset of effects: 6 hours

Onset of clinical results: 24–72 hours

Final stabilization of its clinical action: Up to 14 days

Duration of effect on muscles: 2 weeks to 6 months

Duration of effect on salivation: Up to 6 months

Duration of effect on hyperhidrosis: Up to 12 months

Action of BTX

The physiologic response to BTX injection is observed 6 hours after its administration, and clinical results are seen within 24 to 72 hours after the procedure.[21] While clinical paralysis is observed 24 hours after the injection, the peak of the paralytic effect occurs 14 days later. Depending on individual factors such as doses and postblockage instructions, induced blockage by BTX can last from 2 weeks to 6 months[22] (Box 1-3).

Once BTX is administered, the toxin response is irreversible during the period of time described above. However, eventually the effect is reversed. There are two hypotheses for the reversibility of the BTX effect:

1. Axonal sprouting and muscle reinnervation occur; that is, a new NMJ is formed.
2. Regeneration occurs at the same NMJ altered by the application of BTX.[23]

Subsequently, new SNARE complexes form, thereby preventing the toxin from causing any other effect on the patient.

The duration of BTX-induced blockade, varying from weeks to months, vastly exceeds the recovery time of the action targets of the neurotoxin, which suggests that other intracellular actions are involved in the persistence of its effects. Furthermore, the duration as well as the blocking efficacy is dependent on the doses and formulations of the used serotypes.[22] While the different biochemical cellular events that serve as a basis for this variance are unknown, many factors may contribute:

- Light chain lifetime inside the cytosol
- Turnover (protein renewal) of target SNARE proteins (VAMP, SNAP-25, and syntaxin 1a)
- Secondary biochemical events related to SNARE production and/or peptide release

The metabolic pathway has not been properly documented; however, it may be explained by the presence of proteases that lead to a degradation proteolysis of polypeptide chains present in the molecule.[2]

Biosafety

The toxin biosafety is evidenced by its selective action in the peripheral cholinergic nerve ending inhibiting ACh release. It does not pass the brain barrier or inhibit the release of ACh or any other neurotransmitter in this level. The toxin does not bind to nerve fibers of nerve stems or the postsynaptic region.[2]

Within the muscle, the amount of BTX administered is reduced to about half within approximately 10 hours. Within the 24 hours postinjection, 60% of the substance is excreted through urine.[2]

The Neuromuscular Histology

It is important to review the histology of muscle tissues before using BTX (Fig 1-4).

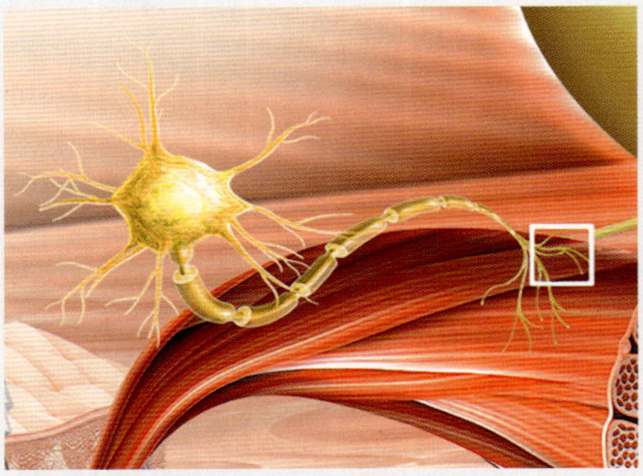

Neuromuscular junction The effects of BTX are especially intense on the hyperkinetic muscles because of the superior number of nicotinic acetylcholine receptors contained therein.

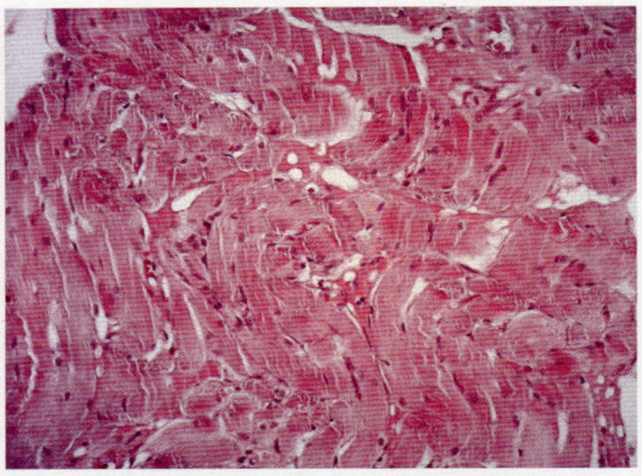

Muscle tissue It is composed of long, multinucleated cells specialized for contractions. Its cytoplasm contains great amounts of contractile protein filaments, primarily actin and myosin. It is a highly vascularized and innervated tissue.

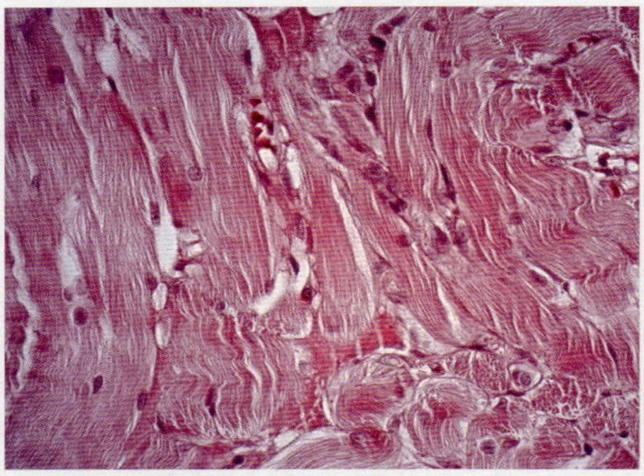

Skeletal muscle Representing most of the muscles in the human body, it is attached to the human skeleton via tendons and is responsible for the performance of various movements, such as walking, running, and holding or manipulating objects.

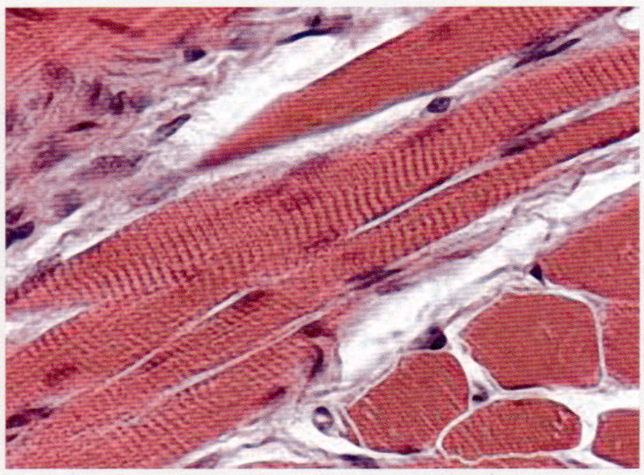

Cardiac muscle Only found in the heart, it has long, cylindric, and striated cells with ramifications. These ramifications connect one cell to another through a structure permeable to an electric impulse called the *intercalated disc*. This disc makes the contraction of the cardiac muscle uniform.

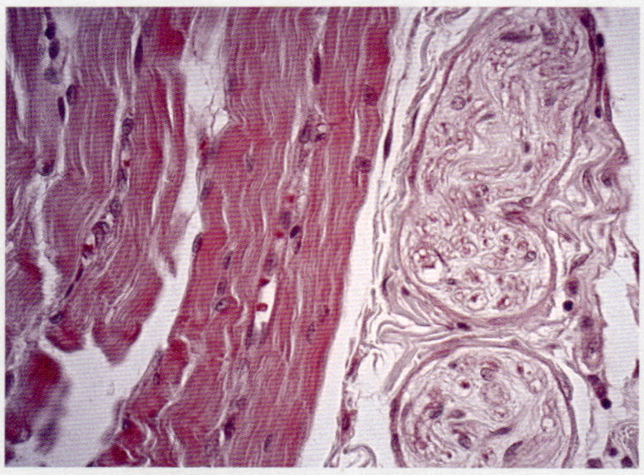

Smooth muscle Found in internal organs such as the intestine, bladder, and uterus, it is responsible for movement characteristics such as peristalsis, elimination of urine, and labor contractions, respectively. It is also found in blood vessels, where it helps to regulate blood pressure.

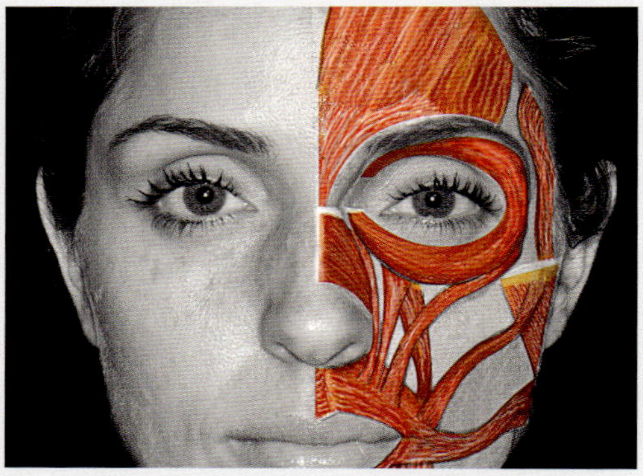

Cutaneous or superficial muscles Situated underneath the skin, these muscles have their origin or attachment at the dermis. They are situated in the head, neck, and hand (hypothenar region).
Deep or subaponeurotic muscles These muscles do not present attachments in the deep layer of the dermis and are inserted in bones. They are located underneath fasciae.

Fig 1-4 Histology of the muscle tissues.

Box 1-4 **Characteristics of BTX-A**

Specificity: The action of this protein specifically occurs in presynaptic neurons of the NMJ.

Temporary irreversibility: The action of BTX-A in the muscle lasts 3 to 4 months. After the third month, a progressive clinical decrease is observed until its total extinction around month 5 or 6.

Immunogenicity: Injections administered less than 3 months apart might cause the "vaccine effect," where the patient no longer responds to the BTX-A injections. A minimum interval of 4 months must be respected.

Diffusion halo: A halo determines the amount of BTX-A diffused around the site injected. The smaller the diffusion halo, the more accurate it is.

Characteristics of BTX-A

Using simple terminology, BTX-A works by reducing the muscle action potential. Its presence in the synaptic cleft decreases the release of the neurotransmitter ACh. Instead of physically sectioning the nerve to weaken a muscle related to it, its tone and strength are chemically reduced, which is a simpler and also temporary process. For this purpose, BTX-A shows some characteristics that make it peculiar, including the following (Box 1-4):

Specificity

BTX-A only affects the muscle tone and contraction power where injected. That is, no other senses are affected by the toxin. Patients will still keep their senses of touch, hearing, smell, sight, and taste. So if the patient presents different symptoms of local muscle hypotonicity after toxin injection, they are not related to BTX-A treatment and may be an adverse event.[24] This specificity provides safety and predictability to professionals using BTX in their patients.

Temporary irreversibility

Once the toxin starts showing its effect, it cannot be reversed until the vesicular activity in the original nerve terminals is restored (reinnervation). If, for instance, when injecting the toxin in the frontal region, an undesired diffusion occurs in the levator palpebrae superioris muscle causing a palpebral ptosis, it is important to understand that this effect is temporarily irreversible. There is no evidence that laser therapy, alpha-adrenergic eye drops, or electric stimulation is able to revert the effect of the toxin.

Immunogenicity

In the manufacturing of BTX in a pharmaceutical laboratory, the stage comprising the purifications is important. Several precipitations in an acid environment are performed to remove ribonucleic acids and other contaminant acids in order to avoid any kind of adverse reactions and to decrease antigenicity.[2]

Immunogenicity refers to the ability of a protein product to elicit antibody formation. As with any therapeutic protein, BTX is regarded as foreign by the host and therefore has the potential to induce an immune response, particularly with repeated administration. This can lead to the development of neutralizing antibodies that may or may not result in secondary treatment failure.[25]

Various factors impact the immunogenicity of botulinum neurotoxins, including product-related factors such as the manufacturing process, the antigenic protein load, and the presence of accessory proteins as well as treatment-related factors such as the overall toxin dose, booster injections, and prior vaccination or exposure.[26]

In clinical practice, it is understood that because the effect of the toxin is temporary, it has to be periodically reinjected to maintain the desired effects. However, it is necessary to wait for a minimum of 4 months between applications. Reinjections in shorter periods might result in the formation of antibodies, which can reduce the duration of BTX's effects or potentially eliminate the effect altogether. Therefore, "touch-ups" should be avoided.[26] Before treatment, the patient should be informed that once the BTX starts to take effect, small asymmetries are likely and are observed even in natural faces. Reinjections to correct asymmetries or readjustments of effects should only be done in cases that really require the procedure. The professional should protect the patient from immunogenicity. Two studies found that patients who developed secondary nonresponse to onabotulinumtoxinA (ONA) received more frequent injections and/or had more booster injections than patients who did not develop resistance.[27,28]

Diffusion halo

Precise location of neurotoxin injection is required to produce the desired clinical results. Temporary disfigurement or functional impairment can occur if the neurotoxin diffuses into adjacent muscle. When injecting BTX-A in the face, it is important to remember that the interface of facial expression muscles is weak due to the lack of fascia. On the other hand, muscles such as the masticatory muscles present a fascia to isolate and individually separate them so that the movements are isolated. While this fascia helps to prevent inflammation from spreading, it also contributes to the muscle-bone attachment. It also protects the muscle from diffusion of toxin.

The origin or attachment of mimetic muscles is located in the dermis, thereby causing skin traction to produce facial expressions. Therefore, the lack of a fascia covering these muscles increases the chance of diffusion when injecting BTX. To achieve a limited action in a specific muscle, it is fundamental to understand and learn how to work with different diffusion profiles of BTX. Choosing a product that allows a higher predictability in terms of results also decreases the possibility of adverse effects. It is also important to consider the dilution to be used and follow the recommendations, because the diffusion depends on the volume to be injected. It is possible to dilute the toxin using different volumes of saline solution; however, using a higher volume of saline solution will increase the chance of diffusion to undesired muscles.

Aoki et al[29] proposed that different diffusion characteristics were attributed to protein complex size and pharmacologic properties, whereby the high molecular weight of ONA limits tissue distribution and explains the reported differences in side effects favoring ONA over abobotulinumtoxinA (ABO). However, more recent studies suggest that this is not the case. These studies compared the diffusion of ONA and ABO by measuring the size of anhidrotic halos following injection of identical volumes into the forehead of patients. Using dose ratios of 1:2.5, 1:3, and 1:4, the authors showed that the area of anhidrosis was larger with ABO in 93% of patients at all dose ratios.[30] Importantly, it has been argued that molecular weight and protein complex size do not affect biologic activity and pharmacologic properties because the BTX-A rapidly dissociates from the complexing proteins (if present) after dilution, drying, and reconstitution of the preparation.[31] A comparison of incobotulinumtoxinA (INCO) with ONA showed no difference in the size of the anhidrotic area produced following injection of the same dose.[32]

These studies also suggest that Dysport (Ipsen) has a greater diffusion halo than Botox (Allergan), and Xeomin (Merz) shows a halo similar to that for Botox.

Frevert[25] evaluated the stability of commercial formulations and found that human serum albumin (HSA) is required to stabilize BTX-A products, with ABO having the lowest content of all. The low amount of HSA in ABO could at least partially explain why not all of the neurotoxin in ABO is bioavailable, depending on the concentration of HSA in the injected volume.[33]

Box 1-5 **Dilution of 100U in 1 mL of saline**

When diluting a 100U vial of BTX (Botox or Xeomin) with 1 mL of saline in order to inject 10U of toxin in a determined muscle, simple algebra can be used to calculate the volume to be administered:

Given: 1.0 mL = 100U

Problem: X mL = 10U

Solution: X = 0.1 mL

When using a 30U syringe, you can see at the bottom that its maximum capacity is 30U and its maximum volume is 0.3 mL. Again, simple algebra can be used to calculate the number of units that would represent 0.1 mL in this dilution:

Given: 0.3 mL = 30U

Problem: 0.1 mL = XU

Solution: X = 10U

CONCLUSION: When using this dilution to obtain 10U, the professional has to inject 10U.

Box 1-6 **Dilution of 100U in 2 mL of saline**

To determine the injection volume when diluting a 100U vial of BTX (Botox or Xeomin) in 2 mL of saline in order to inject 10U of toxin in a determined muscle:

Given: 2.0 mL = 100U

Problem: X mL = 10U

Solution: X = 0.2 mL

You can use the same formula to calculate the number of units that would represent 0.2 mL in this dilution:

Given: 0.3 mL = 30U

Problem: 0.2 mL = XU

Solution: X = 20U

CONCLUSION: In this type of dilution, to obtain 10U, the professional has to inject 20U. This requires an injection double the volume of that obtained with a 1-mL dilution.

Dilution Technique for BTX-A

A preservative-free 0.9% sodium chloride (saline) solution is used to reconstitute lyophilized (freeze-dried) BTX, as preservatives might change the solution pH and affect the toxin potency. The injection becomes painful when distilled water is used for dilution. A good technique for Botox is to use 1 mL of saline to dilute the toxin contained in a 100-unit (100U) vial, or 0.01 mL per unit (Box 1-5). However, several professionals use 2 mL to dilute a 100U vial of BTX-A. In this case, one unit of toxin corresponds to 0.02 mL of solution, meaning that it would be necessary to inject double the volume to obtain 1U (Box 1-6). This procedure may lead to the dispersion of toxin to other nontargeted muscles, thereby causing undesired effects.

Lethal dose 50 (LD50) experiments, whereby toxicity is measured in terms of the amount of a given drug required to kill half of a tested population of laboratory mice after an intraperitoneal injection, define the amount of a drug that will constitute the minimum unit of action—that is, the

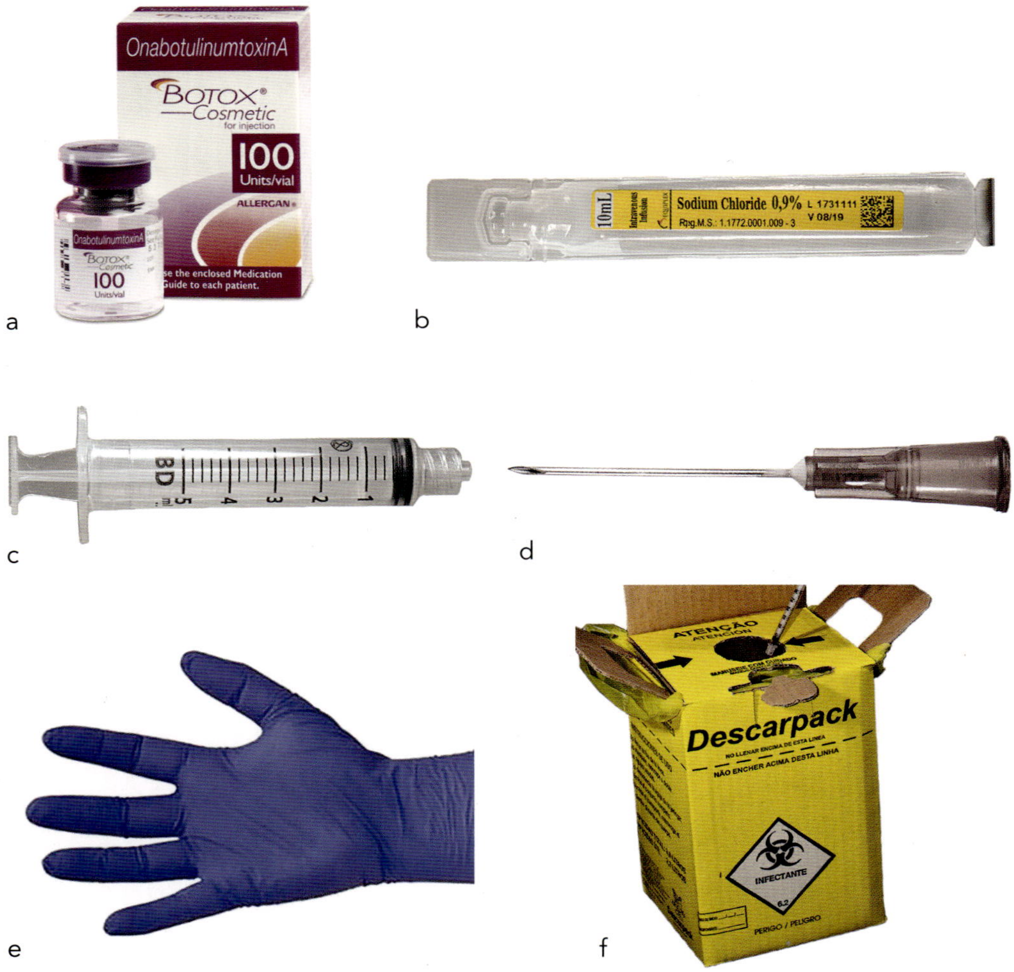

Fig 1-5 *(a)* BTX vial. *(b)* Sterile, preservative-free 0.9% sodium chloride (saline). *(c)* Luer-Lok syringe (in mL). *(d)* 22-gauge needle. *(e)* Sterile gloves. *(f)* Container to discard the needle.

smallest amount of a drug required to promote a minimum effect. Doses of all varieties of BTX are expressed in terms of these units (U), a measure of potency, not milliliters (mL), a measure of volume. A high-volume dilution will result in a less potent solution, meaning that a higher volume of toxin would be necessary to obtain one or more units of BTX. On the other hand, using a small amount of saline solution for dilution will result in a more concentrated and potent solution. With this formulation, the operator would be able to obtain the same number of units with a smaller-volume injection. It is also important to consider that the higher the volume injected, the higher the dispensing of the drug, the level of patient discomfort, and the chances of bruising.

Figure 1-5 shows the armamentarium required for BTX-A dilution, and Fig 1-6 illustrates the procedure. Below are some basic recommendations for this process:

1. Open the box at the recommended site on the side. Do not discard the box.
2. Remove the plastic seal from the vial. Discard it.
3. Do not heat the vial with your hand; instead handle it with the tips of your fingers.
4. Attach a 22-gauge (22G) needle to the Luer-Lok syringe and withdraw the predetermined amount of saline solution required for the dilution.
5. At a 45-degree angle, insert the 22G needle (attached to the syringe) into the rubber stop until the bevel of the needle touches the glass of the vial. Hold the plunger to prevent rapid aspiration of the saline from the syringe, which could cause agitation of the mixture.
6. Do not shake the vial.

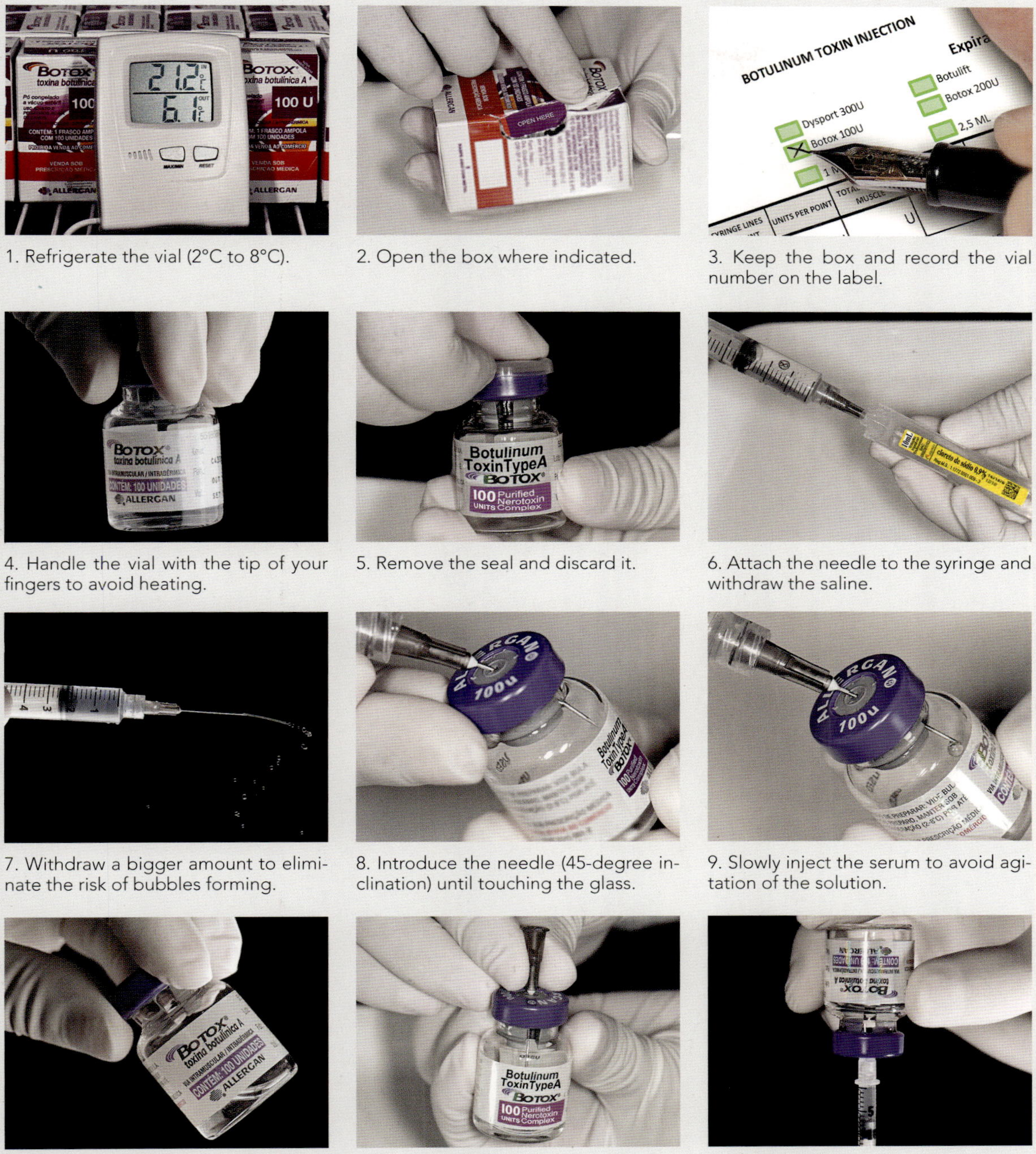

1. Refrigerate the vial (2°C to 8°C).
2. Open the box where indicated.
3. Keep the box and record the vial number on the label.
4. Handle the vial with the tip of your fingers to avoid heating.
5. Remove the seal and discard it.
6. Attach the needle to the syringe and withdraw the saline.
7. Withdraw a bigger amount to eliminate the risk of bubbles forming.
8. Introduce the needle (45-degree inclination) until touching the glass.
9. Slowly inject the serum to avoid agitation of the solution.
10. Slowly rotate the vial to humidify its entire internal surface.
11. Insert, remove, and reinsert the needle to weaken the rubber stop.
12. Turn the vial upside down and draw up the toxin.

Fig 1-6 Step-by-step dilution process.

7. Insert, remove, and reinsert a 22G needle approximately 10 times in the same place in the rubber stop to soften the rubber, which will prevent future injection needles from becoming dull. This will reduce patient pain and bruising during the injection.
8. In case all the diluted toxin is not used, put the vial in the preserved box and refrigerate the solution at 2°C to 8°C. Do not freeze it. Write the day of use on the box.
9. BTX (Botox) can be administered within 72 hours of reconstitution when stored at 2°C to 8°C.

Box 1-7 lists other important considerations for the clinical use of BTX.

Box 1-7 Important considerations for working with BTX

- ❑ Botox is available in 50U, 100U, and 200U vials.
- ❑ Vials should be stored between 2°C and 8°C or at or below –5°C.
- ❑ Diluted solutions can be kept at 2°C to 8°C for up to 3 days.
- ❑ The lethal human dose of Botox is 3,000U.
- ❑ The toxin should only be diluted minutes before its application.
- ❑ When diluting, the saline and the BTX should be at a similar temperature.
- ❑ Do not use the needle to perforate the saline vial, as it may be contaminated by bacteria. Open where indicated.
- ❑ The 0.9% saline should be preservative-free so that it will not change the potency of the BTX.
- ❑ The saline solution should be slowly injected to avoid agitation of the solution and degradation of the BTX.
- ❑ The spaces between the marks are greater in a 30U syringe than in a 100U syringe, making it easier to measure precisely.

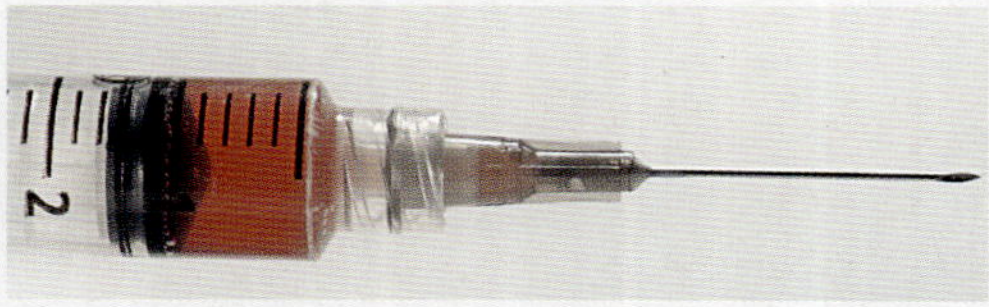

1. Syringe with 1.1 mL of physiologic saline (with dye).

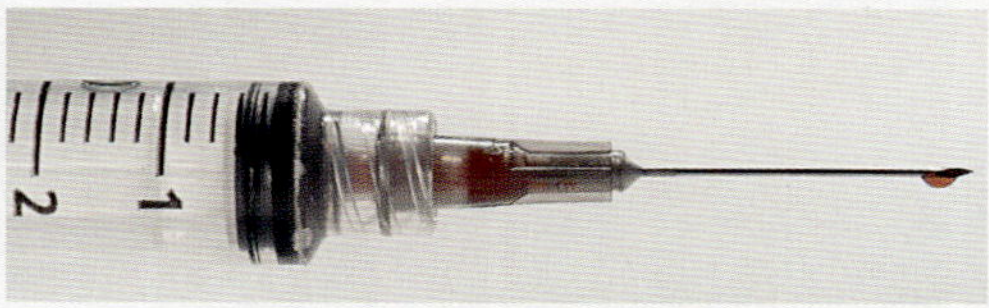

2. Residual liquid in the syringe and hub.

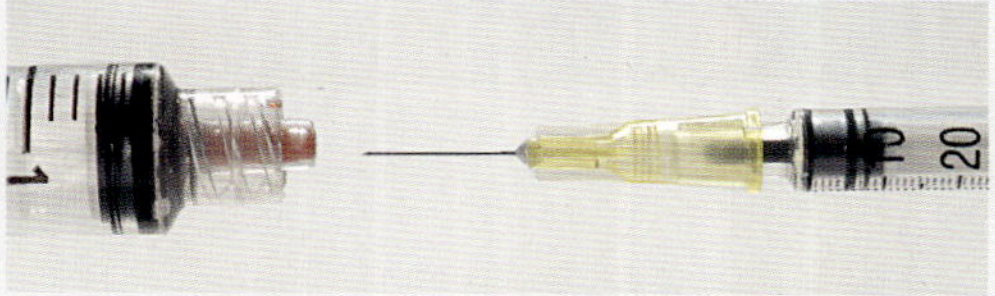

3. Preparing to draw up the residual liquid in the syringe.

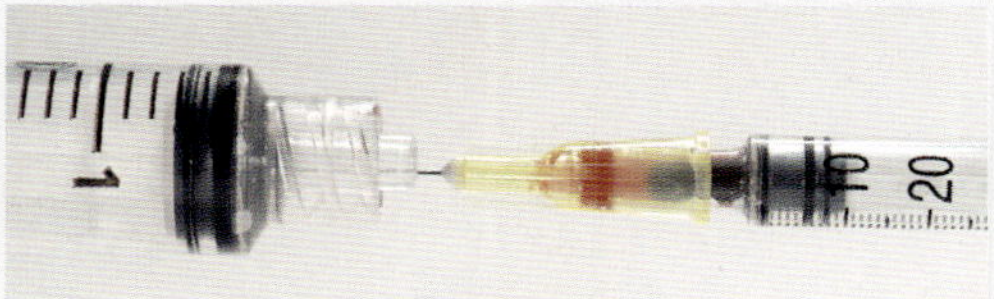

4. Withdrawing the residual liquid.

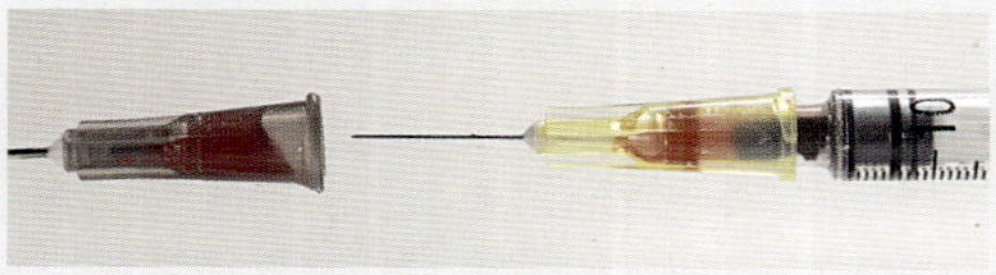

5. Preparing to withdraw the residual liquid from the hub.

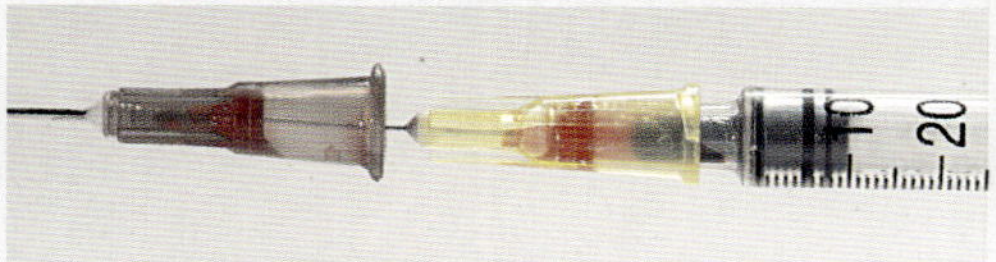

6. Withdrawing the residual liquid from the hub.

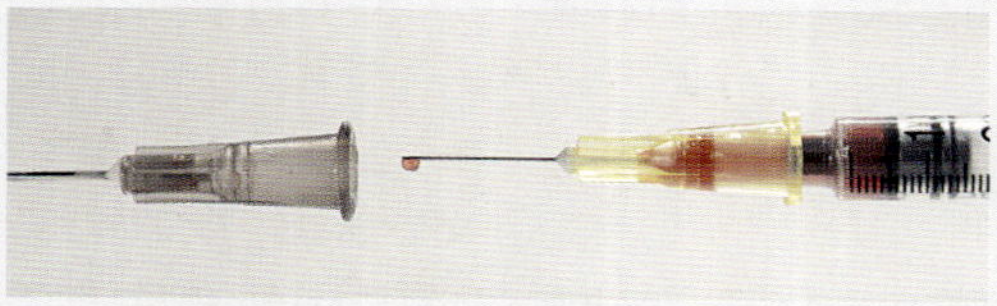

7. Liquid withdrawn from the hub.

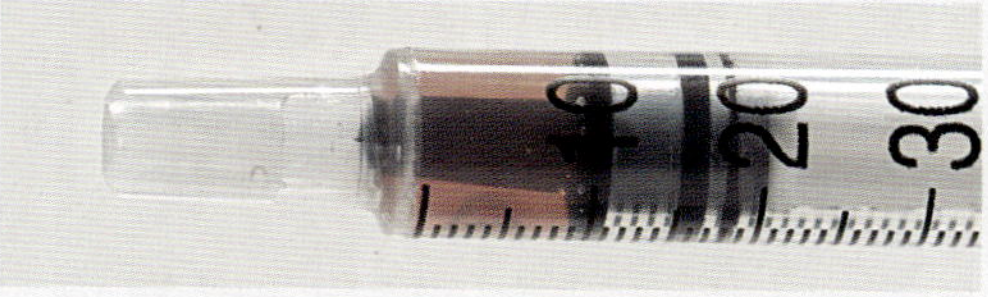

8. Total residual liquid withdrawn from the syringe and hub = 0.1 mL.

Fig 1-7 Compensating for residual liquid.

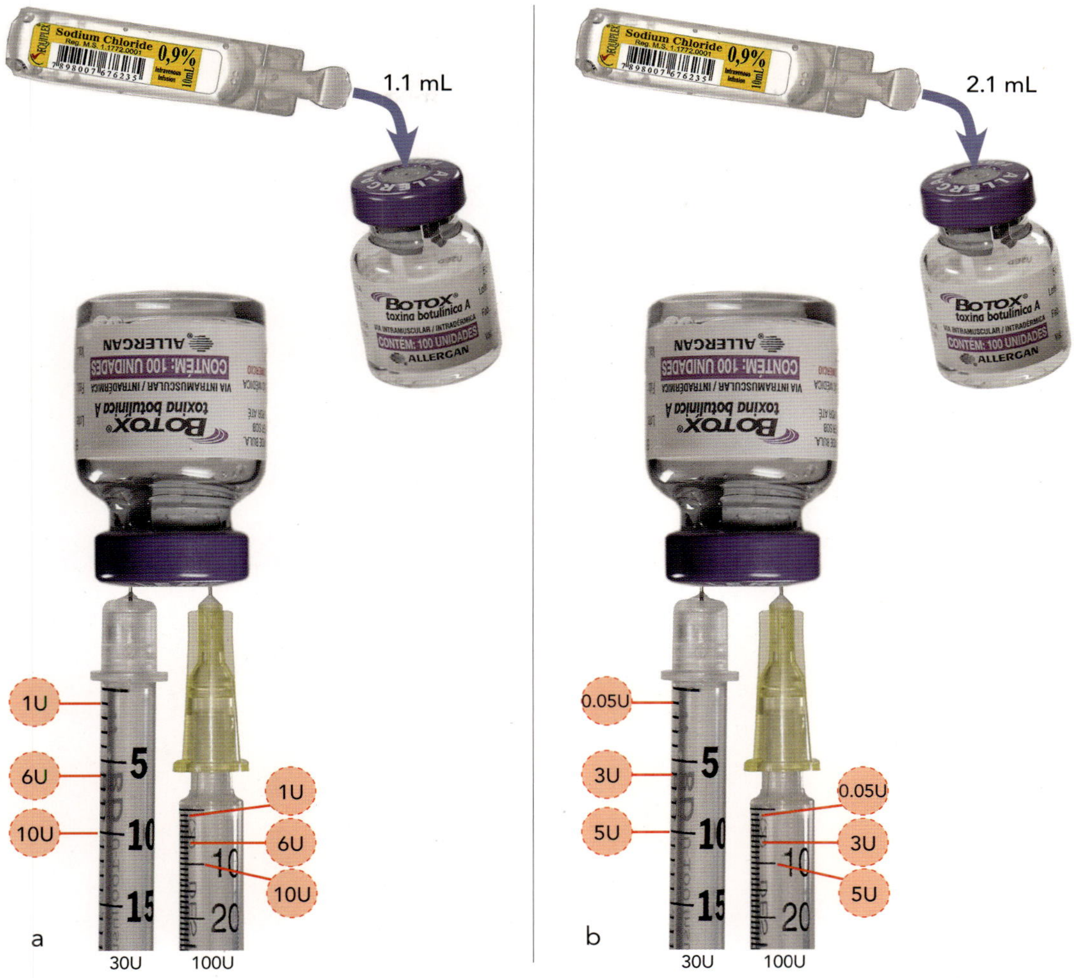

Fig 1-8 *(a)* When diluting 100U of toxin in 1.1 mL of saline, each mark in a 30U or 100U syringe will represent 1U (one toxin unit). *(b)* When diluting 100U of toxin in 2.1 mL of saline, every *two* marks of a 30U or 100U syringe represents 1U (one toxin unit).

Residual liquid

The residual liquid is the amount of saline solution that will not be injected inside the toxin vial because it will be kept inside the syringe and needle used during dilution (Fig 1-7). It is important to compensate for this residual liquid to ensure that no units of BTX are wasted. Therefore, 0.1 mL of sterile physiologic saline may be added to the total volume. That is, if the practitioner plans to dilute the toxin using 1 mL of saline, he or she would draw up 1.1 mL of saline into the syringe, as 0.1 mL will be left in the syringe (see Fig 1-7). If this procedure is not followed, 10% of the dilution in each vial will be wasted, which adds up when you consider a net waste of 1 vial for every 10 vials used. Figure 1-8 illustrates the markings on the syringe when diluting with 1.1 mL and 2.1 mL. It shows that it is easier to use the 30U syringe than the 100U syringe because the space between the marks is greater.

Patient Care

Patient care is an important part of BTX treatment. Figure 1-9 shows the steps involved in a typical appointment.

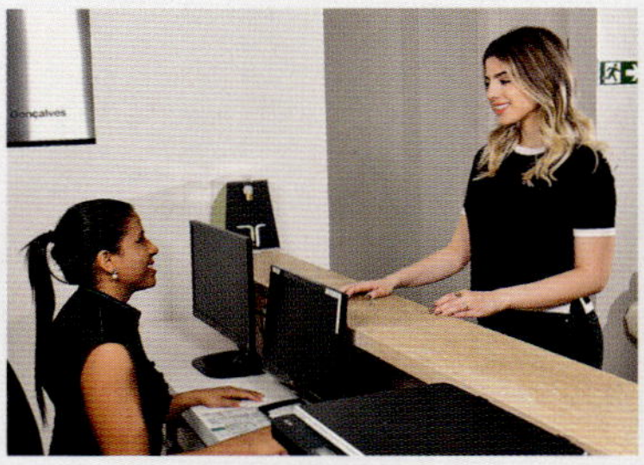

1. The patient is welcomed to the office.

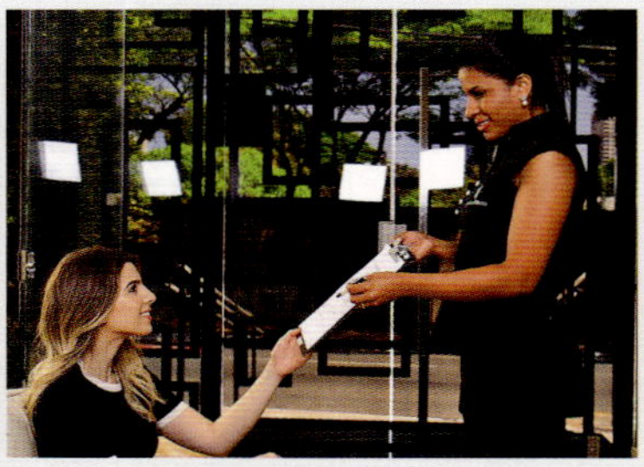

2. The patient is instructed to sit and given the medical history form to fill out.

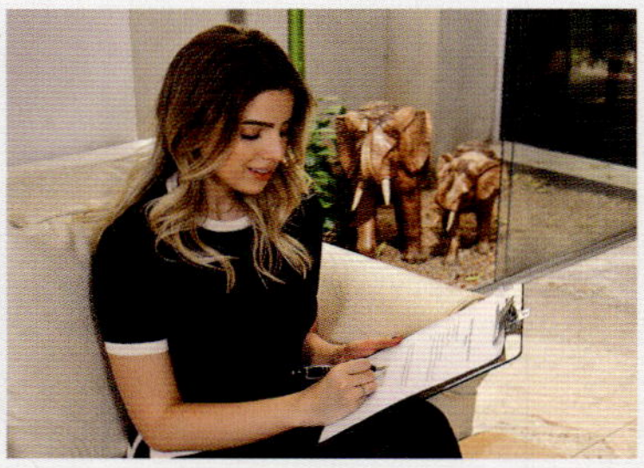

3. The patient fills out the form.

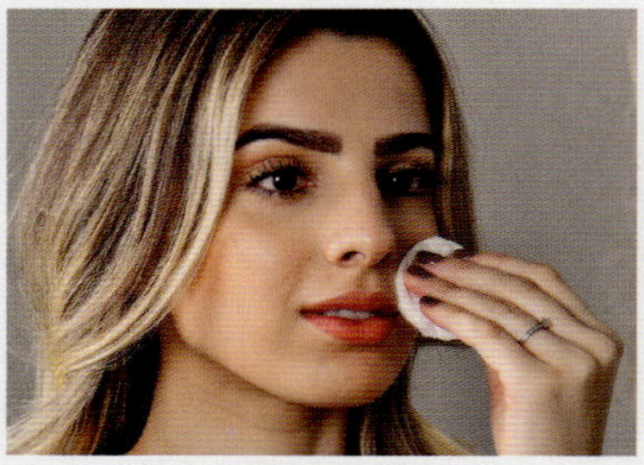

4. The patient is asked to remove all makeup from the face.

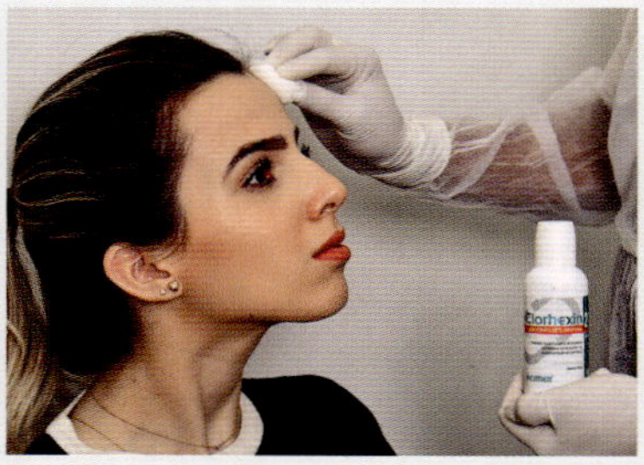

5. An assistant helps the patient clean his or her face.

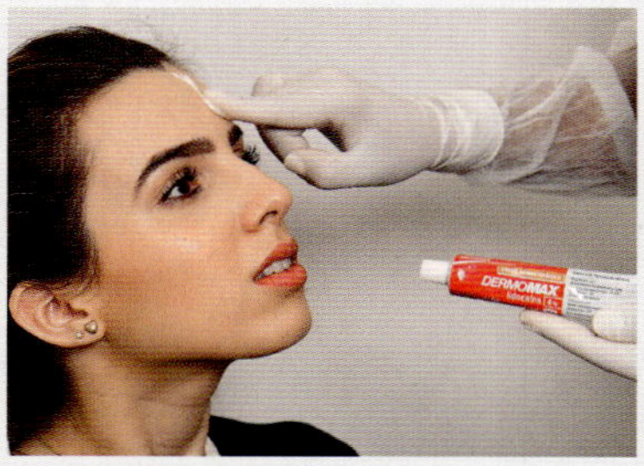

6. An assistant applies topical anesthetic to the face.

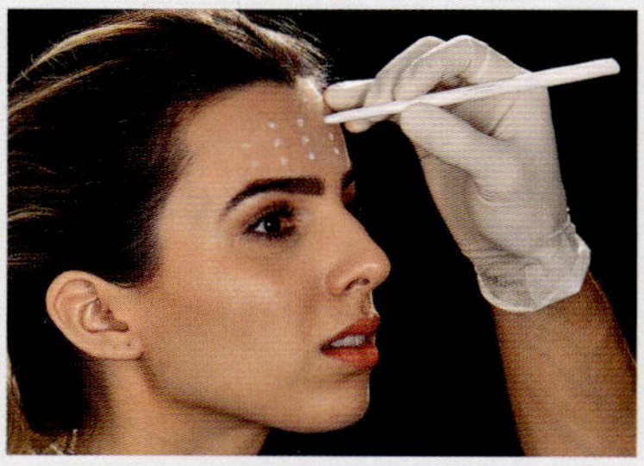

7. A facial analysis is performed, and all injection sites are marked (see protocol for muscle location in chapter 3).

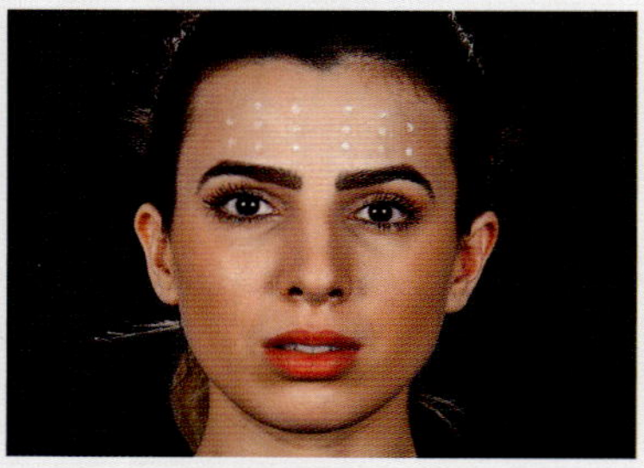

8. A photograph is taken to document the face with the injection sites marked (see protocol photographs in chapter 2).

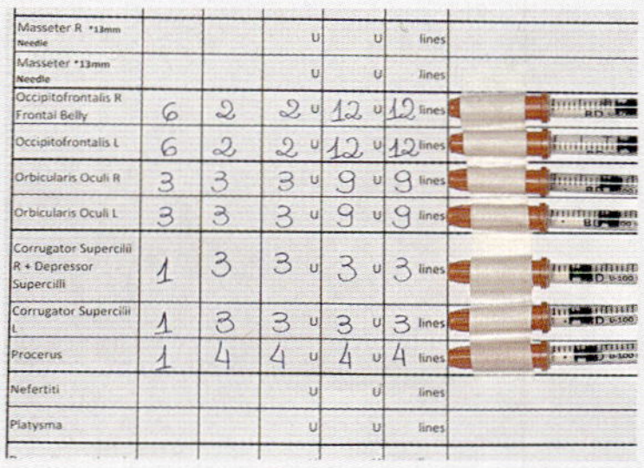

9. The application plan is filled out, and the BTX syringes are prepared and separated (see Fig 1-14b).

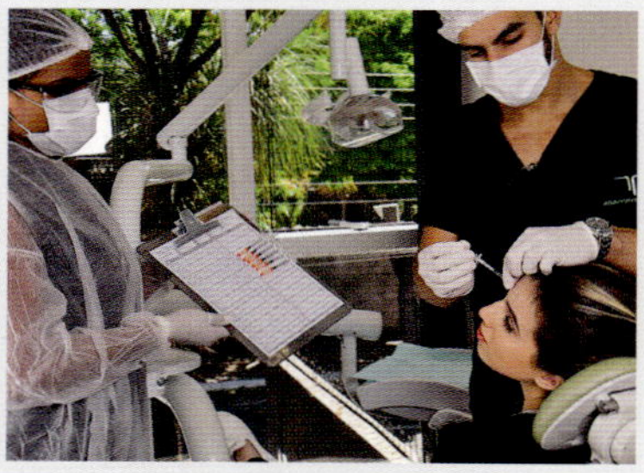

10. The BTX is injected.

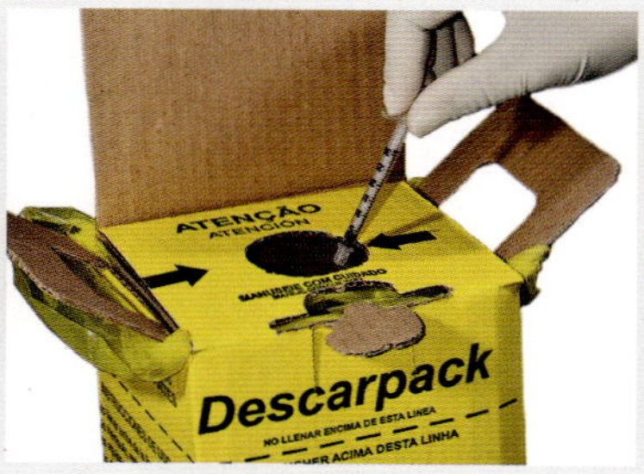

11. The syringes are discarded in a container specifically for piercing/cutting materials.

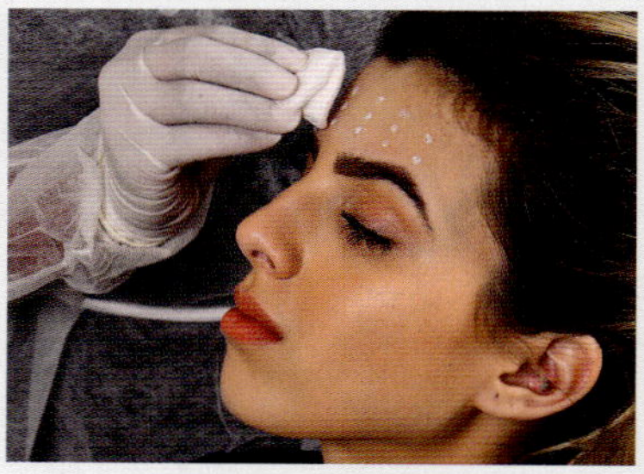

12. An assistant performs a light cleansing of the patient's face.

Fig 1-9 Patient care. Postoperative instructions must be given to the patient after treatment.

Box 1-8 **Indications for treatment with BTX-A (Botox, unless otherwise noted)**

INDICATIONS APPROVED BY THE FDA	OFF LABEL (BOTOX)
Strabismus	Temporomandibular disorders
Blepharospasm	Chronic musculoskeletal pain
Hemifacial spasm	Vaginismus
Cervical dystonia (Botox, Dysport, Xeomin, and NeuroBloc)	Wound healing
Cosmetic use	Diabetic neuropathy
Axillary hyperhidrosis	
Chronic migraine	
Neurogenic detrusor overactivity	
Lower urinary tract disorders	
Gastrointestinal tract disorders	
Spasticity	
Spasmodic dysphonia	
Sialorrhea (drooling)	

(Data from Chen.[34])

General Indications for BTX-A

BTX has been a popular medication for over 20 years and has several different therapeutic uses. Increased research on BTX-A has resulted in new indications for its use (Box 1-8). In general, the chemical denervation is a safe technique showing predictable outcomes.

Therapeutic versus cosmeceutical use

- *Therapeutic use:* Focused on the treatment of diseases. There is a pathology present.
- *Cosmeceutical use:* Focused on the preservation or improvement of physical beauty. There is no pathology.

In clinical practice, treatment with BTX-A cannot always be classified as therapeutic or cosmeceutical. Sometimes the same patient will want and/or require both types of therapy, for example, an aging patient with bruxism who may require therapeutic treatment for the bruxism but who also wants cosmeceutical therapy to smooth expression wrinkles.

Therapeutic use

Therapeutic uses for BTX-A in the face include the following:

- Strabismus
- Blepharospasm
- Hemifacial spasm
- Tension headache
- Bruxism
- Sialorrhea
- Temporomandibular disorder
- Cervical dystonia

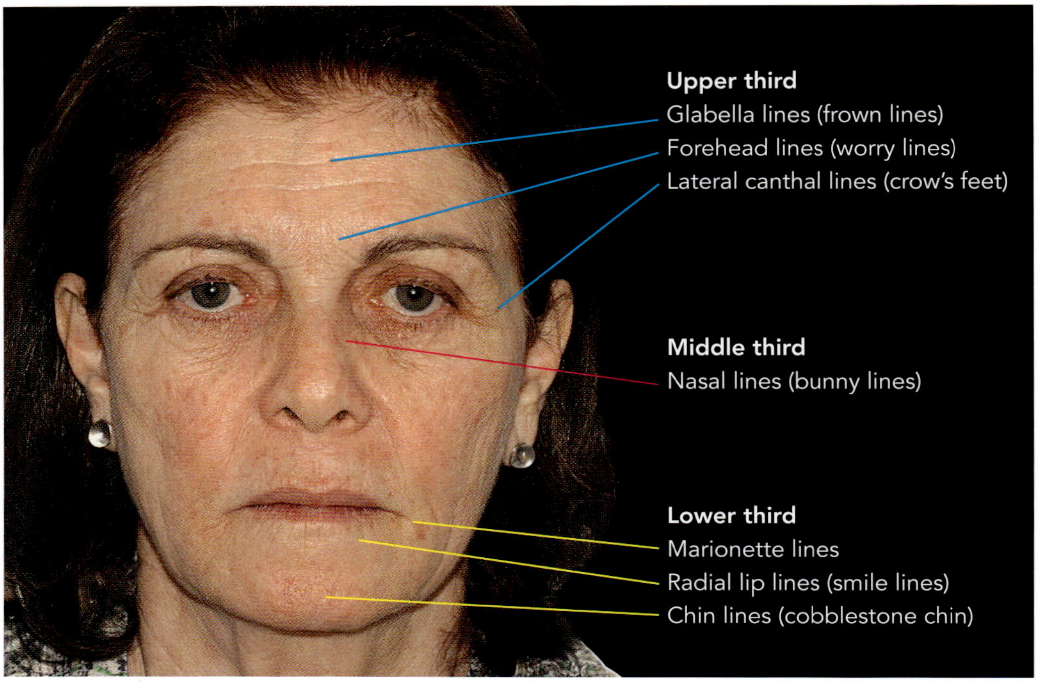

Fig 1-10 Facial wrinkles.

Cosmeceutical use

BTX-A has likely become popular worldwide because of its cosmeceutical use. While most patients understand that its use might improve and/or rejuvenate their physical appearance, its application extends to facial asymmetries resulting from paralysis sequelae or even other facial traumas. In patients living with these conditions, BTX treatment could help restore their self-esteem as well as their social and professional lives.

Cosmeceutical uses for BTX-A in the face include the following:

- Smooth wrinkles related to muscles (occipitofrontal, procerus, corrugator supercilii, nasal, orbicularis oculi, orbicularis oris, mentalis, depressor anguli oris; Fig 1-10)
- Reduce the volume of muscles (nasal, masseter, mentalis, orbicularis oris, platysma)
- Smooth eyelid ptosis
- Improve definition of the jawline
- Lift the eyebrows
- Increase the eye opening
- Reduce the gummy smile
- Elevate the oral commissures

Examples of clinical treatment are illustrated in chapters 2 and 4.

Types of facial wrinkles

Facial wrinkles are caused when muscles attached to the dermis move the skin during facial expressions. When these mimetic muscles contract, the skin is pulled perpendicular to the underlying muscle fibers, leaving it wrinkled. Wrinkles may be classified as dynamic or static (Fig 1-11). When they are formed during facial expression and fade at the end of the muscle dynamics, they

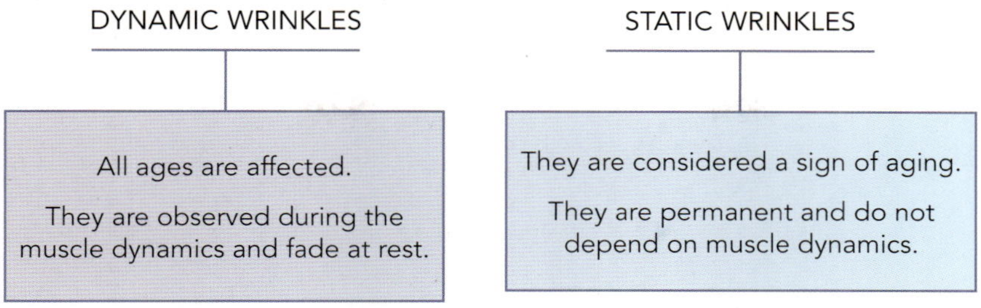

Fig 1-11 Classification of facial wrinkles.

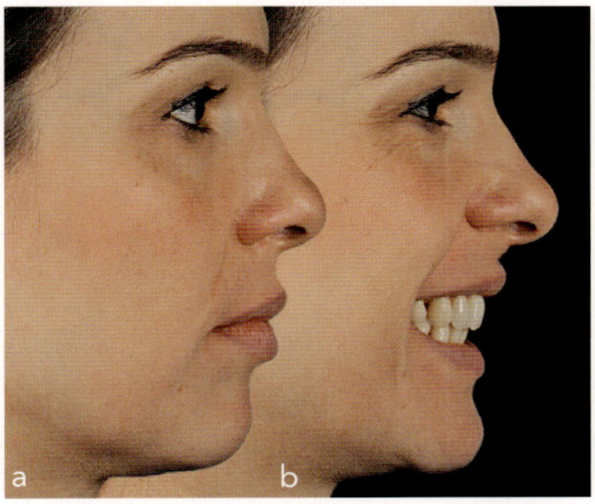

Fig 1-12 *(a and b)* Dynamic wrinkles are formed during mimetics and disappear at the end of the action. At rest, the wrinkles fade away. The lack of wrinkles suggests that this patient is young.

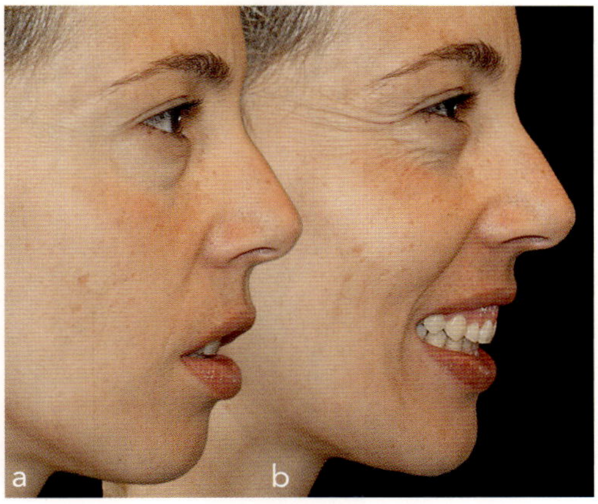

Fig 1-13 *(a and b)* Static wrinkles are formed during facial expressions and do not fade at the end of the muscle action. At rest they are noticeable. The presence of wrinkles suggests that this patient's face is in an aging process.

are classified as *dynamic* (Fig 1-12). However, when they do not fade at rest, they are classified as *static* (Fig 1-13). According to Oriá et al,[35] with aging the skin shows decreased epidermis-dermis thickness, reduced elasticity and secretion of sebum by the sebaceous glands, compromised immunologic response, a decreased number of sweat glands, and reduced vascular tone, with fragility of blood vessels. All of these characteristics associated with repeated skin traction lead to definitive markings (ie, static wrinkles).

It is well known the wrinkles are formed through the action of facial expression muscles. Thus, it is believed that a decrease in muscle action might reduce the number and depth of wrinkles. BTX-A temporarily postpones the wrinkle status from static to dynamic, giving the face a younger aspect. Dynamic wrinkles start to become static around age 30 years, so patients interested in delaying their onset should begin treatment just before then. The procedure must be repeated every 5 months to maintain the results. The main focus of treatment is the upper third of the face (see chapter 2).

The higher the mobility of a skin region, the earlier wrinkles will form. In the upper third, the skin lateral to the eyes tends to show wrinkles because of the sphincter action of the orbicularis oculi. This is an area relatively easily treated with BTX-A. On the other hand, the intense mobility of the muscles in the middle and lower thirds of the face involved with mouth function cause the skin in these areas to show their age more than areas with lower mobility.[36] Due to its complexity, the treatment of the lower third requires more caution and professional expertise.

Box 1-9 shows a checklist of all the facial areas that can be treated with BTX-A.

Box 1-9 **BTX treatment checklist**

TREATMENT AREAS
❑ Glabella lines (frown lines)
❑ Forehead lines (worry lines)
❑ Lateral canthal lines (crow's feet)
❑ Nasal lines (bunny lines)
❑ Marionette lines
❑ Perioral lines (smile lines)
❑ Chin lines (cobblestone chin)
❑ Eyelid ptosis
❑ Voluminous lip skin
❑ Jawline contouring
❑ Eyebrow lifting
❑ Widening of eye opening
❑ Correction of upper gummy smile
❑ Correction of lower gummy smile
❑ Elevation of lip commissures

Contraindications

BTX is a safe drug. No systemic complications resulting from its use have been reported in the literature. However, as with every pharmacologic product, it should be used with caution and following its indications. Box 1-10 details the contraindications and relative contraindications for BTX.

Box 1-10 **Contraindications and relative contraindications for BTX**

DO NOT USE in patients:

Who are pregnant or breastfeeding

With any of the following conditions: myasthenia gravis, amyotrophic lateral sclerosis, myopathies, Lambert-Eaton myasthenic syndrome

Taking certain medications (aminoglycosides, calcium blockers)

With infection in the treatment area

With dermatoses in the treatment area (psoriasis, eczema)

Allergic to any of the components of BTX-A or BTX-B (ie, BTX, human albumin, saline, lactose, sodium succinate)

With herpes eruptions in the treatment area

Use with extreme caution in patients:

Whose livelihoods depend on intact facial movements and expressions (eg, actors, singers, musicians, other media personalities)

Who are psychologically unstable or who have questionable motives and unrealistic expectations

(Data from Small,[37] Sposito,[2] Niamtu,[38] and Patel et al.[39])

Fig 1-14 Side-by-side comparison of the effects of Botox and Xeomin. *(a)* Injection points for Botox *(green)* and Xeomin *(red)*. *(b)* Chart showing the dosages used at each injection point.

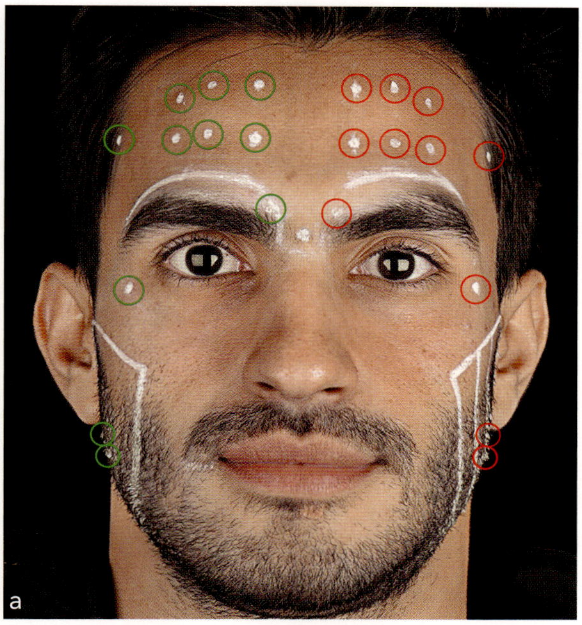

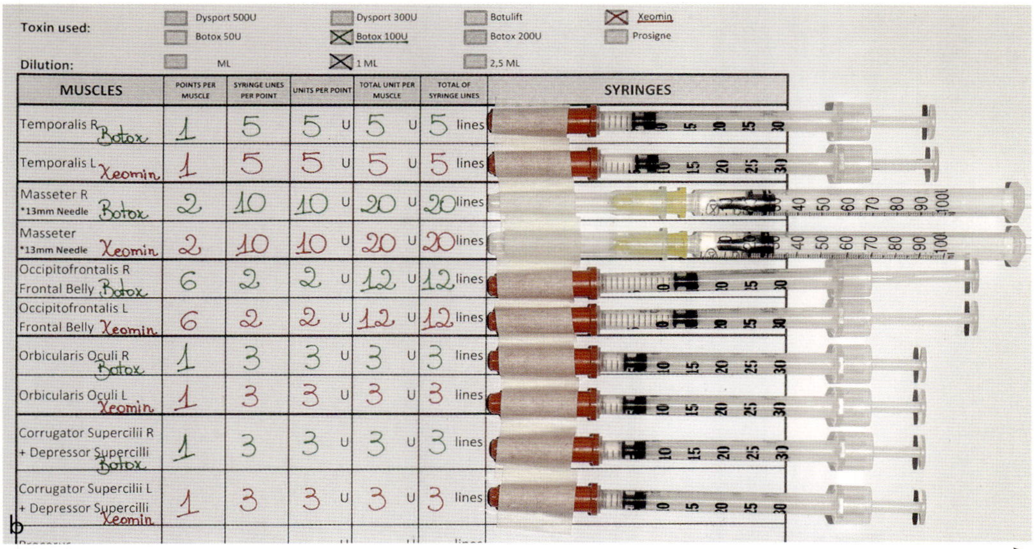

Toxin used: Dysport 500U; Botox 50U; Dysport 300U; [X] Botox 100U; Botulift; Botox 200U; [X] Xeomin; Prosigne

Dilution: ML; [X] 1 ML; 2,5 ML

MUSCLES	POINTS PER MUSCLE	SYRINGE LINES PER POINT	UNITS PER POINT	TOTAL UNIT PER MUSCLE	TOTAL OF SYRINGE LINES	SYRINGES
Temporalis R Botox	1	5	5 U	5 U	5 lines	
Temporalis L Xeomin	1	5	5 U	5 U	5 lines	
Masseter R *13mm Needle Botox	2	10	10 U	20 U	20 lines	
Masseter *13mm Needle Xeomin	2	10	10 U	20 U	20 lines	
Occipitofrontalis R Frontal Belly Botox	6	2	2 U	12 U	12 lines	
Occipitofrontalis L Frontal Belly Xeomin	6	2	2 U	12 U	12 lines	
Orbicularis Oculi R Botox	1	3	3 U	3 U	3 lines	
Orbicularis Oculi L Xeomin	1	3	3 U	3 U	3 lines	
Corrugator Supercilii R + Depressor Supercilli Botox	1	3	3 U	3 U	3 lines	
Corrugator Supercilii L + Depressor Supercilli Xeomin	1	3	3 U	3 U	3 lines	

b

→

Comparison of Botox and Xeomin

In order to evaluate the clinical effect and duration of two different brands of BTX-A, Botox was injected on the right side of the face and Xeomin on the left side of the face of the patient shown in Fig 1-14. The injections were prepared by the author on the same day as they were administered using the same type of syringes and needles and injected at similar inclinations to similar depths. The green circles in Fig 1-14a represent the injection points for Botox, and the red circles are the injection points for Xeomin. After the injections, several photographs were taken to clinically assess the effects of both toxins, mainly at the occipitofrontalis muscle. During each photographic session, the patient was instructed to lift his eyebrows as much as he could.

This experiment showed that Xeomin had a faster onset than Botox, offering an important advantage for therapeutic use in that the patient will notice quicker relief of symptoms. After the effect was completely installed, the action on the muscles was similar and effective for the same amount of time (ie, 52 days).

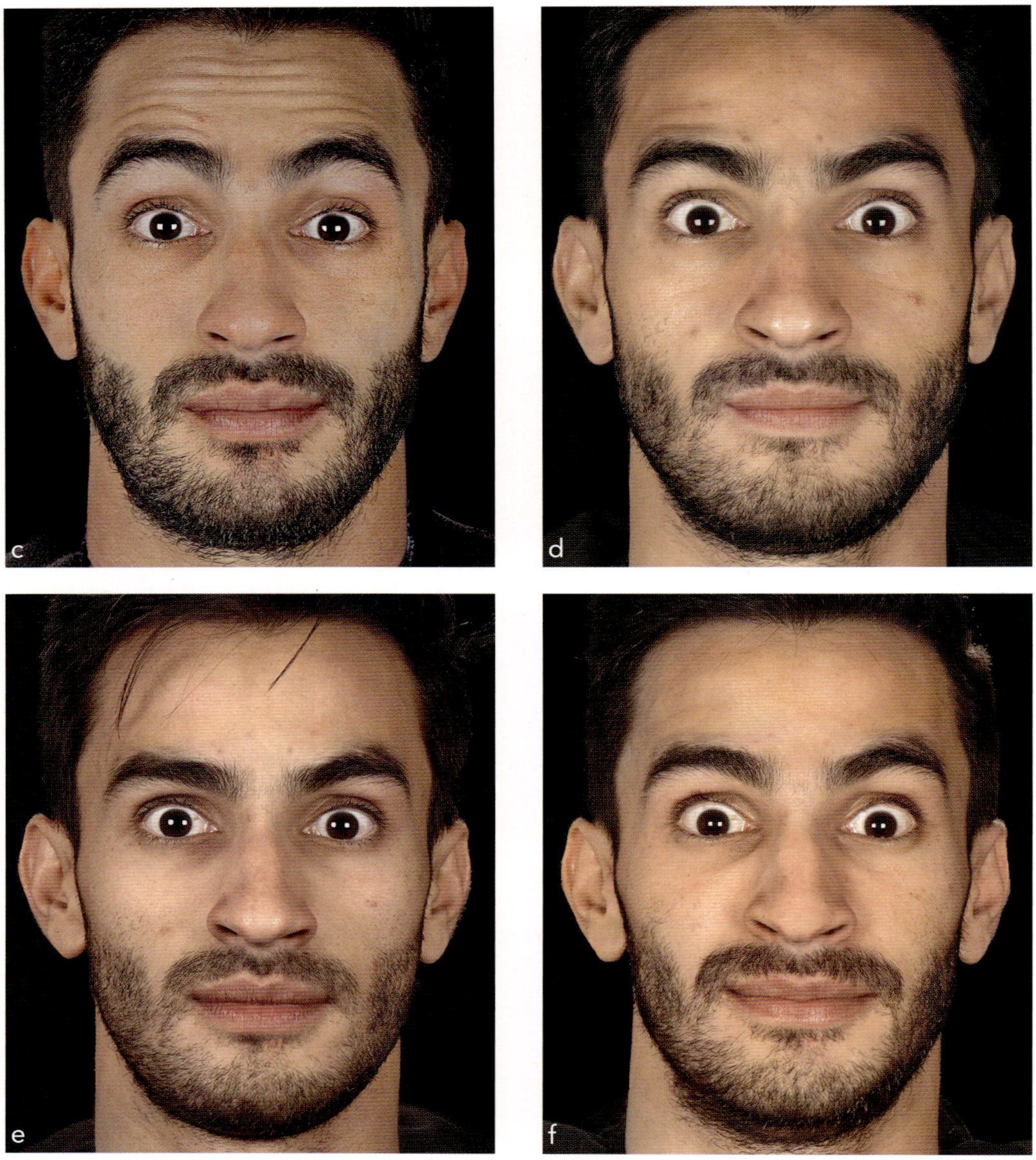

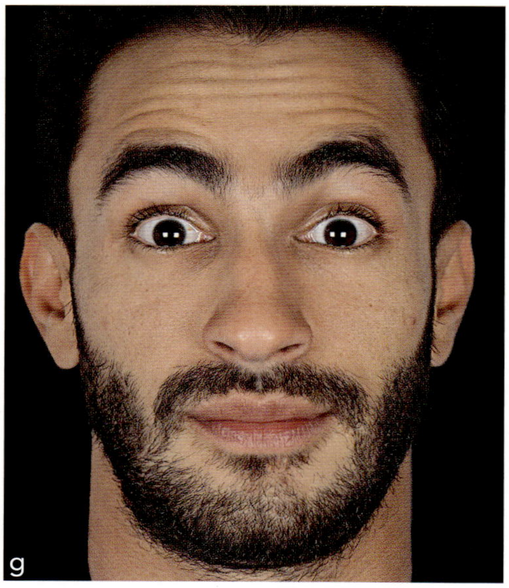

Fig 1-14 *(cont)* *(c)* Pretreatment. *(d)* After 7 days, Xeomin showed a faster onset, indicated by the decreased number of wrinkles on the left side of the face. *(e)* After 21 days, both toxins showed similar results, effectively eliminating all wrinkles. *(f)* After 52 days, both products are still effective. *(g)* After 166 days, both products have worn off, and the patient's dynamic wrinkles have returned.

References

1. Aoki KR. Botulinum toxin: A successful therapeutic protein. Curr Med Chem 2004;11:3085–3092.
2. Sposito MMM. Toxina botulínica tipo A—propriedades farmacológicas e uso clínico. Acta Fisiátr 2004;11(suppl 1):S7–S44.
3. Aoki KR, Guyer B. Botulinum toxin type A and other botulinum toxin serotypes: A comparative review of biochemical and pharmacological actions. Eur J Neurol 2001;8(suppl 5):21–29.
4. Carruthers A, Carruthers J. Botulinum toxin products overview. Skin Therapy Lett 2008;13:1–4.
5. Truong D, Duane DD, Jankovic J, et al. Efficacy and safety of botulinum type A toxin (Dysport) in cervical dystonia: Results of the first US randomized, double-blind, placebo-controlled study. Mov Disord 2005;20:783–791.
6. Factor SA, Molho ES, Evans S, Feustel PJ. Efficacy and safety of repeated doses of botulinum toxin type B in type A resistant and responsive cervical dystonia. Mov Disord 2005;20:1152–1160.
7. Costa J, Espírito-Santo C, Borges A, et al. Botulinum toxin type A therapy for cervical dystonia. Cochrane Database Syst Rev 2005;25:CD003633.
8. Comella CL, Jankovic J, Shannon KM, et al. Comparison of botulinum toxin serotypes A and B for the treatment of cervical dystonia. Neurology 2005;65:1423–1429.
9. Flynn TC, Clark RE 2nd. Botulinum toxin type B (MYOBLOC) versus botulinum toxin type A (BOTOX) frontalis study: Rate of onset and radius of diffusion. Dermatol Surg 2003;29:519–522.
10. Baumann L, Slezinger A, Vujevich J, et al. A double-blinded, randomized, placebo-controlled pilot study of the safety and efficacy of Myobloc (botulinum toxin type B)-purified neurotoxin complex for the treatment of crow's feet: A double-blinded, placebo-controlled trial. Dermatol Surg 2003;29:508–515.
11. Baumann L, Black L. Botulinum toxin type B (Myobloc). Dermatol Surg 2003;29:496–500.
12. Ramirez AL, Reeck J, Maas CS. Botulinum toxin type B (MyoBloc) in the management of hyperkinetic facial lines. Otolaryngol Head Neck Surg 2002;126:459–467.
13. Sadick NS. Prospective open-label study of botulinum toxin type B (Myobloc) at doses of 2,400 and 3,000 U for the treatment of glabellar wrinkles. Dermatol Surg 2003; 29:501–507.
14. Setler PE. Therapeutic use of botulinum toxins: Background and history. Clin J Pain 2002;18(6, suppl):119S–124S.
15. Thakker MM, Rubin PA. Pharmacology and clinical applications of botulinum toxins A and B. Int Ophthalmol Clin 2004;44:147–163.
16. Simpson LL. The action of botulinal toxin. Rev Infect Dis 1979;1:656–662.
17. Gonnering RS. Pharmacology of botulinum toxin. Int Ophthalmol Clin 1993;33:203–226.
18. Neuenschwander MC, Pribitkin EA, Sataloff RT. Botulinum toxin in otolaryngology: A review of its actions and opportunities for use. Ear Nose Throat J 2000;79:788–789,792.
19. Blitzer A, Sulica L. Botulinum toxin: Basic science and clinical uses in otolaryngology. Laryngoscope 2001;111: 218–226.
20. Lam SM. The basic science of botulinum toxin. Facial Plast Surg Clin North Am 2003;11:431–438.
21. Carruthers A, Carruthers J, Cohen J. A prospective, double-blind, randomized, parallel- group, dose-ranging study of botulinum toxin type A in female subjects with horizontal forehead rhytides. Dermatol Surg 2003;29: 461–467.
22. Lew MF, Adornato BT, Duane DD, et al. Botulinum toxin type B: A double-blind, placebo-controlled, safety and efficacy study in cervical dystonia. Neurology 1997;49: 701–707.
23. Hambleton P. Clostridium botulinum toxins: A general review of involvement in disease, structure, mode of action and preparation for clinical use. J Neurol 1992; 239:16–20.
24. Klein AW. Dilution and storage of botulinum toxin. Dermatol Surg 1998;24:1179–1180.
25. Frevert J. Pharmaceutical, biological, and clinical properties of botulinum neurotoxin type A products. Drugs R D 2015;15:1–9.
26. Naumann M, Boo LM, Ackerman AH, Gallagher CJ. Immunogenicity of botulinum toxins. J Neural Transm (Vienna) 2013;120:275–290.
27. Greene P, Fahn S, Diamond B. Development of resistance to botulinum toxin type A in patients with torticollis. Mov Disord 1994;9:213–217.
28. Dressler D, Bigalke H. Botulinum toxin type B de novo therapy of cervical dystonia: Frequency of antibody induced therapy failure. J Neurol 2005;252:904–907.
29. Aoki KR, Ranoux D, Wissel J. Using translational medicine to understand clinical differences between botulinum toxin formulations. Eur J Neurol 2006;13(suppl 4):10–19.
30. Trindade de Almeida AR, Marques E, de Almeida J, Cunha T, Boraso R. Pilot study comparing the diffusion of two formulations of botulinum toxin type A in patients with forehead hyperhidrosis. Dermatol Surg 2007;33 (special issue):S37–S43.
31. Eisele KH, Fink K, Vey M, Taylor HV. Studies on the dissociation of botulinum neurotoxin type A complexes. Toxicon 2011;57:555–565.
32. Sattler G, Callander MJ, Grablowitz D, et al. Noninferiority of incobotulinumtoxinA, free from complexing proteins, compared with another botulinum toxin type A in the treatment of glabellar frown lines. Dermatol Surg 2010;36(suppl 4):2146–2154.
33. Wohlfarth K, Wegner F, Bigalke H, Rummel A. The role of human serum albumin and neurotoxin associated proteins in the formulation of different BoNT/A products. Presented at the TOXINS 2012 conference, Miami Beach, FL, 5–8 December 2012.
34. Chen S. Clinical uses of botulinum neurotoxins: Current indications, limitations and future developments. Toxins (Basel) 2012;4:913–939.
35. Oriá RB, Ferreira FVA, Santana EN, Fernandes MR, Brito GAC. Estudo das alterações relacionadas com a idade na pele humana, utilizando métodos de histo-morfometria e autofluorescência. An Bras Dermatol 2003;78:425–434.
36. Brandt FS, Bellman B. Cosmetic use of botulinum A exotoxin for the aging neck. Dermatol Surg 1998;24: 1232–1234.
37. Small R. Botulinum toxin injection for facial wrinkles. Am Fam Physician 2014;90:168–175.
38. Niamtu J 3rd. Botulinum toxin A: A review of 1,085 oral and maxillofacial patient treatments. J Oral Maxillofac Surg 2003;61:317–324.
39. Patel D, Mehta F, Trivedi R, Thakkar S, Suthar J. Botulinum toxin and gummy smile—A review. IOSR J Dent Med Sci 2013;4:1–5.

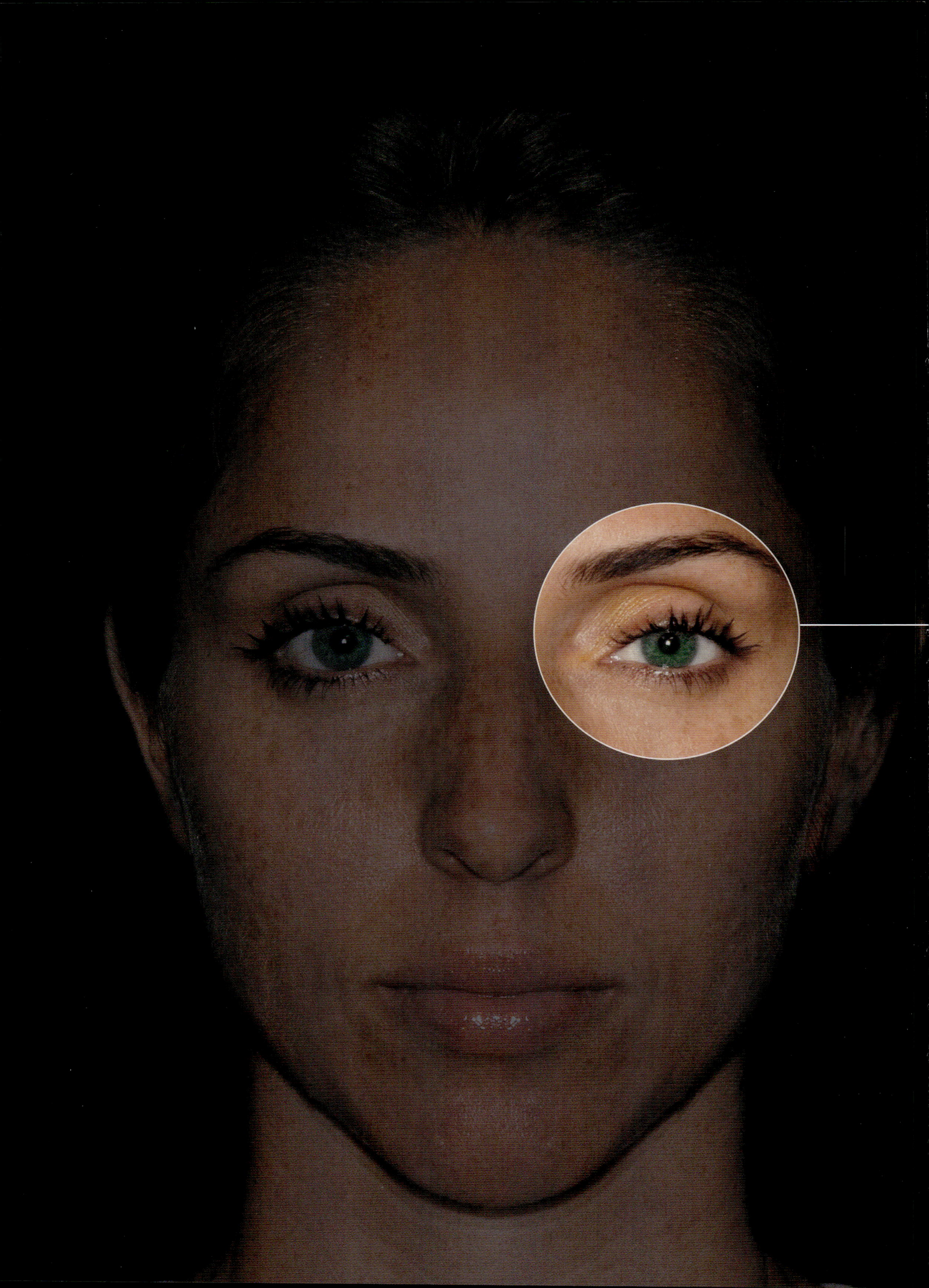

CHAPTER

02

Facial Analysis and Photographic Documentation

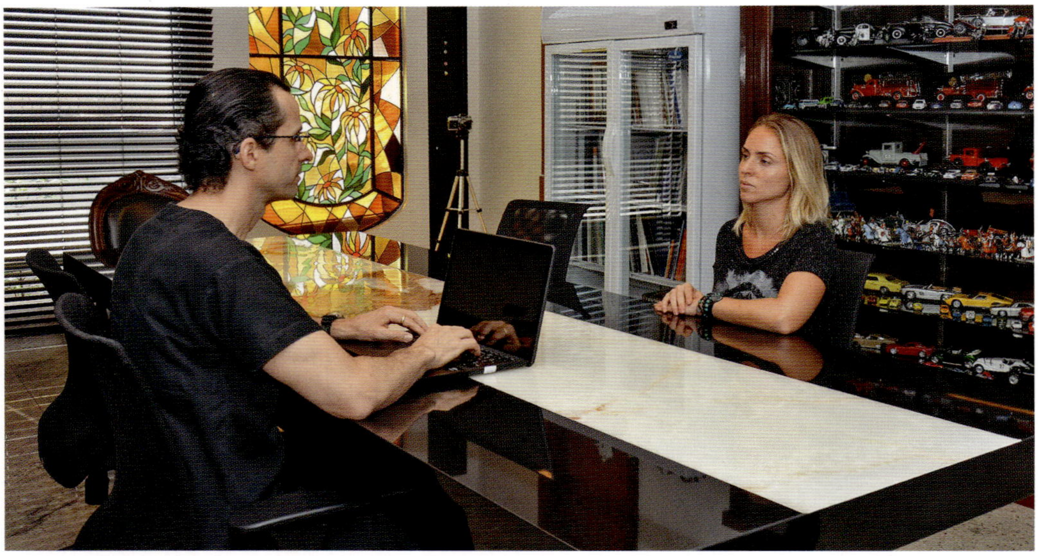

Fig 2-1 First impression. During the initial patient consultation, the clinician should record all facial aspects with the muscles at rest as well as the problems that might arise during the natural smile and speech.

Dentistry goes beyond treating the oral cavity and smile. A complete facial analysis and use of esthetic references allow the professional to identify changes that can be made to establish facial harmony.

During the first appointment, the patient should fill out a medical history form at the front desk. The clinician should then review this history with the patient considering the following:

- Main complaints
- History of present medical conditions (location, onset, evolution, previous treatments, and possible causes)
- Dental history, including all relevant previous treatments not related to the main complaint
- Medical history, including all medical conditions and medical interventions
- Personal and social history, including oral hygiene, parafunctional habits, and diet habits (sugar, acid)

It is important for the clinician to observe the patient at rest, when speaking, and when smiling during this consultation (Fig 2-1). All spontaneous facial expressions should also be observed and recorded. This will allow the clinician to fully evaluate the patient's face and determine any asymmetries or hyperkinetic muscles.

Complete Facial Analysis

The facial analysis should be as thorough as possible. A complete diagnosis will provide the most effective treatment plan. Therefore, all aspects of the face—the positive and the negative—should be considered from multiple perspectives:

- Frontal view at rest and smiling
- Profile view at rest and smiling
- Photographs of frontal view at rest and smiling
- Photographs of profile view at rest and smiling
- In case of asymmetries during speech, video of the patient speaking

Each facial characteristic and its possible correction should be recorded.

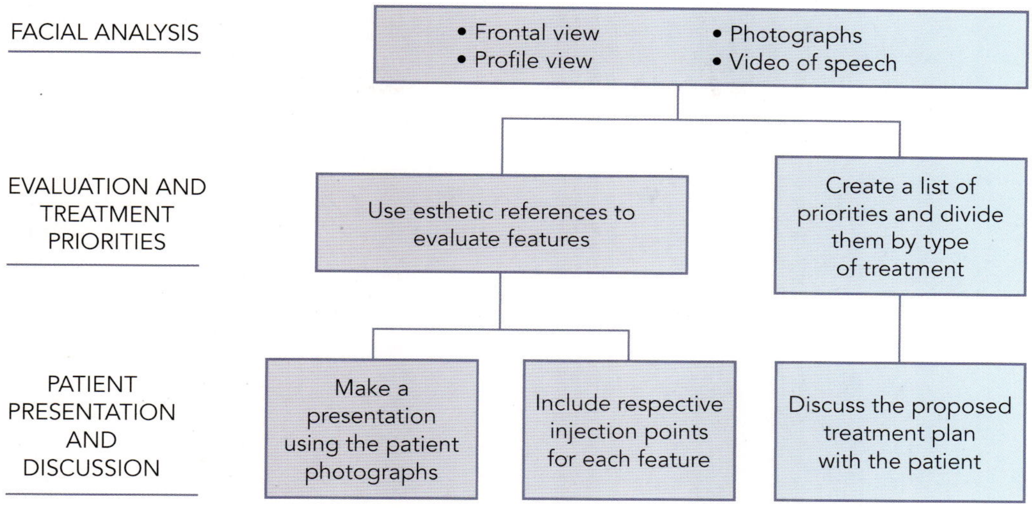

Fig 2-2 Facial analysis and patient presentation.

The clinician should continue the facial analysis with the following steps:

1. Evaluate the findings according to several esthetic references.
2. Create a numbered list of priorities. At the top of the list should be the least esthetic features that require the most attention. This list will help to explain the treatment priorities to the patient.
3. Subdivide the list of characteristics by type of treatment: therapeutic, structural, and aging. Any therapeutic treatment is most important, followed by structural. A frequent mistake is to only consider the aging process of the patient.
4. Make a presentation using the patient photographs and respective injections points.
5. Discuss the treatment plan with the patient. This should be an interactive discussion. Sometimes patients are surprised when looking at their own photographs because they are used to looking at themselves only through a mirror, which provides fewer details than a photograph. This conversation will provide the clinician the opportunity to readjust the plan according to the patient's desires for treatment.

Figure 2-2 summarizes this process.

Photographic Documentation

Photography can be used in dentistry for many different reasons, including assisting the clinician during initial examination of the patient; helping with diagnosis; evaluating treatment over time; storing legal documentation; capturing digital material for publication; educating patients or students; communicating with patients and professional team members, colleagues, and technicians; and finally, marketing. Each of these applications enhances and elevates the status of the practice as well as improves delivery of care to patients.[1]

Regardless of clinical experience, the treatment plan should never be based on a clinician's intuition. Instead, it should be guided by esthetic, facial, and dental analysis.

Evaluation of esthetic references should be performed over the photographs of the patient. Rulers, masks, and projections can be placed over the images and used as tools for facial analysis. This should be done when the patient is not present.

Photographs taken during the first appointment help the operator to perform facial analysis and can be used to help the patient understand the treatment plan and diagnosis. The clinician can also obtain facial data by performing measurements directly on the patient's face. This is faster and more practical than using images for the measurements, which are scale representations. At least one actual measurement on the patient's face should be recorded when the patient is present so that the other measures can be proportionally performed using an image.

Studio infrastructure

It is important to equip the dental office with a photographic studio to ensure that any photograph taken is good quality and captures the necessary information. A proper photographic studio includes the following (Fig 2-3):

- Two medium-sized soft boxes to diffuse a smooth and regular light to the patient's face. They should be slightly longer than the vertical measurement of the patient's face and neck. Avoid smaller light sources because they tend to concentrate the light at the center of the face. Modern digital cameras are able to remotely command the soft box, shooting with no need for cables.
- One hair light to delineate head contour, thereby improving the contrast with the black background. Black backgrounds are neutral and do not compete with the face. Position this light above or below the face so that the device is not displayed.
- Three tripods to support the flash units and hair light devices. They should be positioned higher than a tall standing patient.
- One black background with its own support to standardize the photographs. Avoid a white background, as it will compete with the face because it is brighter than the skin. A matte background is preferred to avoid shadowing.

Preparing the patient

Certain procedures must be performed before photographs are taken to ensure that the photographs capture the necessary information:

1. Remove all makeup from the face, because it blocks the visualization of the skin. Keep the face dry at all times to avoid reflexes from the flash. → *Provide makeup removers and cotton pads.*
2. Neutralize the hair by tying it up and using headbands. → *Provide the most discreet type of headband.*
3. Ask the patient to remove all jewelry (eg, earrings and necklaces) to eliminate the distraction. → *Focus on the anatomical aspects of the face.*
4. Instruct the patient to look horizontally and not tilt or turn the head. → *Consider the patient's height and indicate on the wall or the flash unit where he or she should look.*

Facial photographs should be taken with the lips closed, with the lips relaxed, and with the patient smiling (Fig 2-4).

Protocol

Frontal and profile facial views should be captured (Figs 2-5 and 2-6). Facial views should also be taken with the patient sitting to diagnose wrinkles, grooves, and volume deficiencies (Figs 2-7 and 2-8).

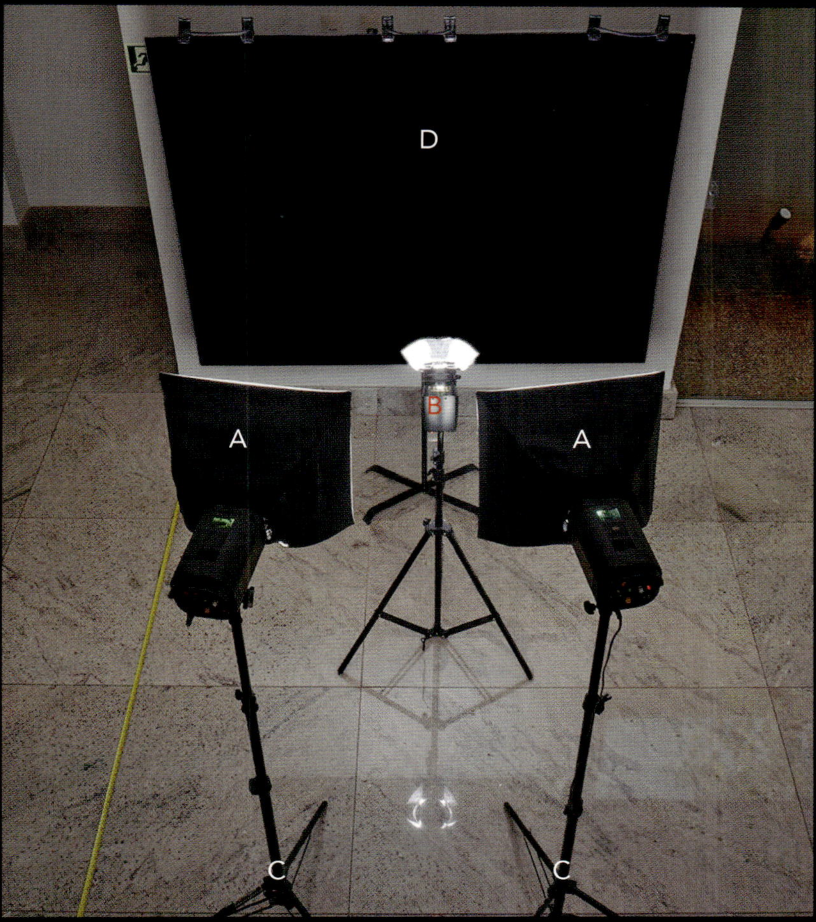

Fig 2-3 Studio infrastructure. A, soft box. B, hair light. C, tripod. D, black background.

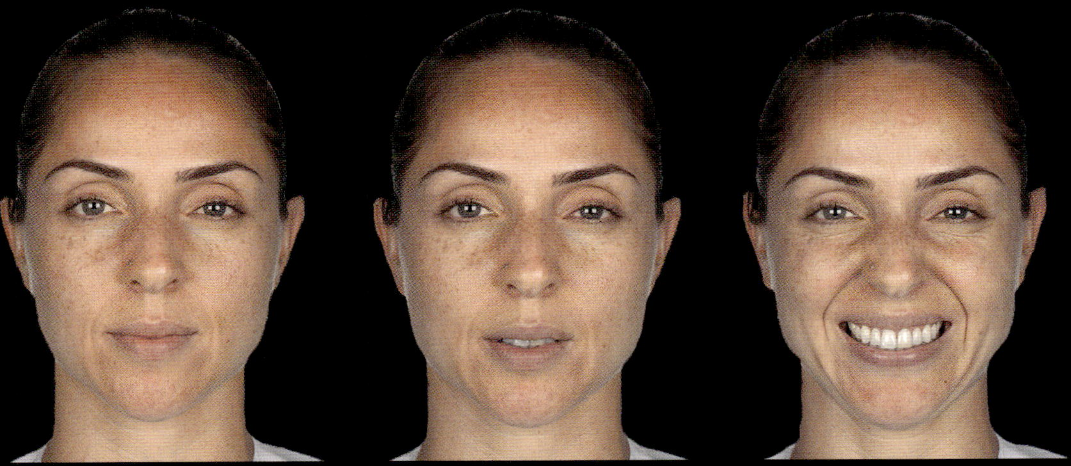

Lips closed: Instruct the patient to avoid moving the face so that the facial muscles will not be activated. Also instruct him or her to slightly close the lips.

Lips relaxed: Instruct the patient to keep the same position but relax the lips. Ask the patient to breathe through his or her mouth.

Smile: Ask the patient to smile as spontaneously as possible. The photographer should also smile and say something funny to encourage a natural smile. Ask the patient not to incline the head sideways when smiling.

Fig 2-4 Facial photographs.

Frontal view

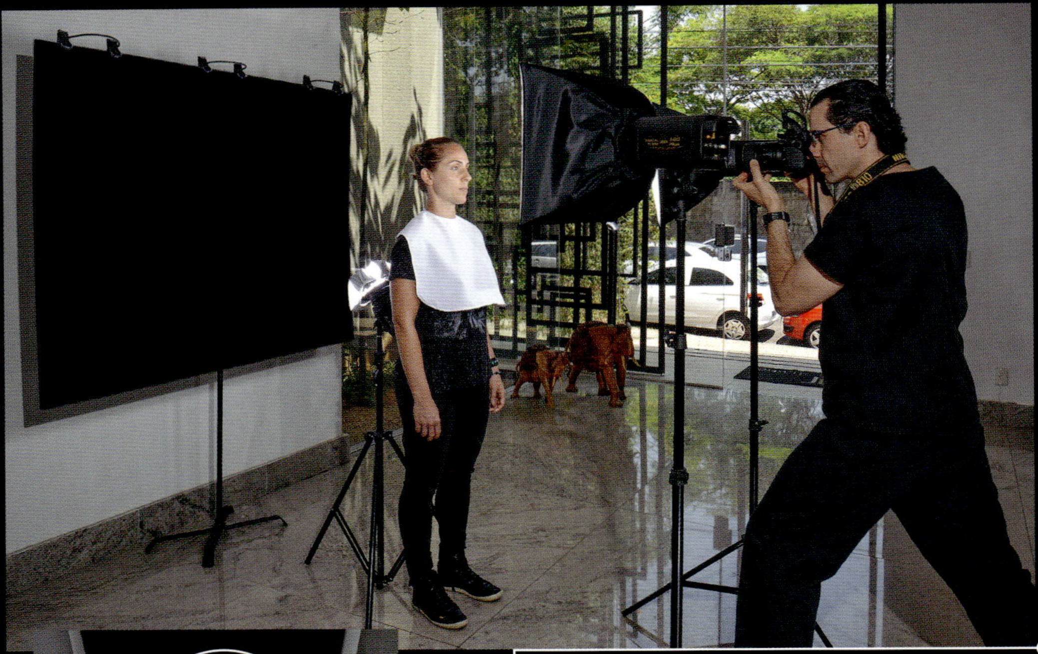

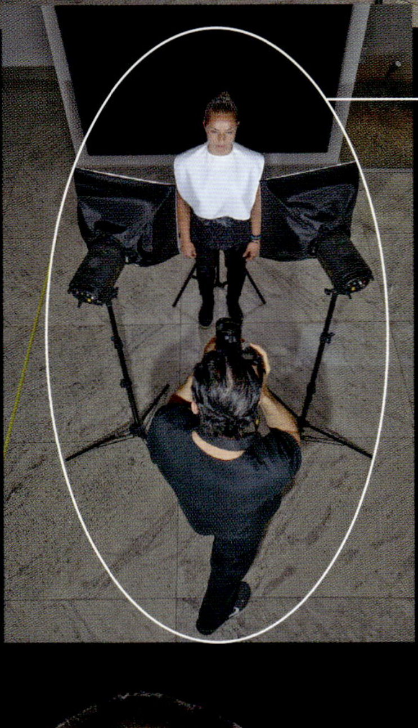

Fig 2-5 The photographer should bend the knees so that the camera is parallel to the ground and at the same level as the patient's face. The flashes are positioned almost perpendicular to the face.

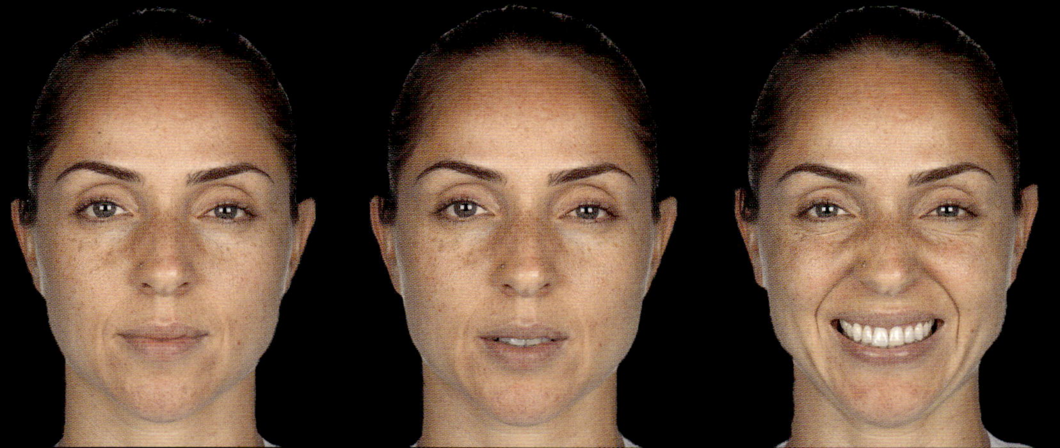

Profile view

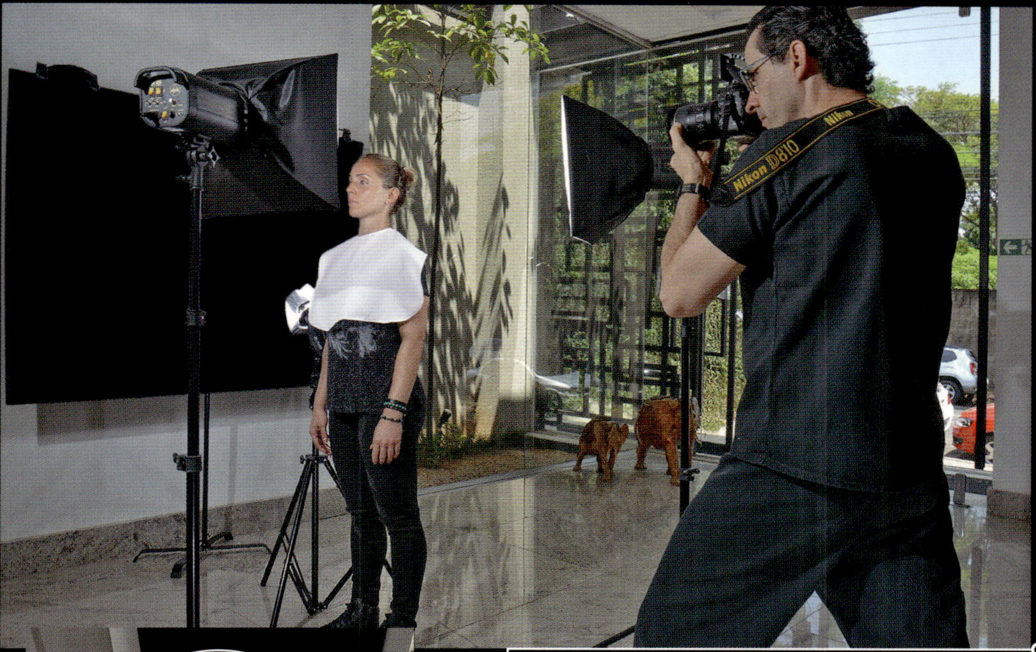

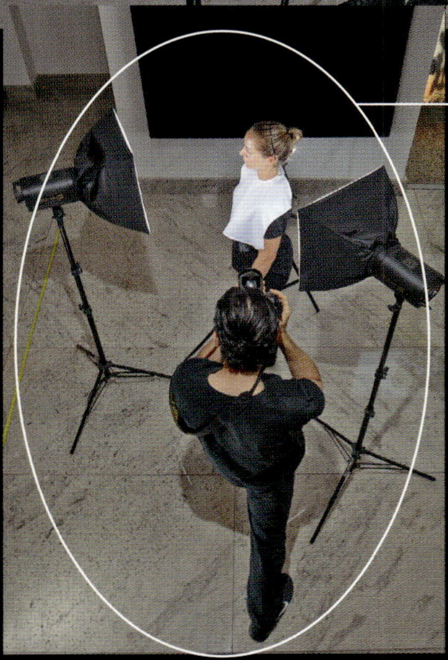

Fig 2-6 Only one flash is moved laterally, almost perpendicular to the frontal plane of the face.

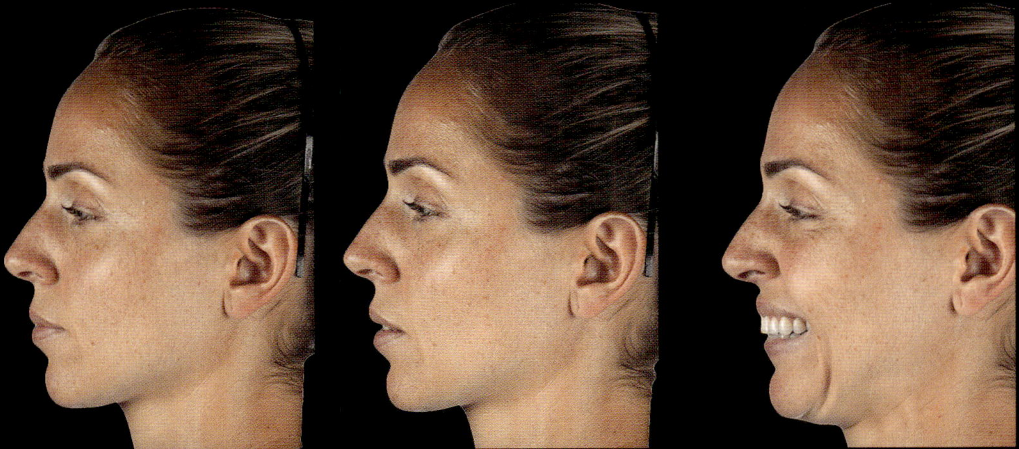

Sitting view ("shower technique")

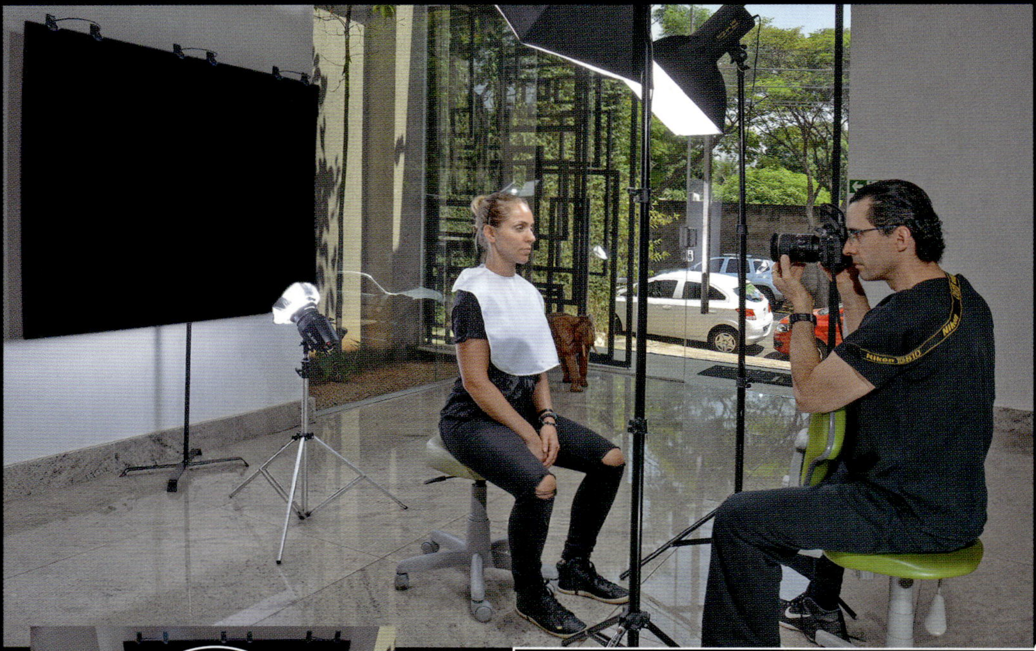

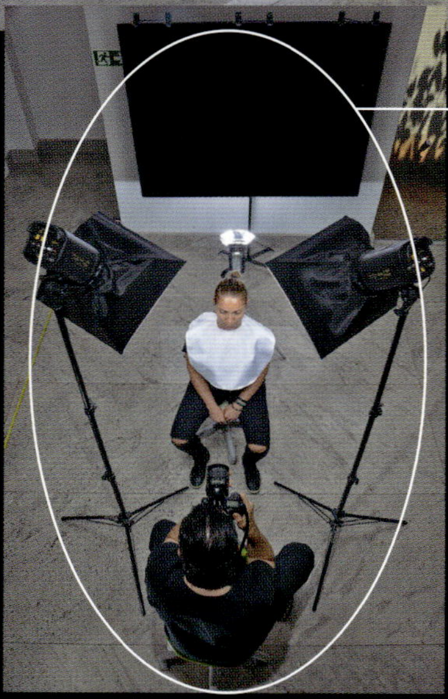

Fig 2-7 The patient should sit on a stool so that his or her face is below the flash. The seat should not have a back support so that the patient can keep the head in a natural position.

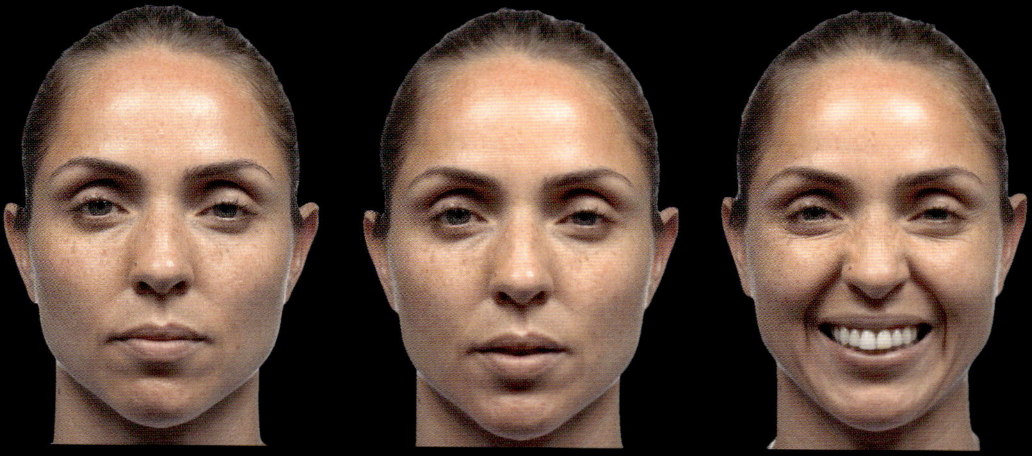

Flash positioning

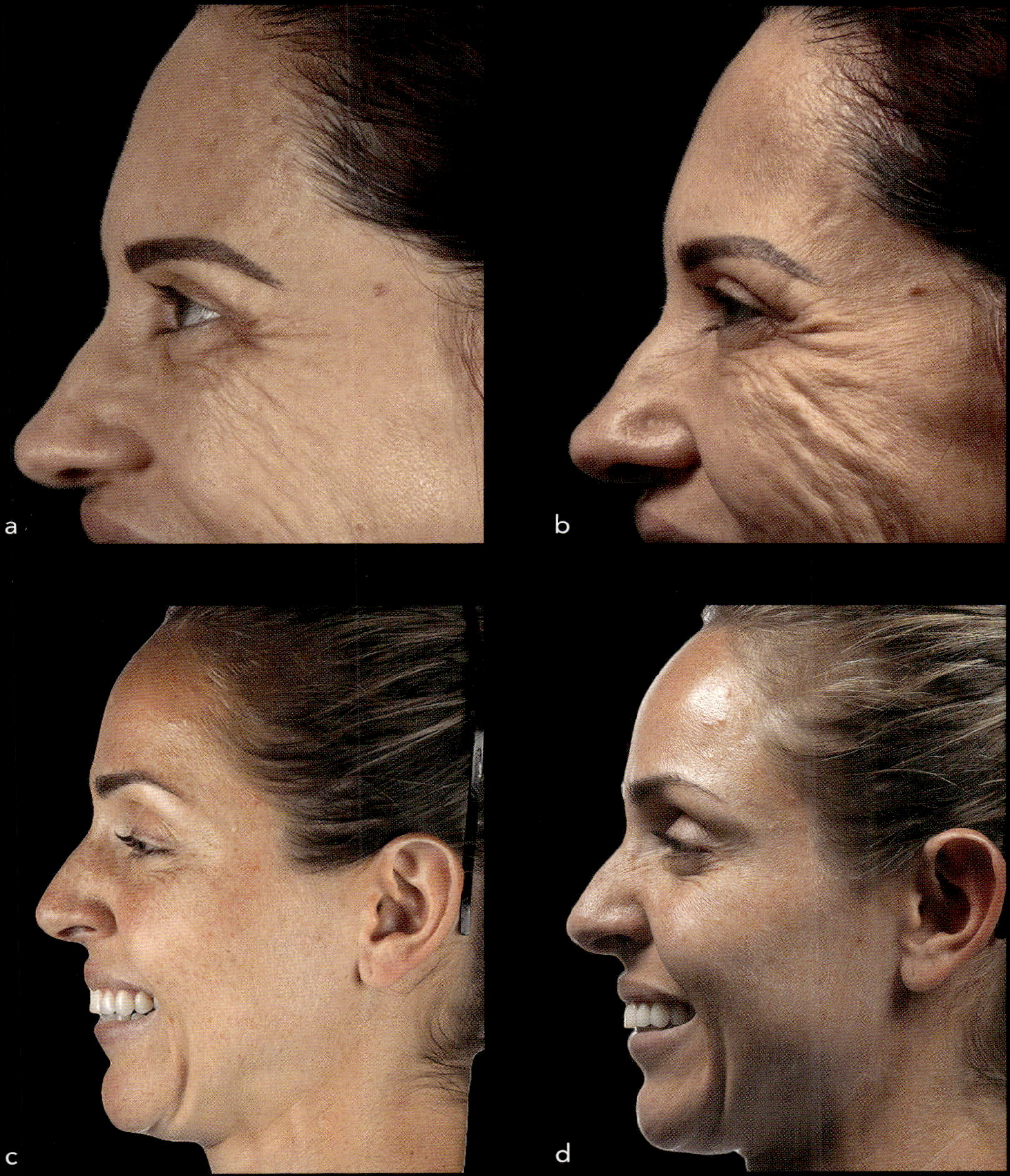

Fig 2-8 Flash positioning is important when taking photographs to diagnose wrinkles, grooves, and volume deficiencies. *(a and c)* Photographs used for diagnosis with the flashes positioned in a conventional way, that is, at the same height as the patient's face. *(b and d)* Photographs taken on the same day but with the flashes positioned above the patient's face, similar to a shower technique. Note that although the photographs show some dark areas, dynamic wrinkles at the orbicularis oculi and nasal muscles are clearly visible.

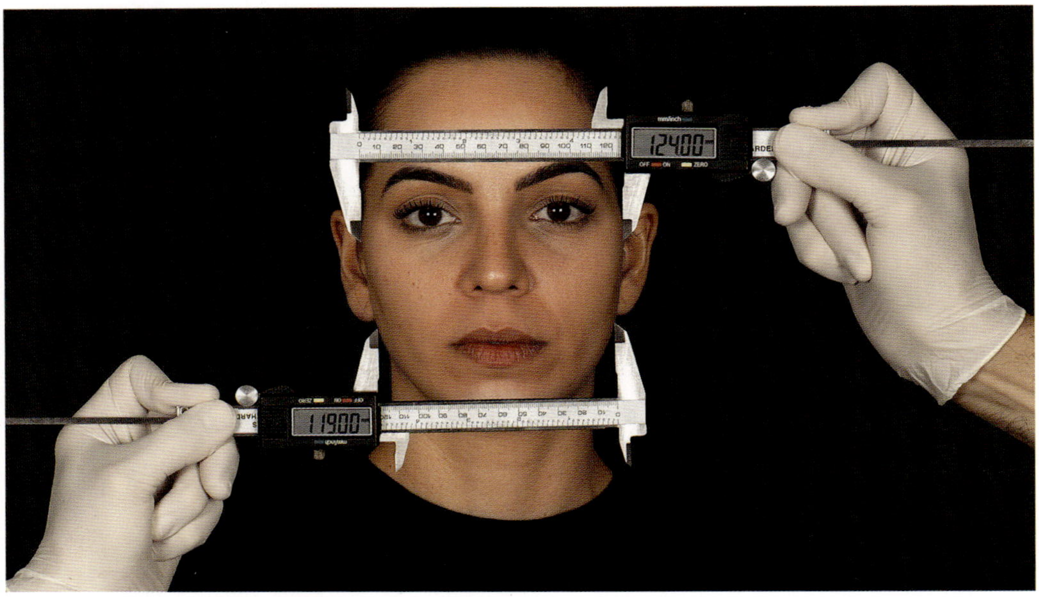

Fig 2-9 Examples of facial measurement. Note the correct measurement of the bizygomatic and bigonial distances. The difference between these two measurements must be at least 4%. A smaller number could mean masseter muscle hypertrophy. A difference of 12% is esthetically very pleasant.

Clinical Examination

Ricketts[2] described *esthetics* as the study of beauty. Dierkes[3] stated that beauty of the face might be defined as a state of harmony and balance of facial proportions, that is, a balanced relationship among skeletal structures, teeth, and soft tissue.

In order to provide more objective guidelines regarding the perception of smile esthetics, numerous studies were performed using digital image manipulation.[4] Characteristics that were better elucidated with this technology include the following:

- The smile arc[5,6]
- The optimal amount of gingival display[7–9]
- The ideal amount of buccal corridors[4,10]
- The prominence of dental and gingival asymmetries[5,11]
- The influence of maxillary anterior diastemata[11–13]
- The impact of midline and long axis deviations[5,7,11]
- The importance of maxillary incisor size, proportion, and symmetry[13–17]

Several anthropometric measurements[18] are extremely important when performing facial and smile analysis, including the bizygomatic distance and the bigonial distance (Fig 2-9):

- *Bizygomatic distance:* From the right to the left zygion, the most lateral points on the right and left sides of the zygomatic arches—that is, the widest part of the face (see Fig 2-11). For females, this distance is 65% to 70% of the face length measured from the middle of the hairline to menton. For males, it is 65% of the face length.
- *Bigonial distance:* From the right to the left gonion, the most external and prominent angle of the right and left side of the jaw—that is, the lowest facial width (see Fig 2-11).

Box 2-1 shows the facial aspects to evaluate during the clinical examination, based on the literature and the author's clinical experience. Each of these is explained in detail in the sections that follow.

Box 2-1 **Facial aspects to evaluate during the clinical examination**

Face shape: Triangular, square, or oval. Observe if the patient shows a lack of harmony.

Bizygomatic distance: The measurement is made at the widest point.

Temporomandibular joints: Observe for signs of temporomandibular disorders, sounds (clicking and popping), deviations, limitations, and reduction. Palpate the temporomandibular joints as well as masseter and temporal muscles.

Dental exposure: Anterior and posterior, at rest and while smiling.

Dynamic wrinkles: Note when these wrinkles become accentuated. Inject the toxin as a preventive measure.

Static wrinkles: Record all of them. Toxin is injected for correction.

Buccal corridor and commissure asymmetries: Evaluate the face in a static view and during muscle dynamics. See chapter 4 for examples in clinical cases.

Definition of the jawline: Observe if the body and angle of the mandible are outlined. See chapter 4 for examples in clinical cases.

Hyperkinetic muscles: Note the hyperkinetic muscles (see chapter 4).

Nasal tip mobility: Assess during smile and speech, asking the patient to pronounce the letter M several times. See chapter 4 for examples in clinical cases.

Width of jaw and buccal corridor: The patient's eye could be a reference for this evaluation.

Face Shape

The size, shape, and arrangement of the maxillary anterior teeth are the most influential factors for a harmonious appearance, particularly when the face is viewed from the front.[19] These teeth normally dominate during a person's smile.[17,20] Fornaziero and Souza[21] established a correlation between the buccal outline of the maxillary central incisor and the face shape and observed a predominance of triangular maxillary anterior teeth as well as triangular faces. Table 2-1 illustrates the three basic face shapes and their characteristics.

How to determine face shape

Sit in front of the patient and ask him or her to relax all facial muscles. Mark a point at the widest part of the zygomatic bone (bizygomatic distance), another point at the angle of the jaw, and a third point at the lateral aspect of the chin. Draw a line connecting the first and third points (see examples in Table 2-1).

Observing the second point in relation to the neck, the face shape can be determined as follows:

- *Triangular:* The second point is anterior to the junction between the neck and jawline (inside the neck area).
- *Square:* The second point is above the junction between the head and neck (outside the neck area).
- *Oval:* The second point is located exactly at the junction of the head and neck.

Table 2-1 Face shapes and their characteristics

	TRIANGULAR	SQUARE	OVAL
Characteristics	• Shows a bizygomatic distance that is markedly greater than the bigonial distance. • More feminine face shape. • Can be altered in cases of hypertrophic masseters, turning it square. • Generally gives the impression of a delicate, young face.	• Shows a bizygomatic distance that is slightly greater than the bigonial distance. • More masculine face shape. • A bigonial distance greater than the bizygomatic distance might mean masseter hypertrophy. • Generally gives the impression of a strong face.	• Shows a roundness observed between the zygomatic bone and gonial angle. • More childlike face. • Check indication for a bichectomy, which is rare. • Generally gives the impression of a childlike face because of the big cheeks characteristic of children.
Advantage	It adds more value to the patient's mouth because the smaller cheeks avoid competition with the mouth.	It helps to define a better limit of the head/neck, which is an important criterion for beauty.	The face is smoother and more curved.
Disadvantage	Aging and/or overweight patients quickly lose definition of the jawline.	It decreases the dominance of the mouth because the lower third is wide.	A slight malar depression is not observed between the zygomatic bone and the two gonial angles, which in other face shapes accentuates the mouth. Women with this face shape often wear blush to give the impression of this depression.
Male examples	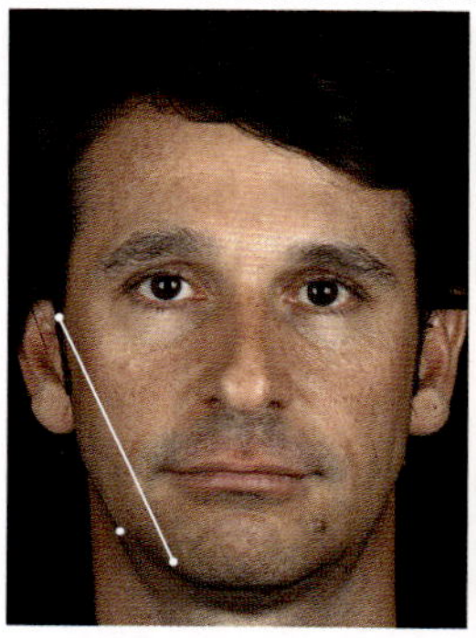	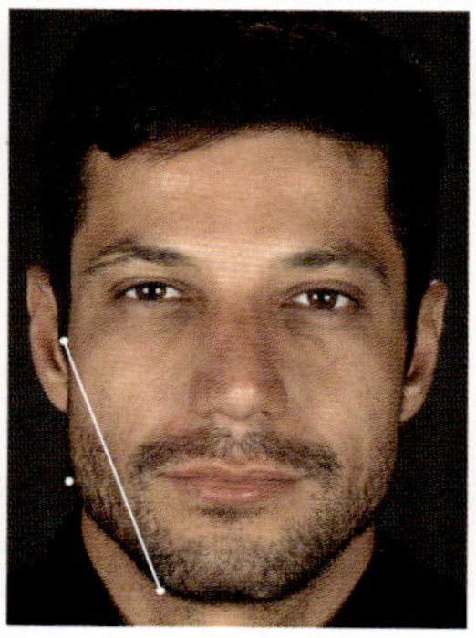	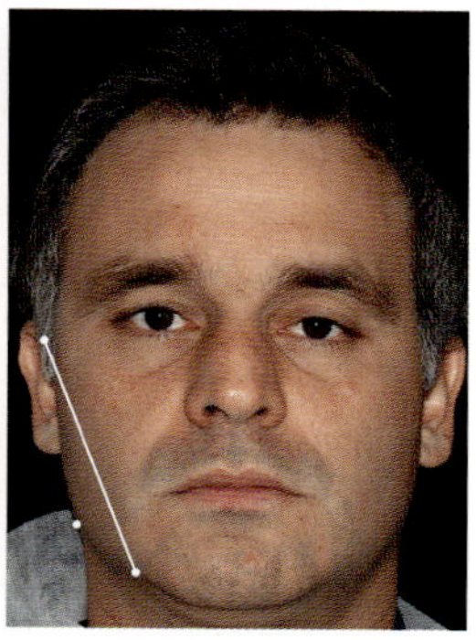
Female examples	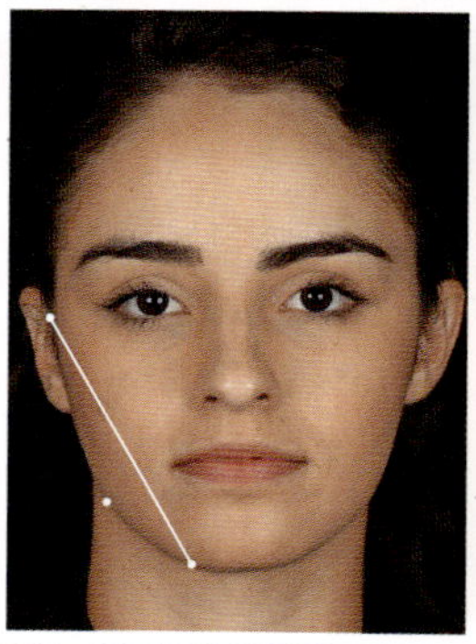	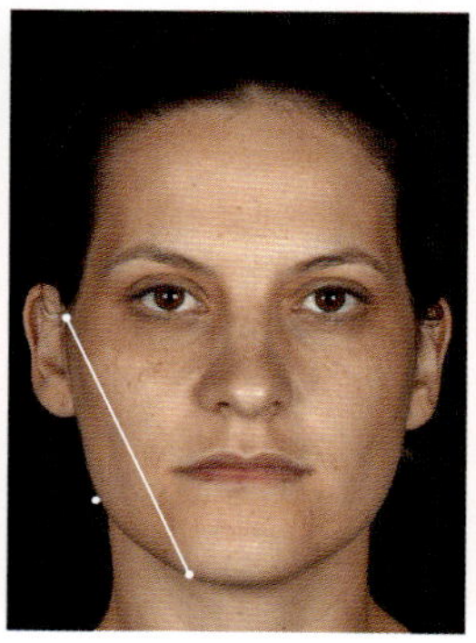	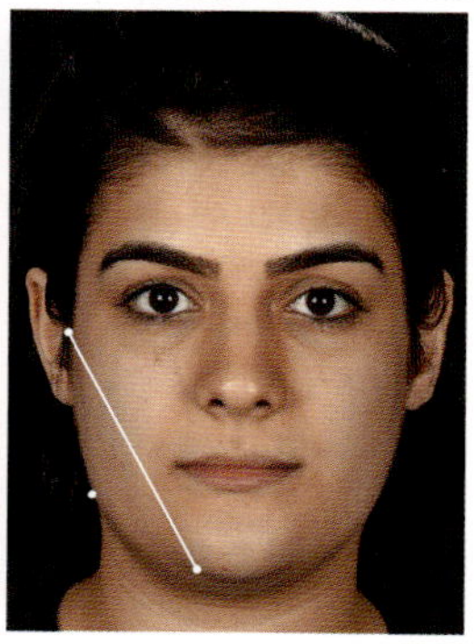

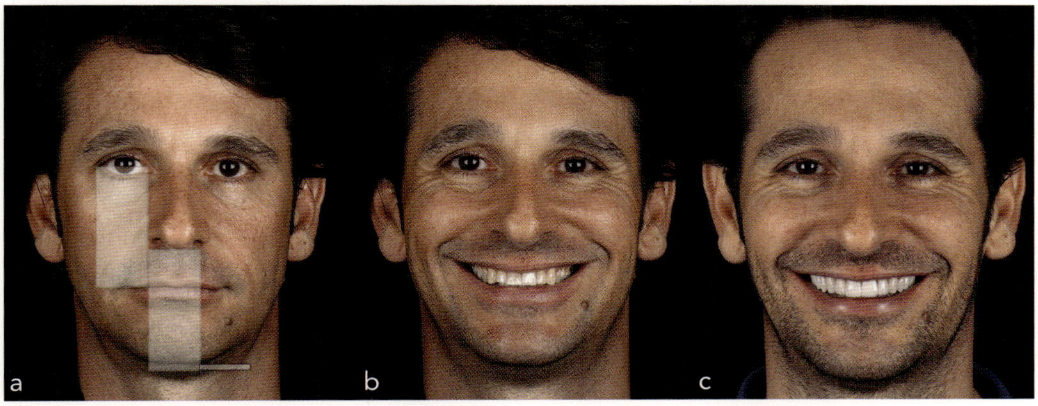

Fig 2-10 *(a)* Patient with decreased OVD. Rectangles of equal length are used to verify if the distance from the lateral palpebral fissure to the buccal commissure is the same as that from the nasolabial angle to the base of the chin. *(b and c)* Smile views before and after treatment. Note that the OVD has been increased with BTX injections and dental restorations.

Observing the line drawn between the points, the face shape can be determined as follows:

- *Triangular:* Between the most superior and most inferior point, the side of the face is almost straight, with no noticeable angle located at the level of the second point.
- *Square:* Between the most superior and most inferior point, the side of the face is angled, with an abrupt change of direction, with a more noticeable angle located at the level of the second point.
- *Oval:* Between the most superior and most inferior point, the side of the face is round, with a curvilinear path and no noticeable angle at the second point.

Decreased occlusal vertical dimension

Facial analysis of the patient pictured in Fig 2-10a revealed a bilateral clicking at the temporomandibular joint (TMJ) and a slight decrease in the occlusal vertical dimension (OVD), assessed using a Willis compass.

Rectangles of equal length are used to verify if the distance from the lateral palpebral fissure to the buccal commissure is the same as that from the nasolabial angle to the base of the chin. This measurement should be taken in the following clinical situations: *(1)* when the lower third of the face is shortened, *(2)* in the presence of parafunctional signals and symptoms, and *(3)* before extensive rehabilitations.

HOW COULD BOTULINUM TOXIN (BTX) HELP?

By decreasing the tonus of the main mandibular elevator muscles to allow the restoration of the OVD. In these cases, the injection should be administered preoperatively to help with the increase of the OVD, intraoperatively if the dental rehabilitation will take more than 4 months, and postoperatively to maintain the effect as long as parafunction is present. In cases of temporomandibular disorder (TMD) associated with parafunctional oral habits, excessive force during maxillary elevation could harm the stomatognathic system. Therefore, reducing the strength of the mandibular elevator muscles might work as an adjuvant therapy to existing treatments.[22,23]

TREATMENT PERFORMED:

1. Ten units (10U) of Botox (Allergan) were injected at two points in each masseter muscle, and 5U were injected at one point in each temporalis muscle.
2. The OVD was increased using direct resin composite restorations on the mandibular posterior teeth.
3. Ceramic veneers were bonded to the maxillary teeth (second premolar to second premolar) to obtain anterior guidance with an overbite (minimum of 2 mm and maximum of 4 mm).
4. Labial and malar augmentation were performed.

Figures 2-10b and 2-10c show the pretreatment and posttreatment smile views.

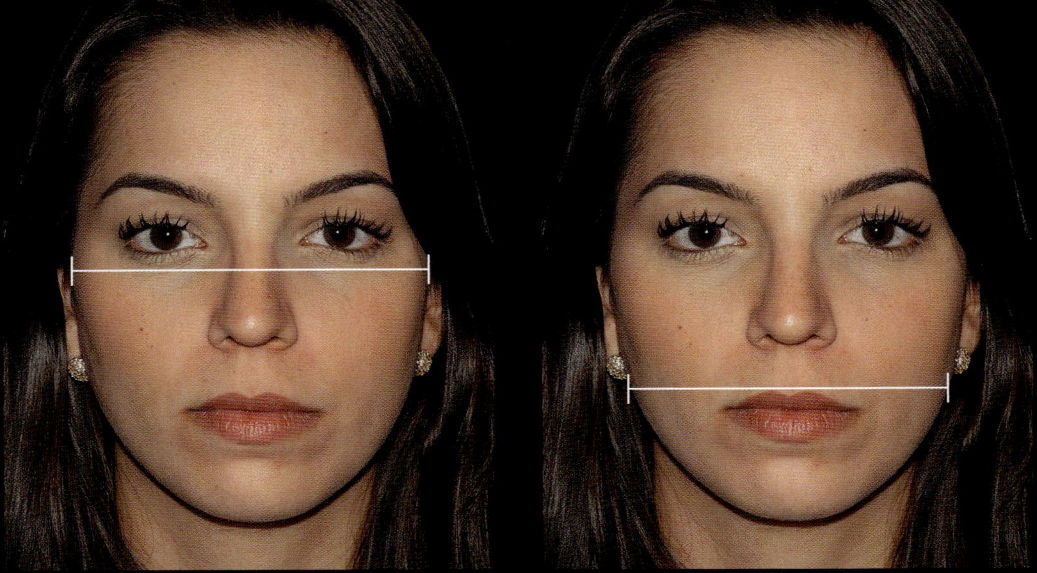

Fig 2-11 Bizygomatic distance and bigonial distance. The bigonial distance is approximately 12% shorter than the bizygomatic distance.

Bizygomatic Distance

Facial width is defined as the maximum distance between the most external points of the malar prominences (zygomatic width).[24,25] The largest part of the face is the zygomatic width, or bizygomatic distance. The bigonial distance is approximately 30% shorter than the bizygomatic distance.[26] The author observes that beautiful women show a difference of 12% between these two measurements, while a small number is found in men's faces because men have larger masseter muscles. The bizygomatic distance should be visually and numerically greater than the bigonial distance[27,28] (Fig 2-11).

Increased width of lower third of the face

Facial analysis of the patient pictured in Fig 2-12a showed that the bizygomatic distance was not remarkably greater than the bigonial distance. The patient reported left unilateral chewing and parafunctional habits.

Horizontal lines are drawn at the widest point between the zygomatic bones and gonial angles. This measurement should be taken in the presence of signs and symptoms of parafunctional habits.

HOW COULD BTX HELP?
After toxin injection, the volume of the masseter muscle is decreased, leading to a narrowing of the lower third. Injecting a higher dose of toxin in the mandibular elevators on the side the patient prefers to chew will tend to encourage chewing on the other side.

TREATMENT PERFORMED:

1. 10U of Botox were injected at two points in the right masseter muscle, and 5U were injected in the right temporalis muscle. On the left side, injections were given in the same muscles at doses of 50% higher.
2. The central incisors were lengthened with direct resin to improve anterior guidance.
3. The nasolabial fold was filled.
4. Deoxycholic acid was used to reduce fat at the submental region (double chin).

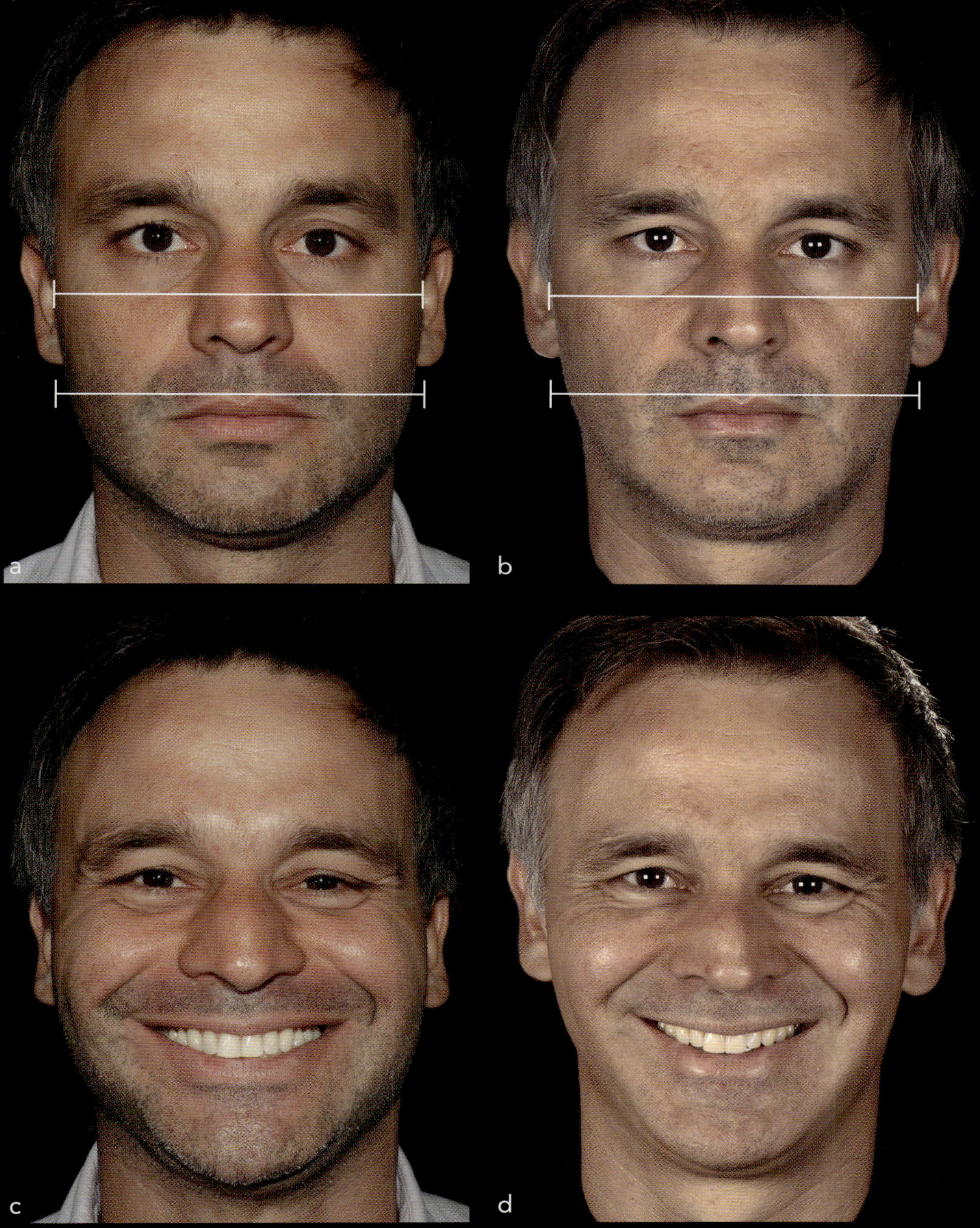

Fig 2-12 *(a)* Patient with increased width of the lower third. Note that the bigonial distance is almost the same as the bizygomatic distance. Also note the asymmetry (wider on left side of the face). *(b)* Measurements after BTX injection. Note the reduction in the bigonial distance and symmetry achieved in the lower third. *(c and d)* Smile views before and after treatment.

Figure 2-12b shows the patient after treatment. The left side of the face, previously a little wider than the right side, became symmetric after the injection (Figs 2-12c and 2-12d). The patient also reported that he began chewing on both sides.

With injections into the masseter muscle, it is important to inform the patient prior to treatment that the lower third of the face will likely be narrower after injection. Even a slight decrease in the definition of the jawline should make the face more esthetically pleasing, but the patient should be prepared for this change.

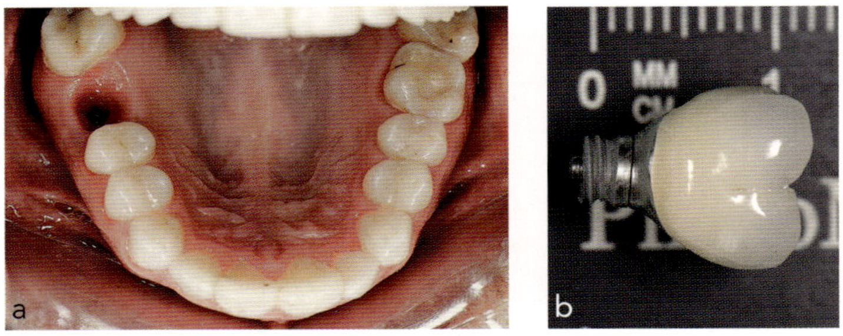

Fig 2-13 *(a and b)* Example of parafunction: Rare fracture of a Brånemark implant caused by clenching. The implant and its crown were functional for 10 years.

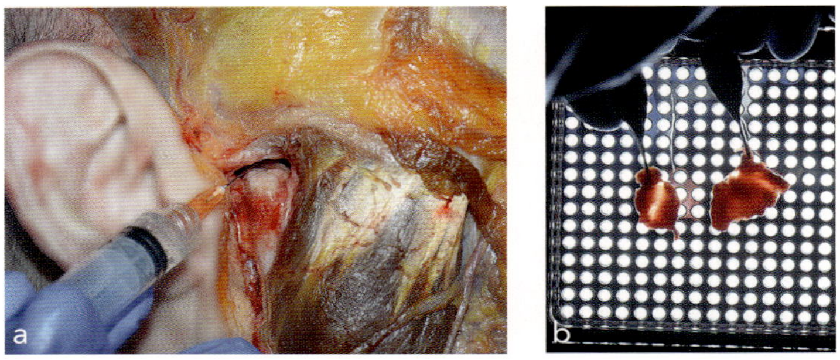

Fig 2-14 *(a)* Cadaver showing TMJ after synovium aspiration. *(b)* The articular disc on the left belonged to a cadaver whose teeth were worn out by attrition. The disc on the right was from a patient with preserved teeth.

Temporomandibular Joints

Any signs or symptoms of TMD should be evaluated and recorded during the clinical examination. These include the following[29,30]:

- Facial pain
- Tension headaches
- Dental loss related to parafunction
- Tooth and/or restoration fracture (Fig 2-13)
- Incisor or canine attrition (Fig 2-14)
- Dental mobility
- Cracks in dental enamel
- Abfraction
- Diastema opening
- A concave occlusal surface in the mandibular second molars
- Articular sounds (clicking)
- Linea alba in the buccal mucosa
- A tongue edge marked by the anatomical shapes of the teeth
- Bone exostosis (torus)
- A decrease in the lip vermilion volume
- Asymmetry and/or hypertrophy of the masseter muscles
- Apical and/or periodontal bone resorptions

HINT:
A good-quality stethoscope should be used to check the TMJ during movement, enabling an early diagnosis.

Kim et al[29] point out that successful TMD treatment starts from correctly differentiating the origin of symptoms. Because myofascial pain and limited mouth opening are the most frequent symptoms of masticatory muscle disorders, directing treatment at the muscular components of TMD could yield therapeutic gains.[31] Therefore, noninvasive conservative treatments such as counseling, a soft diet, behavioral medicine, physiotherapy, oral appliances, pharmacotherapy, and BTX injections are reported to be effective as first-line therapies for extra-articular pathologic conditions.[32]

Intra-articular pathologic conditions such as internal derangement and osteoarthritis could also benefit from the reversible interventions used to treat myofascial pain. Patients with acute pain, however, may require intra-articular injection of lidocaine, hyaluronic acid, or even a corticosteroid.[33] When the symptoms and pain surpass the effectiveness of these techniques, surgical approaches such as arthrocentesis, arthroscopy, and arthroplasty may be performed to treat anatomical pathology.

After the introduction of commercial brands of BTX-A (Botox, Dysport [Ipsen]), its injection therapy on orofacial muscles became a valuable adjunct in managing myofascial components of TMD.[22,30,34,35] Supporting literature dates back three decades, with successes reported in various therapeutic applications since the 1980s.[36] While clinical injection of BTX-A in the masticatory musculature of TMD patients can be considered a useful supportive treatment option for controlling complex TMD and alleviating its associated symptoms, more randomized controlled studies with larger sample sizes and longer follow-up periods are necessary in order to scrutinize and evaluate the full effects of BTX-A injections.

Dental Exposure

At rest

When the lips are at rest and slightly open, part of the clinical crowns of the central incisors should be displayed without any papillae showing. Women generally have shorter upper lips than men (an average of 19.5 mm in young women and 22 to 24 mm in young men), so this central incisor display averages 3.4 and 1.91 mm, respectively.[25] For maxillary lateral incisors, a smaller exposure is ideal, and the mesiobuccal aspect of the crown should be more exposed than the distobuccal. The maxillary canines may not be exposed at all or perhaps just the tip of the crown.

If the papilla between the maxillary central incisors is exposed or if more than the tip of the maxillary canine is exposed while the lips are at rest, the patient may have a gummy smile. The possible treatment could be injection of BTX into the muscles that lift the upper lip. However, before this diagnosis is made, it is fundamental to observe the upper lip during a smile.

Mandibular teeth should not be too exposed when the lips are at rest; this display should be smaller than that of the maxillary teeth. Greater exposure of the mandibular central incisor clinical crowns might mean one of the following:

- The patient is aging, with labial ptosis. This can be treated with fillers at the mentolabial sulcus.
- Dentoalveolar extrusion of the mandibular anterior teeth. This can be corrected with orthodontics.
- Hyperkinetic depressor labii inferioris. This can be treated with BTX injections in these muscles.

Figure 2-15 illustrates an ideal dental exposure at rest and an unesthetic dental exposure at rest.

During a smile

During a smile, the lower edge of the upper lip vermilion should touch the neck of the maxillary central incisors, hiding part of the neck but leaving the central papilla visible. Gingival exposure of up to 3 mm around the maxillary central incisors is considered acceptable.[7] An exposure exceeding 3 mm is considered a gummy smile. One of the possible treatments for gummy smile is the injection of BTX into the muscles responsible for elevating the upper lip. However, it is important to observe the upper lip at rest before any decisions are made.

Ideally, the clinical crowns of the maxillary premolars or at least their papillae should be entirely exposed. Lack of exposure could mean that the depressor anguli oris muscle and/or posterior fibers of the platysma are hyperkinetic.

The clinical crowns of the mandibular teeth should barely be visible during a smile. An exposure of the mandibular teeth greater than that of the maxillary teeth is considered unesthetic because it decreases the dominance esthetically required for the maxillary teeth during a smile. The display of gingiva around mandibular teeth is considered esthetically unpleasant, characterizing a lower gummy smile. The hyperkinetic activity of the depressor labii inferioris might explain this kind of smile.

Figure 2-16 illustrates an ideal dental exposure during a smile and an unesthetic dental exposure during a smile.

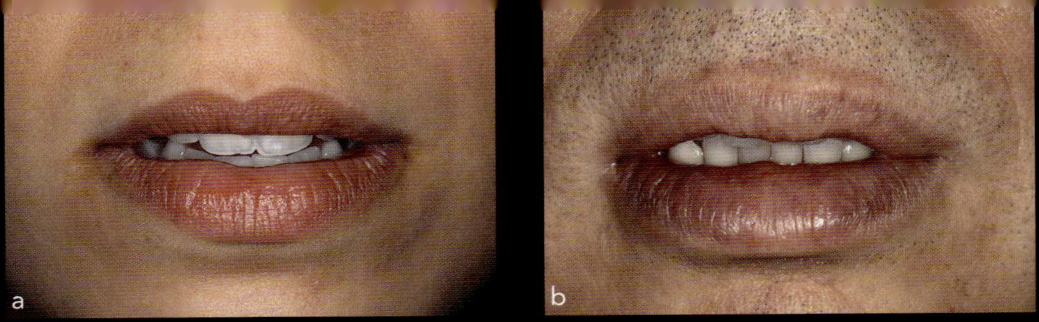

Fig 2-15 Ideal *(a)* and unesthetic *(b)* dental exposure at rest.

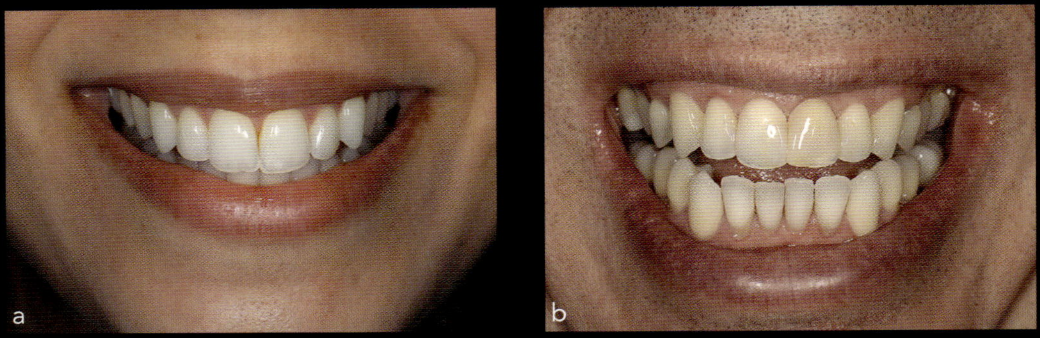

Fig 2-16 Ideal *(a)* and unesthetic *(b)* dental exposure during a smile.

Improper dental exposure

Facial analysis of the patient pictured in Fig 2-17a showed a face that looked too long due to an excessive dental display while smiling. During a smile, a greater display of clinical crown length of the maxillary anterior teeth should be visible compared with the mandibular teeth.[37] While the desired gingival exposure in relation to the neck of the maxillary central incisor is zero, up to 3 mm is considered acceptable. The mandibular teeth should not be exposed much at all.[25] If the mandibular teeth are more exposed than the maxillary teeth and/or there is exposure of mandibular gingival tissue, treatment should be considered.

HOW COULD BTX HELP?

Bilateral injection of BTX in the depressor labii inferioris decreases the depressing action of this muscle, thereby lifting the horizontal level of the lower lip, hiding the mandibular gingiva, and decreasing the exposure of mandibular anterior teeth at rest and during a smile.

TREATMENT PERFORMED:

1. 2U of Botox were injected at two points in the depressor labii inferioris, one on the right side and the other on the left side, for a total of 4U (Fig 2-17b).
2. Filler was injected in the upper lip to bring it forward in the profile view and reduce the slight gummy smile (Fig 2-17c).
3. Filler was injected in three regions of the menton to visually integrate it with the face, making it firmer and lifting its horizontal level (Fig 2-17d).
4. Preparationless direct composite resin veneers were placed (Fig 2-17e).

Figure 2-17f shows the posttreatment smile. The results address preventive, esthetic, and functional aspects of the face:

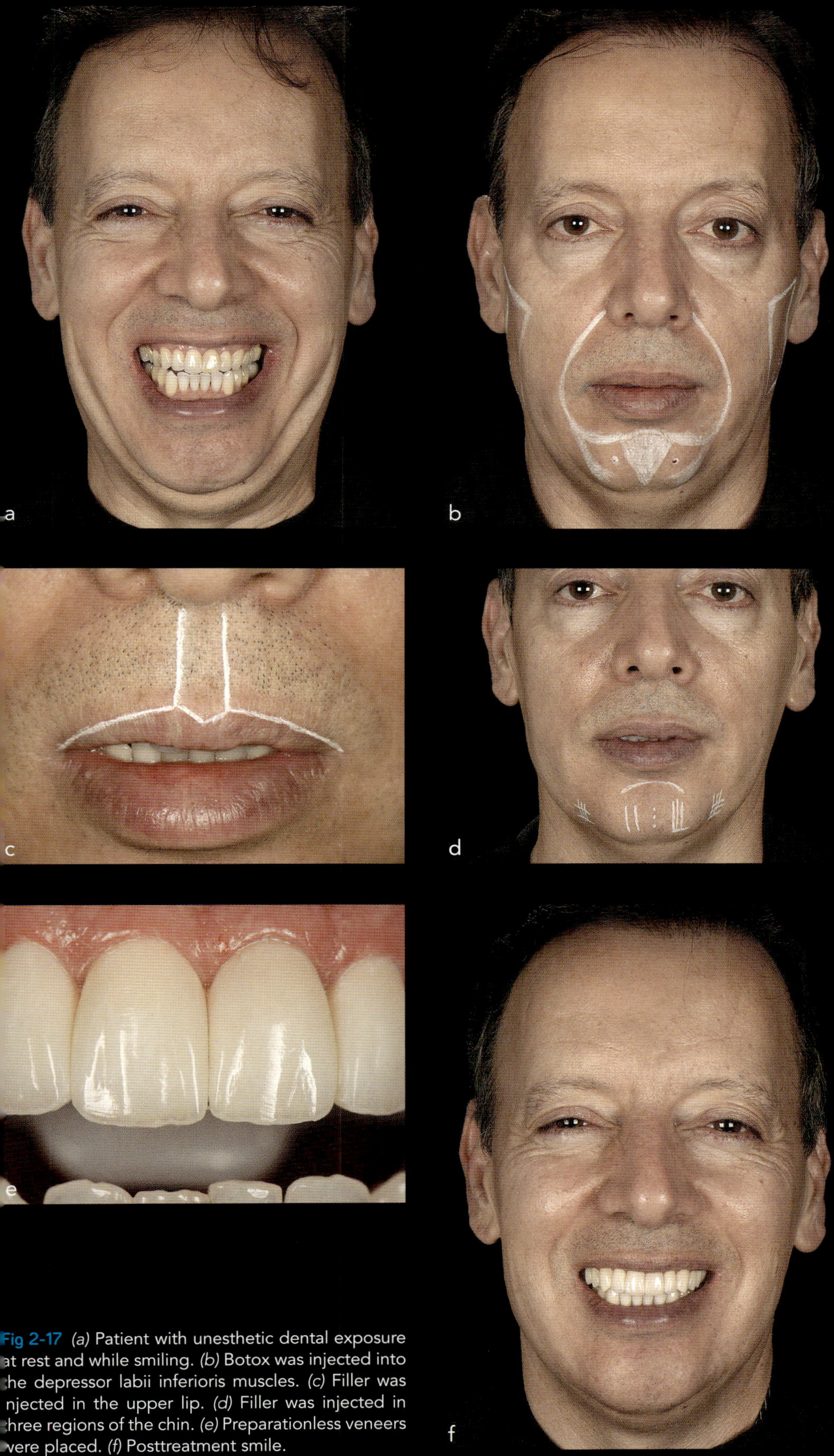

Fig 2-17 *(a)* Patient with unesthetic dental exposure at rest and while smiling. *(b)* Botox was injected into the depressor labii inferioris muscles. *(c)* Filler was injected in the upper lip. *(d)* Filler was injected in three regions of the chin. *(e)* Preparationless veneers were placed. *(f)* Posttreatment smile.

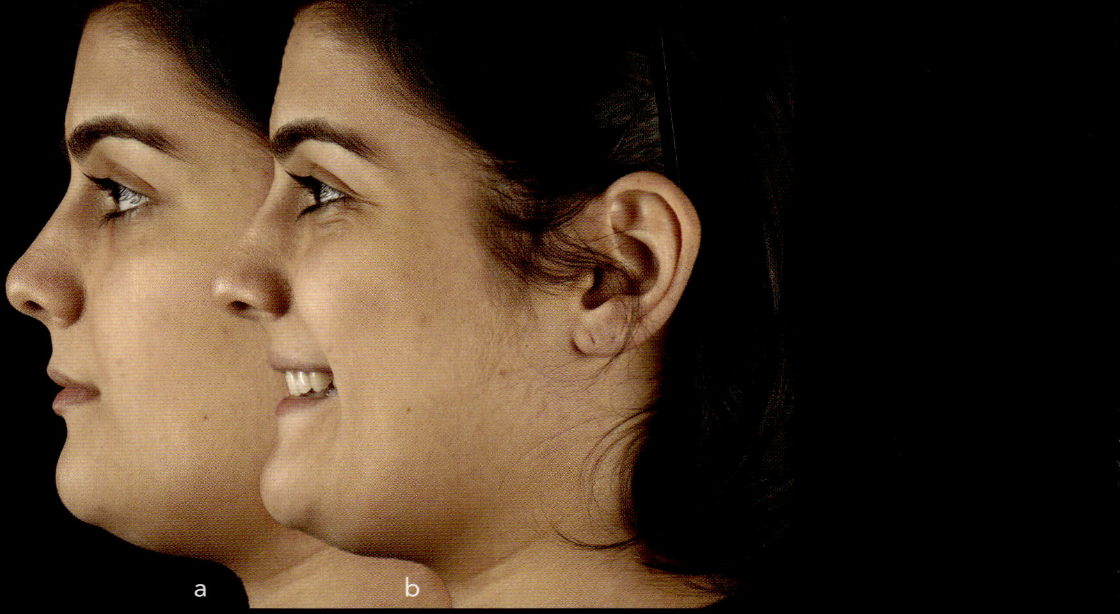

Fig 2-18 *(a and b)* Dynamic wrinkles around the eye with smiling. These wrinkles did not require treatment because they faded when the patient relaxed her face.

- *Preventive*: In many cases of lip incompetence, the mentalis muscle becomes hyperkinetic, forcing the lower lip against the upper lip. This damages the lip vermilion, which could show an accelerated loss of volume, thereby adversely affecting its position in relation to the lower lip (behind lower lip in profile). This was avoided by lifting the horizontal level of the lower lip through BTX injection in both depressor labii inferioris muscles.
- *Esthetic*: There was an apparent decrease in the excessive facial length, resulting in a more esthetic face. Fillers allowed for integration of the chin with the face, which were previously separated by grooves and depressions. The perception of a double chin was also reduced, as the lower lip was previously too low and pushed the neck skin backward.
- *Functional*: An improvement in labial seal was observed, favoring nasal breathing.

Dynamic Wrinkles

Spontaneous facial expressions such as speech and smiles are used to evaluate and classify wrinkles as static or dynamic. Forced facial expressions of "scared" and "angry" are used to mark injection points, using the wrinkles as reference (see chapter 3).

To diagnose dynamic wrinkles, ask the patient to make spontaneous facial expressions such as smiling and talking and observe and/or photograph the formation of wrinkles. Wrinkles formed during facial expressions that fade away as soon as the muscle action is over are considered *dynamic wrinkles*[38,39] (Fig 2-18). Their formation starts around the age of 28 years. Wrinkles should be treated as soon as they are observed at rest (static wrinkles). A magnifier might be used for the examination.

For the patient pictured in Fig 2-19, a magnifier was used to observe static wrinkles after spontaneous facial expressions. These wrinkles should be treated as soon as they are recognized and before they become easily noticeable as a preventive treatment.[38,39] In this case, the smoothing of periorbicular wrinkles was aided by treating the gummy smile. Only 2U of BTX were injected in two points of the orbicularis oculi muscle.

HOW COULD BTX HELP?
Because one of the causes of facial wrinkles is the action of muscles involved with facial expression, BTX can be injected in the muscle as soon as it starts marking the skin to prevent these lines from becoming permanent prematurely.

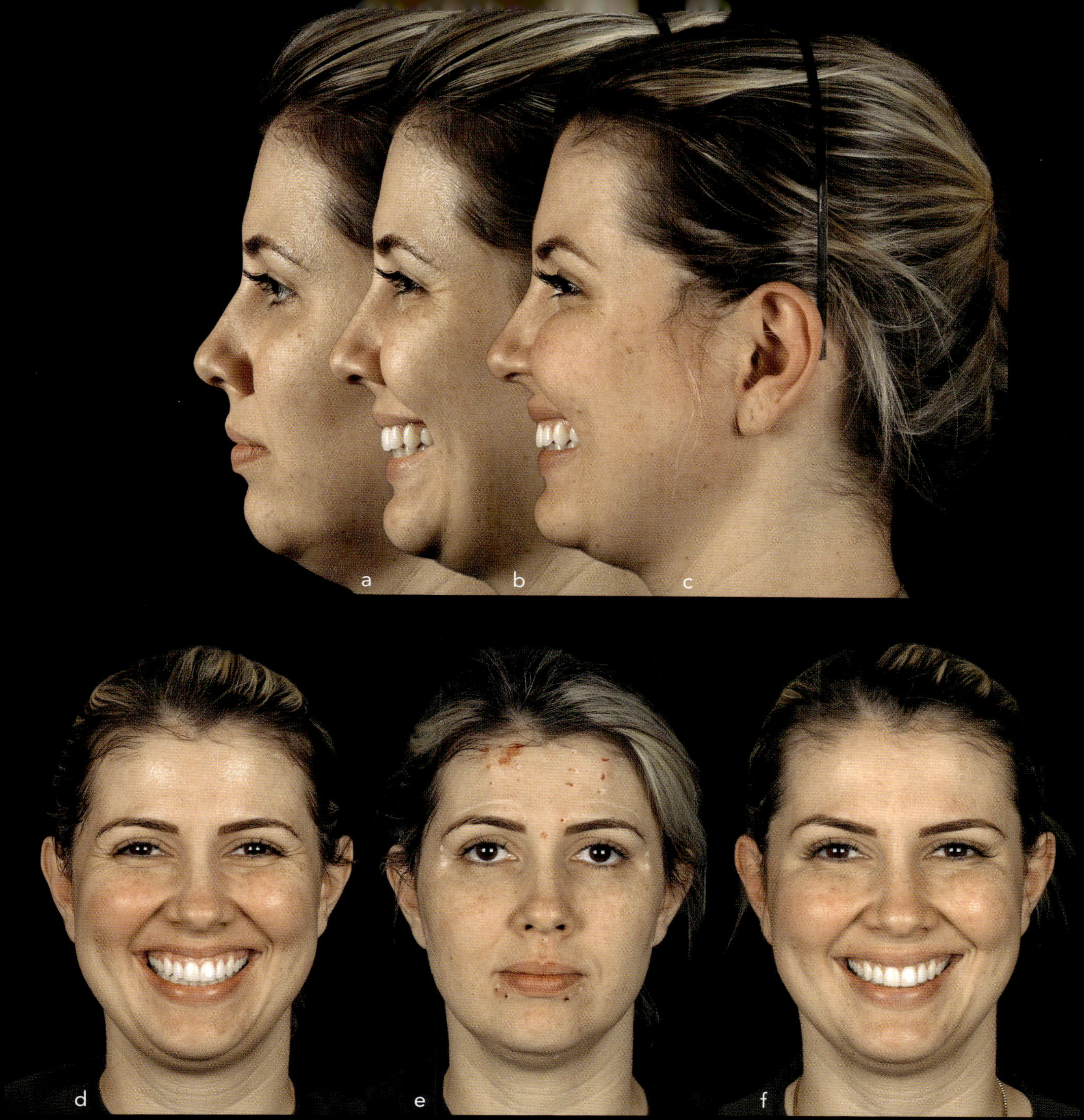

Fig 2-19 *(a to f)* This patient's dynamic wrinkles around the eyes were beginning to set in as static wrinkles, so they were treated with BTX. Her gummy smile was also treated with BTX injection in the depressor septi nasi muscle, further reducing the wrinkles at the eyes. The final view shows markedly fewer dynamic wrinkles *(f)*.

During a smile, the horizontal level of the lower lip is lifted, and consequently the malar region is also lifted, thereby pushing the lower eyelid upward and the eyes more closed. This causes the formation of periorbital wrinkles. In this case, the amplitude of this movement was reduced due to the injection of toxin in the depressor septi nasi muscle to decrease the gummy smile. The horizontal level of the upper lip was therefore lifted less, resulting in fewer wrinkles around the eyes.

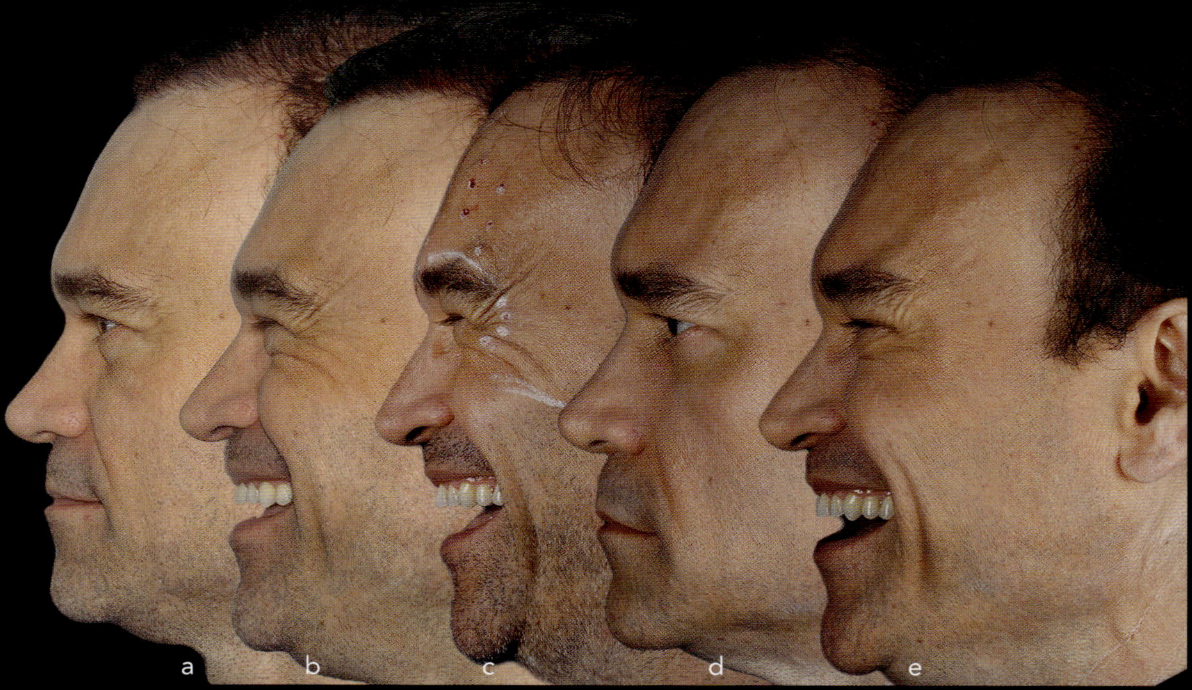

Fig 2-20 *(a to e)* This patient's periorbital wrinkles were present even when the face was at rest, so treatment with BTX was performed to smooth them. *(f and g)* Restorations were placed on the maxillary anterior teeth to elongate the crowns and give the face a more dolichofacial appearance. *(h and i)* Comparison of pretreatment and posttreatment smiles. Note the younger-looking appearance after treatment.

Static Wrinkles

Static wrinkles are wrinkles observed while the facial muscles are at rest.[38,39] Areas of the face with more mobility have an earlier onset of wrinkles compared with other areas. Treatment should be performed before dynamic wrinkles become static. The earlier the treatment of these wrinkles is performed, the better the result will be. In the patient pictured in Fig 2-20, the result was obtained with bilateral injections of 2U of Botox in each point at the orbicularis oculi muscle.

> **HOW COULD BTX HELP?**
> The toxin should be bilaterally injected at the orbicularis oculi muscle. The BTX will decrease the sphincter action of this muscle at the lateral of the eye socket and make the skin smoother during a smile, resulting in a younger-looking appearance.

Figures 2-20h and 2-20i show the patient before and after treatment. In addition to BTX injection in the orbicularis oculi muscle to treat the static wrinkles around the eyes, treatment included BTX injection in the occipitofrontalis, procerus, and corrugator muscles to reverse the "pity face" (see chapter 4) through a brow arching. Bilateral masseter injections were used as coadjuvant therapy for the treatment of bruxism, and injections in the platysma were used for better definition of the jawline. The maxillary anterior teeth were elongated with restorations to make the face more dolichofacial. This dolichofacial effect was also achieved by narrowing the face through the bilateral chemodenervation of the masseter muscles. After treatment, arching of the eyebrow tractioned the skin lateral to the eye socket upward, further smoothing the periorbital wrinkles.

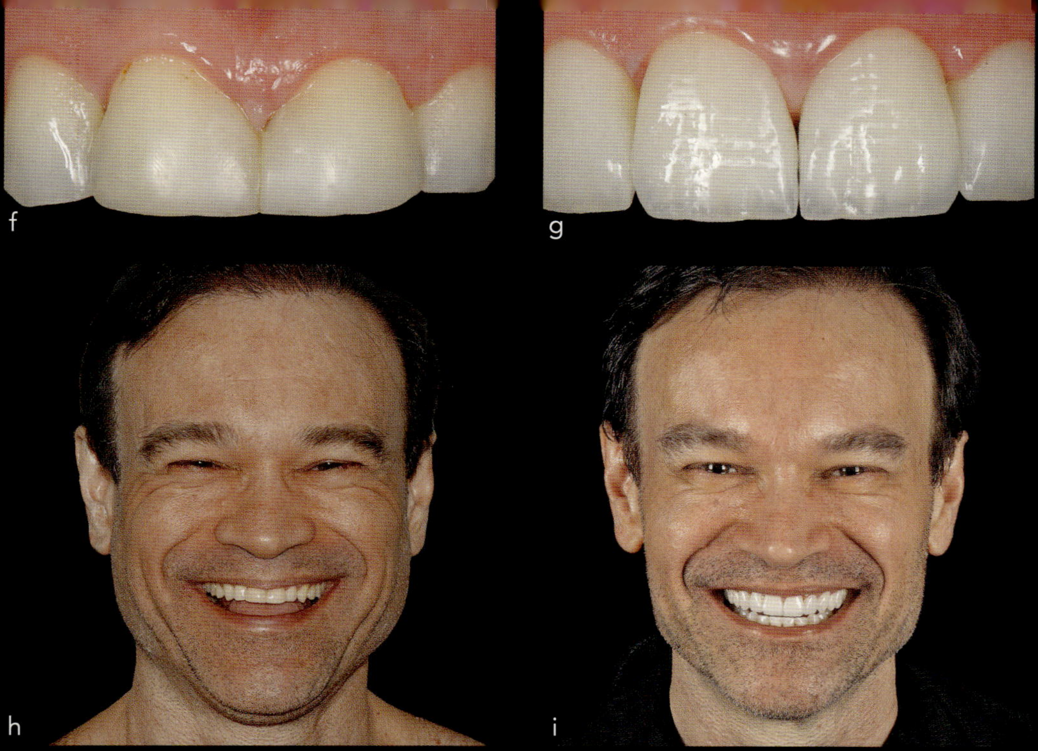

f g h i

Buccal Corridor and Commissure Asymmetries

The buccal corridor is the small space between the buccal surface of the maxillary first molar and the buccal mucosa. The buccal corridors should ideally be symmetric, but they can be asymmetric for a number of reasons:

- Unsuccessful BTX injection
- Facial paralysis
- Facial spasms
- Wide or narrow maxilla (natural or as a result of dental treatment)

Buccal corridor asymmetry can result from BTX injection into the anterior masseter bundle when the risorius muscle is affected by the diffusion. When injected into the orbicularis oculi, BTX can diffuse into the zygomaticus major muscle and cause buccal corridor asymmetry.

The *buccal commissure* refers to the angle of the mouth. Ideally the mouth should be level on both sides. If the buccal commissures are not level, the muscle to be treated depends on the exposure of the maxillary premolars. If the clinical crowns of these teeth are hidden by the upper lip, BTX should be injected into the depressor anguli oris muscle. If there is a gummy smile around the premolars, BTX should be injected into the levator anguli oris muscle.

The patient shown in Fig 2-21a has asymmetric buccal corridors and uneven buccal commissures. BTX was used to correct these asymmetries (Fig 2-21b).

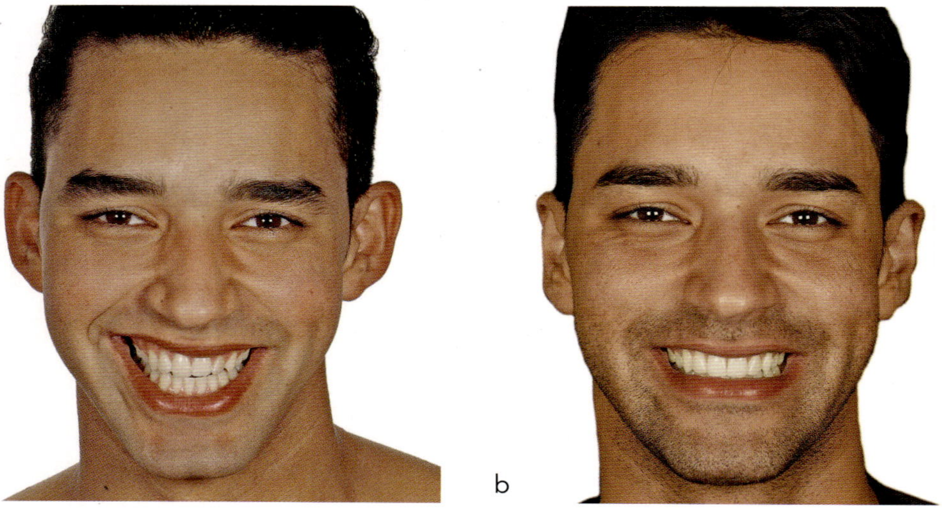

a b

Fig 2-21 *(a and b)* Patient with buccal corridor and commissure asymmetries before and after treatment with BTX.

Definition of the Jawline

The jawline is an important characteristic of the face. More defined jawlines are generally seen as esthetic. Therefore, the junction of the neck and the submandibular region should be observed during the clinical examination.[25] A visible outline of the mandible from the base of the chin up to the gonial angle should be noted. The absence of this definition makes the patient look older.[40–42]

In such cases where this definition is absent and the patient elects treatment, ask the patient to contract the neck several times. If you are able to feel movement of the platysma, that is where the toxin should be injected. If this movement cannot be felt, most likely there is fat accumulation that will make any BTX treatment ineffective.

> **HOW COULD BTX HELP?**
> A hyperkinetic platysma muscle shows more contraction than the normal muscle, forming a bridge between the neck and the mandible that makes the transition between these two structures indistinct. Injection of BTX into the platysma muscle will reestablish its normal tonus and consequently the definition of the jawline.[40–42]

The patient pictured in Fig 2-22 had little definition of the jawline and a sagging facial appearance. BTX was therefore used to restore the tonus of the platysma and add definition back to the jawline.

TREATMENT PERFORMED:

1. Besides treating the upper third of the face to smooth out the wrinkles and level asymmetric eyebrows, 3U of BTX were injected at two points in each hyperkinetic platysmal band.
2. 2U of BTX were injected at the mentalis muscle using the intraoral technique.
3. Deep filling was also performed at the malar region.

Figure 2-22d shows that the double chin was eliminated, and Fig 2-22b shows that a more continuous view of the jawline up to the gonial angle was observed. At the upper third, the eyebrows were leveled, resulting in a smoother look (see Fig 2-22d).

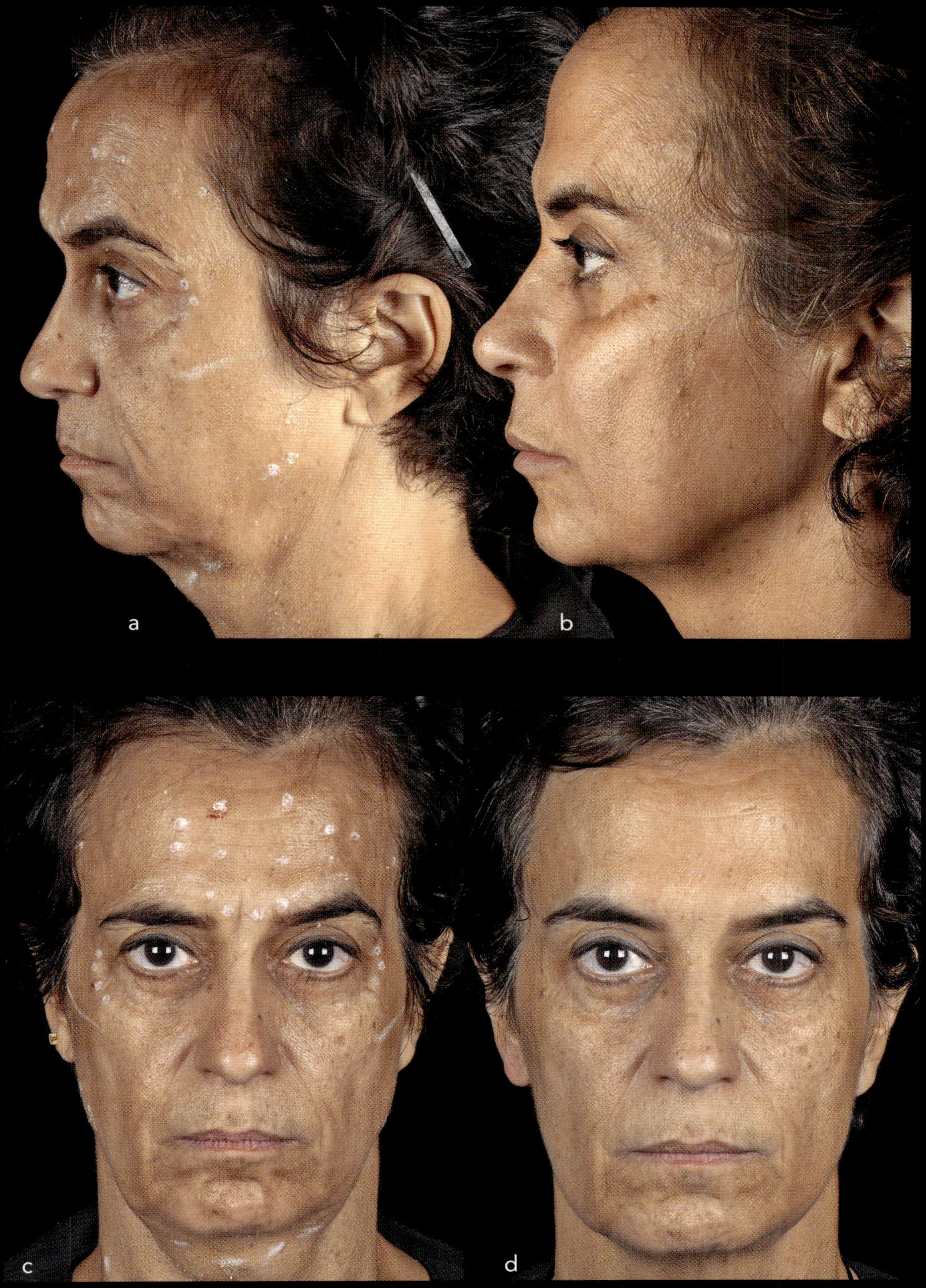

Fig 2-22 *(a to d)* Patient with little jaw definition before and after treatment with BTX.

Hyperkinetic Muscles

During speech, facial structures should be symmetric to the vertical and horizontal planes. Socially, asymmetries are perceived not only as anti-esthetic but also as a sign of disease.[43,44] Therefore, during the clinical examination, any sign of inadequate exposure of the mandibular teeth or gingival tissue as well as any asymmetries during speech should be observed (see chapter 4). If asymmetry is noted, a video of the patient speaking should be recorded and screenshots exported to confirm the diagnosis and aid the treatment plan (see Figs 2-23a to 2-23c).

Possible causes for asymmetries observed during spontaneous speech include Bell's palsy, hemifacial spasms, idiopathic cases, or, as in Fig 2-23, sequelae from surgeries. In this case, the patient had an ameloblastoma removed from the right side of the mandible. While the tumor was benign, its removal caused damage to the right inferior alveolar nerve, mandibular marginal nerve, and cervical ramus of the facial nerve. This caused paresthesia in the right mandibular teeth and paralysis of the right depressor labii inferioris, right depressor anguli oralis, and right platysma muscles. Consequently, the contralateral muscles became hyperkinetic.

HOW COULD BTX HELP?

Some asymmetries can be observed when one or more muscles are hyperkinetic. Identify each of the muscles involved with the asymmetries and include them in the BTX treatment plan. For the first treatment, use small doses; if necessary, increase the doses in future treatments. This is important to understand the patient's response to treatment. High unilateral doses might cause greater effects than desired. The basic concept is to decrease the activity of the muscles that are not paralyzed so that both sides will be the same.

TREATMENT PERFORMED:

1. The large depression of the left lower lip was treated with 2U of BTX injected in the depressor labii inferioris on the left side.
2. Because the patient squeezed the eyes during speech, 2U of BTX were injected at two points of each orbicularis muscle.
3. The slight depression of the left buccal commissure causing horizontal asymmetry was treated with 1U of BTX injected at the left depressor anguli oris muscle.
4. In addition to the hyperkinetic muscles, the patient reported having bruxism. This was treated with 15U of BTX at two points in the left masseter muscle and 5U at one point in the left temporalis muscle. The right masseter was not treated because it was surgically detached through bone resection.

Figure 2-23d shows the exact points where the BTX was injected. A comparison of Figs 2-23a and 2-23e shows the difference it made during speech.

The results address social, functional, and esthetic aspects of the face:

- *Social*: After treatment, the asymmetry is no longer observed during speech. This was a great benefit for this patient because he is a professor at a dental school.
- *Functional*: The control of bruxism was essential to keep the titanium plate fixation that connected the remaining parts of the jaw after surgery.
- *Esthetic*: The patient's appearance was softened through the relaxation of the orbicularis oculi muscle, and the dental exposure during speech and smiling was improved (no exposure of posterior mandibular teeth).

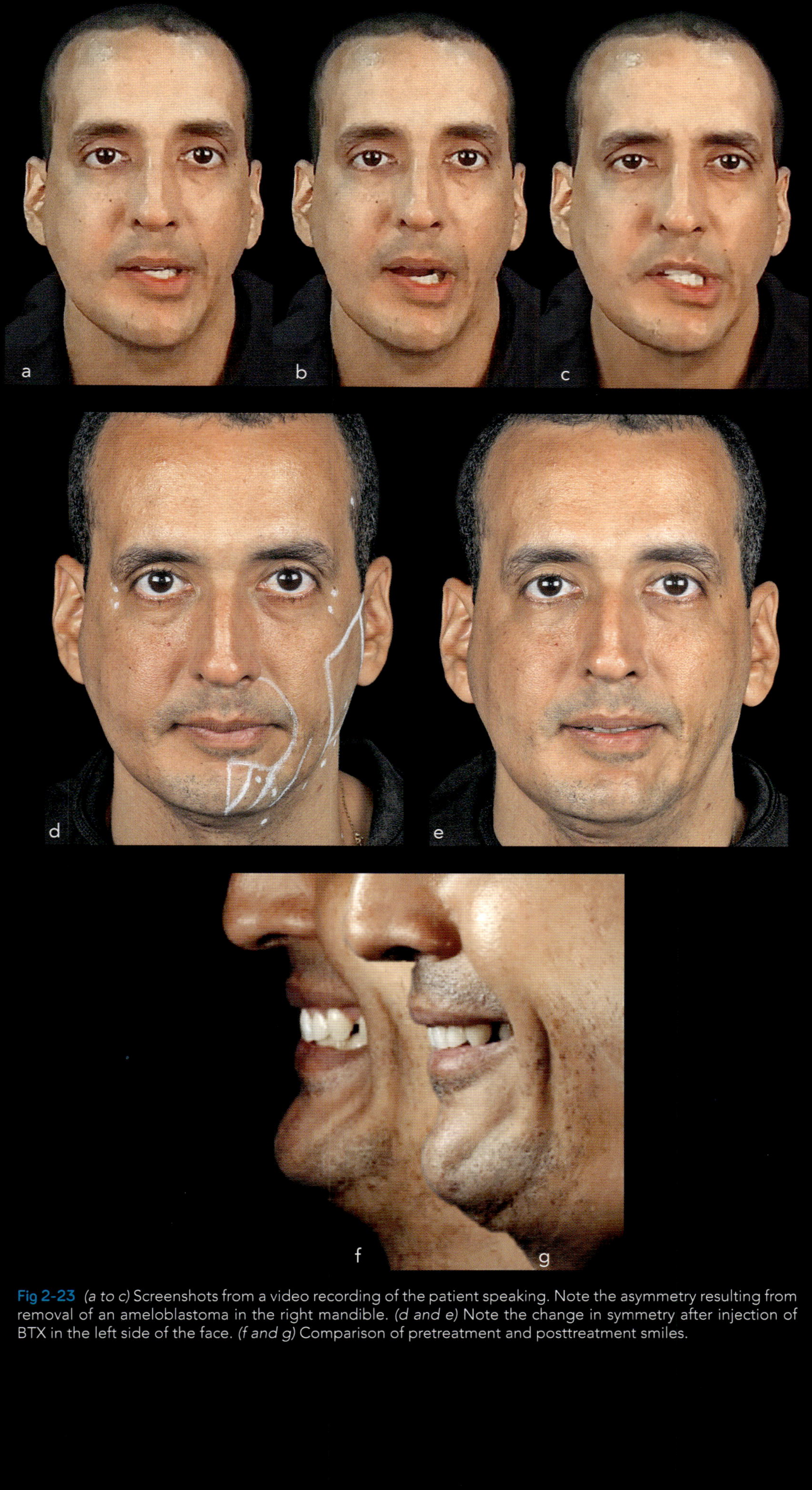

Fig 2-23 *(a to c)* Screenshots from a video recording of the patient speaking. Note the asymmetry resulting from removal of an ameloblastoma in the right mandible. *(d and e)* Note the change in symmetry after injection of BTX in the left side of the face. *(f and g)* Comparison of pretreatment and posttreatment smiles.

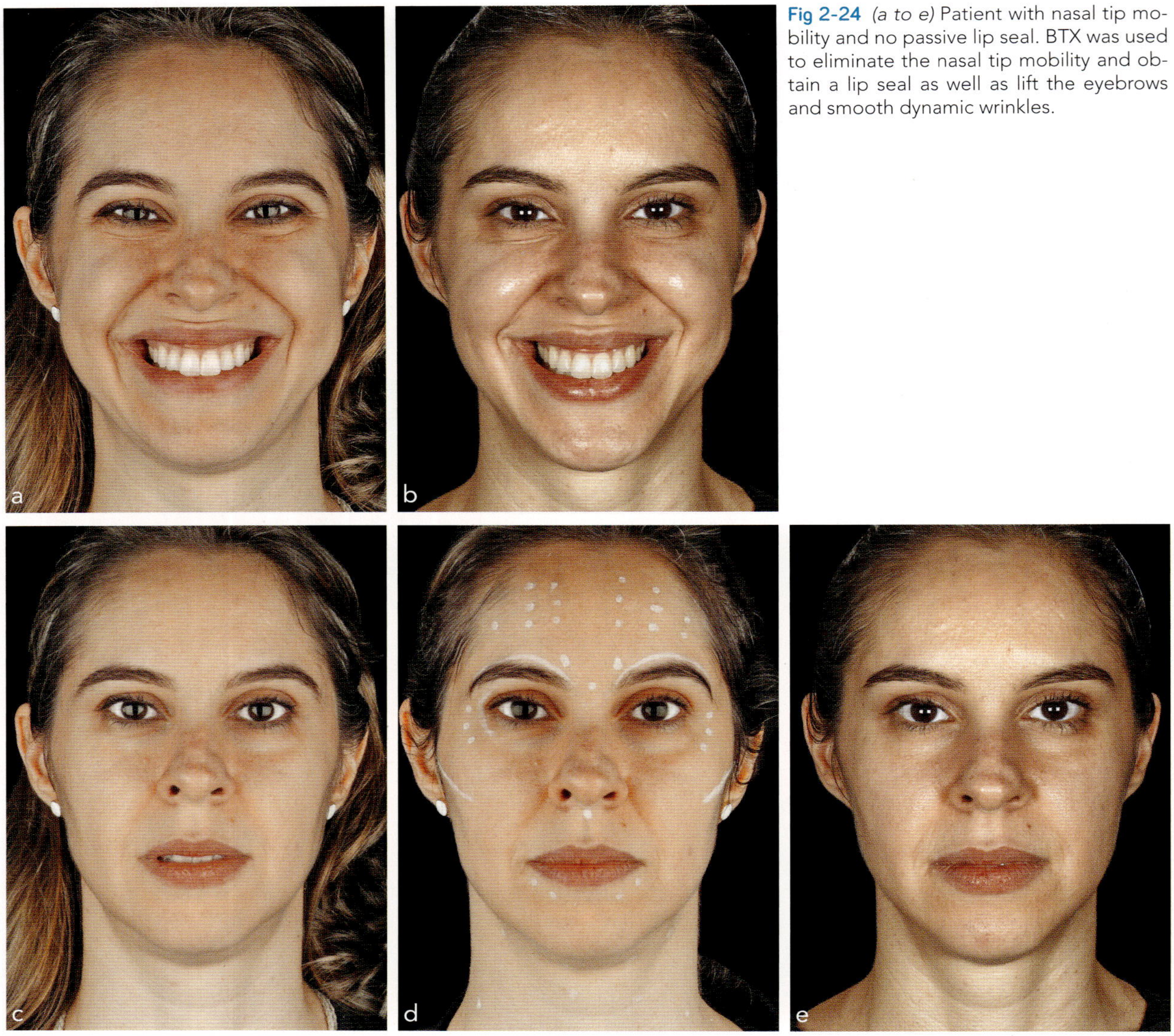

Fig 2-24 *(a to e)* Patient with nasal tip mobility and no passive lip seal. BTX was used to eliminate the nasal tip mobility and obtain a lip seal as well as lift the eyebrows and smooth dynamic wrinkles.

Nasal Tip Mobility

The tip of the nose should not move much during speech. If it does, the depressor septi nasi muscle is most likely hyperkinetic. BTX can be injected to correct this mobility, but it should only be injected if the patient has a gummy smile. In such cases, the BTX will prevent the depressor septi nasi muscle from depressing the nasal tip during upper lip movement (ie, pulling it down), thereby eliminating the gummy smile. If BTX injection is not performed in such cases, the patient's nasal tip may become flattened or concave in the future, and/or the patient may develop a horizontal fold in the skin of the upper lip.[45]

To assess for this during the clinical examination, ask the patient to pronounce the letter M several times. Mobility will be easily observed if present. When there is an excessive movement of the nasal tip during speech, treatment with BTX should be considered.

The patient pictured in Fig 2-24 had nasal tip mobility during speech. In addition, there was no passive lip seal while her muscles were at rest (see Fig 2-24c). Lip seal could only be obtained by the action of the orbicularis oris muscle and mentalis muscle. In patients like this who can only achieve lip seal with activation of these muscles, the shape of the lips may change from round to flat.

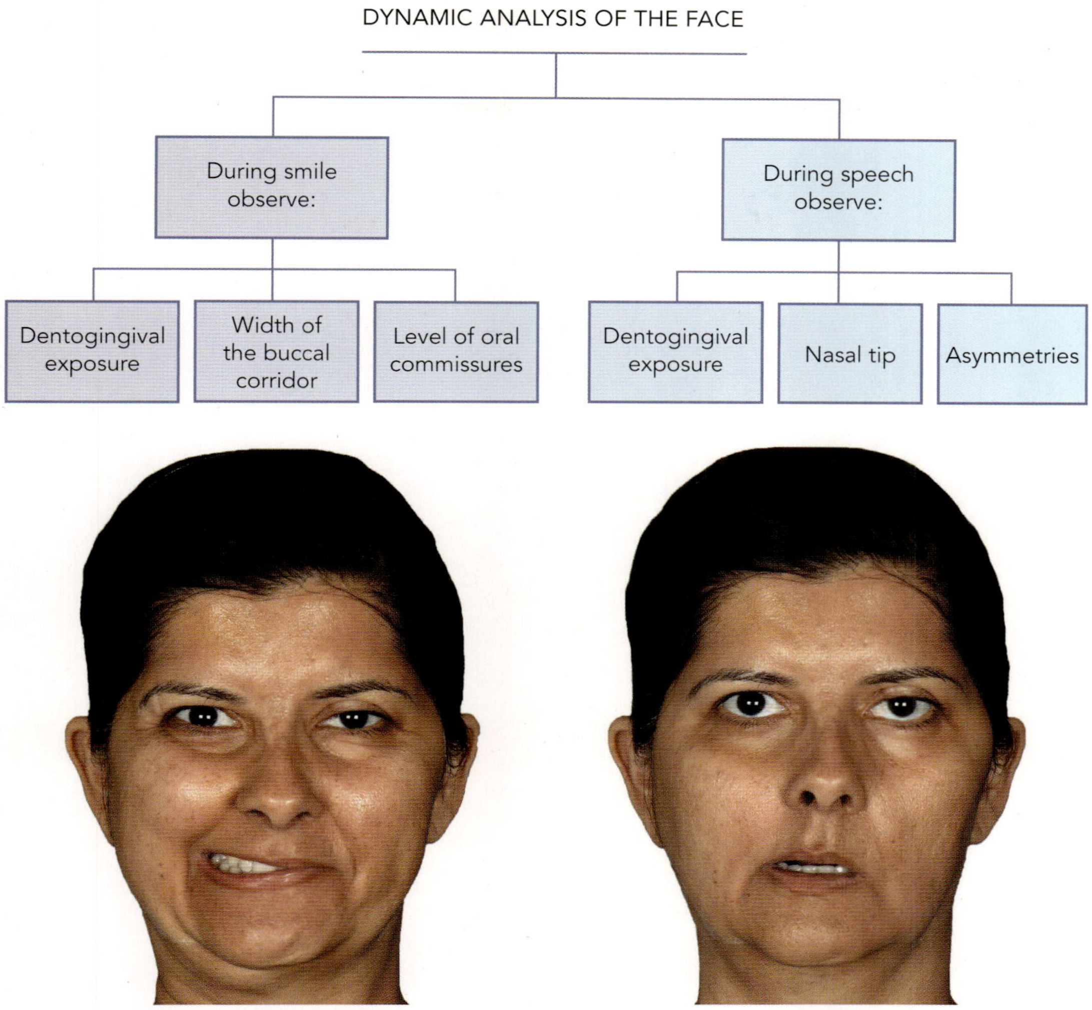

Asymmetric patient during a smile

Asymmetric patient during speech

Fig 2-25 Dynamic analysis of the face includes analysis of the patient during a smile and during speech.

TREATMENT PERFORMED:

1. The intense movement of the nasal tip when pronouncing the letter M and the lack of passive labial seal were treated with 2U of BTX injected into the depressor septi nasi muscle.
2. The double chin was treated with 1U of BTX injected at 10 points in the platysma muscle.
3. The volume of the lower lip was restored with 1U of BTX injected at four points in the orbicularis muscle of the lower lip. It decreased the volume of the orbicularis muscle.

Remaining injections were administered in the upper third of the face to lift the eyebrows and smooth out dynamic wrinkles (see clinical examples in chapter 4). Figures 2-24b and 2-24e show the final results. The patient now has passive lip seal and decreased movement of the nasal tip during speech, the gummy smile and double chin have been eliminated, the upper third has been smoothed, and the lips show better contour.

Figure 2-25 summarizes dynamic analysis of the face.

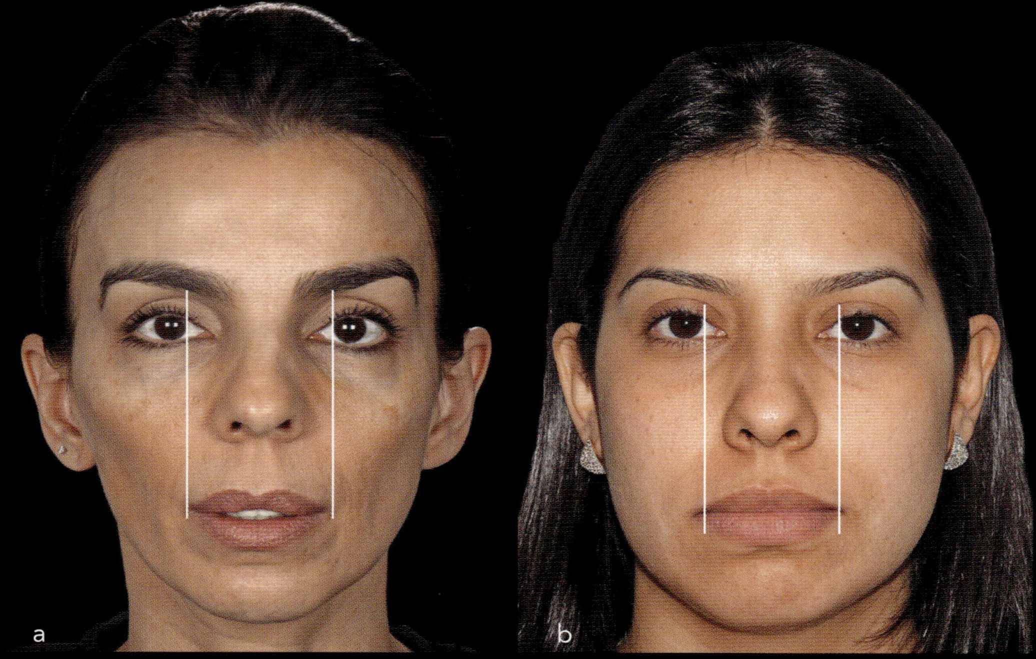

Fig 2-26 *(a)* The mouth is proportional to the face, because the vertical line tangent to the iris is also tangent to the oral commissures. *(b)* The mouth is dominant, because at rest the oral commissures are beyond the vertical line tangent to the iris.

Width of Jaw and Buccal Corridor

With the face at rest, the width of the mouth can be evaluated by drawing a vertical line tangent to the iris (Fig 2-26):

- If the line is lateral to the commissure, the mouth is *narrow*, or slightly small in relation to the face.
- If the line goes through the commissure, the mouth is *proportional* to the face, and the width is correct in relation to the face (see Fig 2-26a).
- If the line is medial to the commissure, the mouth is wide and *dominant* (see Fig 2-26b).

The clinician can use this information to assess oral asymmetries at rest and decide whether to correct them by increasing muscle tonus. The prosthodontist and orthodontist will be able to use these results to identify the ideal width of the central incisor clinical crowns. In the case of a narrow mouth, the smallest average should be used for clinical crown width (8.3 mm for females, 8.6 mm for males). When the mouth is proportional to the face, the average clinical crown width should be used (8.6 mm for females, 8.9 mm for males). In the case of a dominant mouth, the highest average should be used for central incisor clinical crown width (8.9 mm for females, 9.2 mm for males).

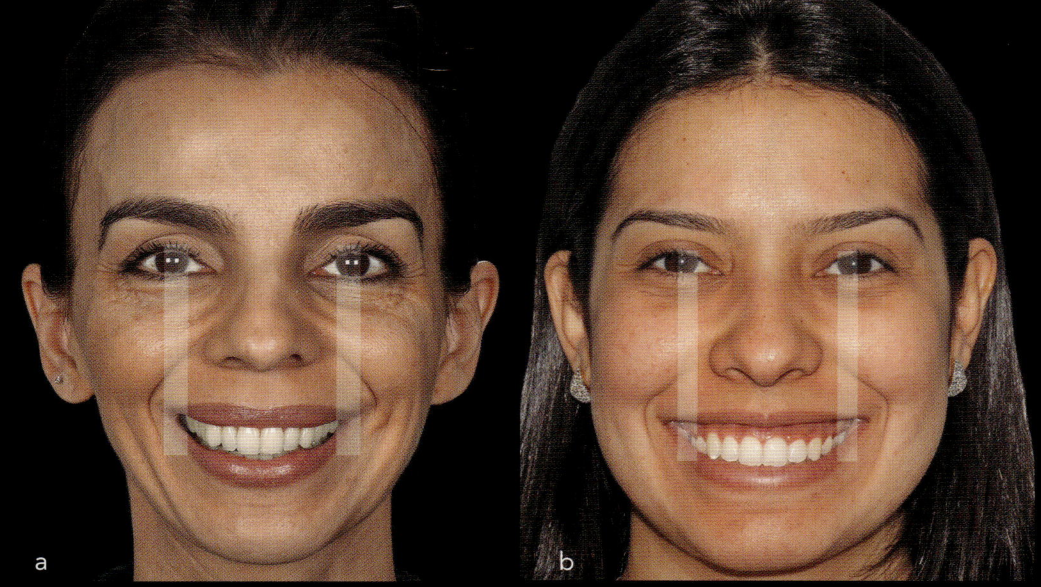

Fig 2-27 *(a)* The mandible width is ideal for this type of face because the internal line of the rectangle touches the maxillary first molar. The black space that characterizes the buccal corridor inside the rectangle is easily observed. The amplitude of the smile is proportional because the external line of the rectangle touches the oral commissure. *(b)* The maxilla is very large because the first molar trespasses the internal line of the rectangle. The buccal corridor is not observed within the rectangle. The smile is very wide as evidenced by the invasion of the commissures into the external line of the rectangle.

The iris mesial to pupil distal rule evaluates the width of the jaw and buccal corridor as well as the amplitude of the commissures during a smile. This evaluation is performed by drawing a rectangle wide enough to touch the mesial of the iris and the distal of the pupil (Fig 2-27):

- If the internal line touches the buccal surface of the maxillary first molar (this tooth cannot be inside the rectangle), the maxillary arch width is proportional to the face (see Fig 2-27a).
- If there is black space inside the rectangle, the patient shows a buccal corridor. If not, a bichectomy could be considered.
- If the external line of the rectangle touches the commissure, the smile has the correct amplitude for the face.

The clinician can use this information to assess oral asymmetries during the smile and decide whether to correct any hyperkinetic muscles. The orthodontist or surgeon might also use this information to identify the ideal width of the maxillary arch, using the buccal surface of the maxillary first molar as a reference. The surgeon will be able to evaluate the buccal fat pad in case the buccal corridor is absent, the dental technician can position the posterior teeth in the wax-up, and the clinician can select the correct thickness for veneers to adjust the maxillary dental arch width.

References

1. Casaglia A, De Dominicis P, Arcuri L, Gargari M, Ottria L. Dental photography today. Part 1: Basic concepts. Oral Implantol (Rome) 2016;8:122–129.
2. Ricketts RM. The biologic significance of the divine proportion and Fibonacci series. Am J Orthod 1982;81: 351–370.
3. Dierkes JM. The beauty of the face: An orthodontic perspective. J Am Dent Assoc 1987;special issue:89E–95E [erratum 1988;116:614].
4. Parekh SM, Fields HW, Beck M, Rosenstiel S. Attractiveness of variations in the smile arc and buccal corridor space as judged by orthodontists and laymen. Angle Orthod 2006;76:557–563.
5. Ker AJ, Chan R, Fields HW, Beck M, Rosenstiel S. Esthetics and smile characteristics from the layperson's perspective: A computer-based survey study. J Am Dent Assoc 2008;139:1318–1327.
6. Gul-e-Erum, Fida M. Changes in smile parameters as perceived by orthodontists, dentists, artists, and laypeople. World J Orthod 2008;9:132–140.
7. Kokich VO Jr, Kiyak HA, Shapiro PA. Comparing the perception of dentists and lay people to altered dental esthetics. J Esthet Dent 1999;11:311–324.
8. Kokich VO, Kokich VG, Kiyak HA. Perceptions of dental professionals and laypersons to altered dental esthetics: Asymmetric and symmetric situations. Am J Orthod Dentofacial Orthop 2006;130:141–151.
9. Suzuki L, Machado AW, Bittencourt MAV. An evaluation of the influence of gingival display level in the smile esthetics. Dental Press J Orthod 2011;16:37–39.
10. Nascimento DC, Dos Santos ER, Machado AW, Bittencourt MAV. Influence of buccal corridor dimension on smile esthetics. Dental Press J Orthod 2012;17:145–150.
11. Correa BD, Bittencourt MAV, Machado AW. Influence of maxillary canine gingival margin asymmetries on the perception of smile esthetics among orthodontists and laypersons. Am J Orthod Dentofacial Orthop 2014; 145:55–63.
12. Machado AW, Moon W, Campos E, Gandini LG Jr. Influence of spacing in the upper lateral incisor area on the perception of smile esthetics among orthodontists and laypersons. J World Fed Orthod 2013;2:169–174.
13. Rosenstiel SF, Rashid RG. Public preferences for anterior tooth variations: A web-based study. J Esthet Restor Dent 2002;14:97–106.
14. Bukhary SM, Gill DS, Tredwin CJ, Moles DR. The influence of varying maxillary lateral incisor dimensions on perceived smile esthetics. Br Dent J 2007;203:687–693.
15. Wolfart S, Thormann H, Freitag S, Kern M. Assessment of dental appearance following changes in incisor proportions. Eur J Oral Sci 2005;113:159–165.
16. King KL, Evans CA, Viana G, BeGole E, Obrez A. Preferences for vertical position of the maxillary lateral incisors. World J Orthod 2008;9:147–154.
17. Menezes EBC, Bittencourt MAV, Machado AW. Do different vertical positions of maxillary central incisors influence smile esthetics perception? Dental Press J Orthod 2017;22:95–105.
18. Farkas LG. Anthropometry of the Head and Face, ed 2. New York: Raven, 1994:1–77.
19. Ward DH. Proportional smile design using the recurring esthetic dental (red) proportion. Dent Clin North Am 2001;45:143–154.
20. Sandeep N, Satwalekar P, Srinivas S, Reddy CS, Reddy GR, Reddy BA. An analysis of maxillary anterior teeth dimensions for the existence of golden proportion: Clinical study. J Int Oral Health 2015;7:18–21.
21. Fornaziero CC, Souza MHS Jr. Odontologia estética: Estudo das dimensões e formas dos incisivos superiores. JBD, Rev Íbero-Am Odontol Estét Dent Oper 2003;2: 291–300.
22. Bogucki ZA, Kownacka M. Clinical aspects of the use of botulinum toxin type A in the treatment of the masticatory system. Adv Clin Exp Med 2016;25:569–573.
23. De la Torre Canales G, Câmara-Souza MB, do Amaral CF, Garcia RC, Manfredini D. Is there enough evidence to use botulinum injections for bruxism management? A systematic literature review. Clin Oral Investig 2017;21:727–734.
24. Viazis AD. Avaliação do tecido mole. In: Atlas de Ortodontia: Princípios e aplicações clínicas. São Paulo: Santos, 1996:49.
25. Suguino R, Ramos AL, Terada HH, Furquim LZ, Maeda L, Filho OGS. Análise facial. Dental Press de Ortopedia Maxilar 1996;1:86–107.
26. Arnett GW, Bergman RT. Facial keys to orthodontic diagnosis and treatment planning—Part II. Am J Orthod Dentofacial Orthop 1993;103:395–411.
27. Fradeani M. Análise estética: Uma abordagem sistemática para o tratamento protético. São Paulo: Quintessence, 2006.
28. Shivhare P, Shankarnarayan L, Basavaraju SM, Gupta A, Vasan V, Jambunath U. Intercanine width as a tool in two dimensional reconstruction of face: An aid in forensic dentistry. J Forensic Dent Sci 2015;7:1–7.
29. Kim HS, Yun PY, Kim YK. A clinical evaluation of botulinum toxin-A injections in the temporamandibular disorder treatment. Maxillofac Plast Reconstr Surg 2016;38:5.
30. Patel AA, Lerner MZ, Blitzer A. IncobotulinumtoxinA injection for temporomandibular joint disorder. Ann Otol Rhinol Laryngol 2017;126:328–333.
31. von Lindern JJ, Niederhagen B, Bergé S, Appel T. Type A botulinum toxin in the treatment of chronic facial pain associated with masticatory hyperactivity. J Oral Maxillofac Surg 2003;61:774–778.
32. Guarda-Nardini L, Manfredini D, Salamone M, Salmaso L, Tonello S, Ferronato G. Efficacy of botulinum toxin in treating myofascial pain in bruxers: A controlled placebo pilot study. Cranio 2008;26:126–135.
33. Bjørnland T, Gjaerum AA, Møystad O. Osteoarthritis of the temporomandibular joint: An evaluation of the effects and complications of corticosteroid injections compared with injection with sodium hyaluronate. J Oral Rehabil 2007;34:583–589.

34. Connelly ST, Myung J, Gupta R, et al. Clinical outcomes of Botox injections for chronic temporomandibular disorders: Do we understand how Botox works on muscle, pain, and the brain? Int J Oral Maxillofac Surg 2017;46: 322–327.
35. Keenan JR. Unclear results for the use of botulinum toxin therapy for TMD pain. Evid Based Dent 2015;16:122.
36. Ludlow CL, Hallett M, Rhew K, et al. Therapeutic use of type F botulinum toxin. N Engl J Med 1992;326:349–350.
37. Subtelny JD. A longitudinal study of soft tissue facial structures and their profile characteristics, defined in relation to underlying skeletal structures. Am J Orthod Dentofacial Orthop 1959;45:381–507.
38. Schlessinger J, Gilbert E, Cohen JL, Kaufman J. New uses of abobotulinumtoxinA in aesthetics. Aesthet Surg J 2017;37(suppl 1):S45–S58.
39. Sapra P, Demay S, Sapra S, Khanna J, Mraud K, Bonadonna J. A single-blind, split-face, randomized, pilot study comparing the effects of intradermal and intramuscular injection of two commercially available botulinum toxin A formulas to reduce signs of facial aging. J Clin Aesthet Dermatol 2017;10:34–44.
40. Jabbour SF, Kechichian EG, Awaida CJ, Tomb RR, Nasr MW. Botulinum toxin for neck rejuvenation: Assessing efficacy and redefining patient selection. Plast Reconstr Surg 2017;140:9e–17e.
41. Gassia V, Beylot C, Béchaux S, Michaud T. Botulinum toxin injection techniques in the lower third and middle of the face, the neck and the décolleté: The "Nefertiti lift" [in French]. Ann Dermatol Venereol 2009;136(suppl 4): S111–S118.
42. Levy PM. Neurtotoxins: Current concepts in cosmetic use on the face and neck—Jawline contouring/platysma brands/necklace lines. Plast Reconstr Surg 2015;136(5, suppl):80S–83S.
43. Cooper L, Nduka C. Botulinum toxin treatment for facial palsy: A systematic review. J Plast Reconstr Aesthet Surg 2017;70:833–841.
44. Sahan A, Tamer F. Restoring facial symmetry through non-surgical cosmetic procedures after permanent facial paralysis: A case report. Acta Dermatovenerol Alp Pannonica Adriat 2017;26:41–42.
45. Kouwenhoven ST, van Kester MS, Genders RE. The wingman flap: Bilateral closure of a supra-tip defect of the nose. J Am Acad Dermatol 2017;76:e57–e58.

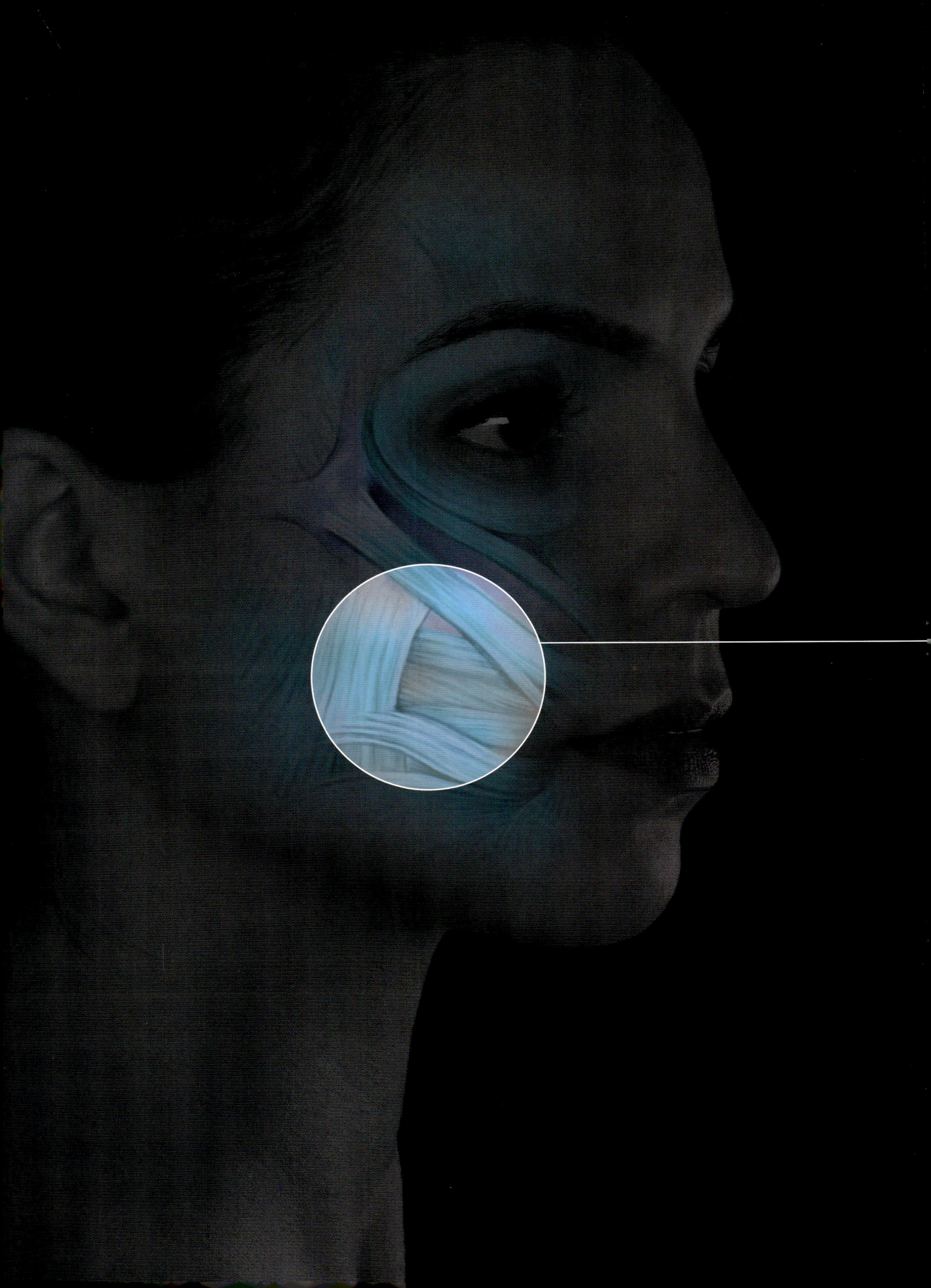

CHAPTER 03

Muscles: Injection Technique and Location

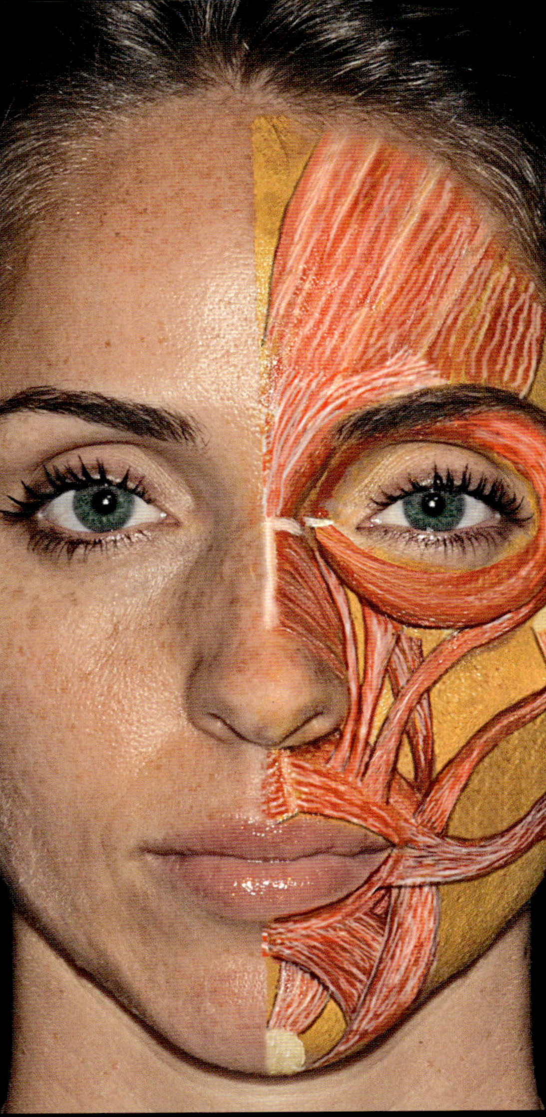

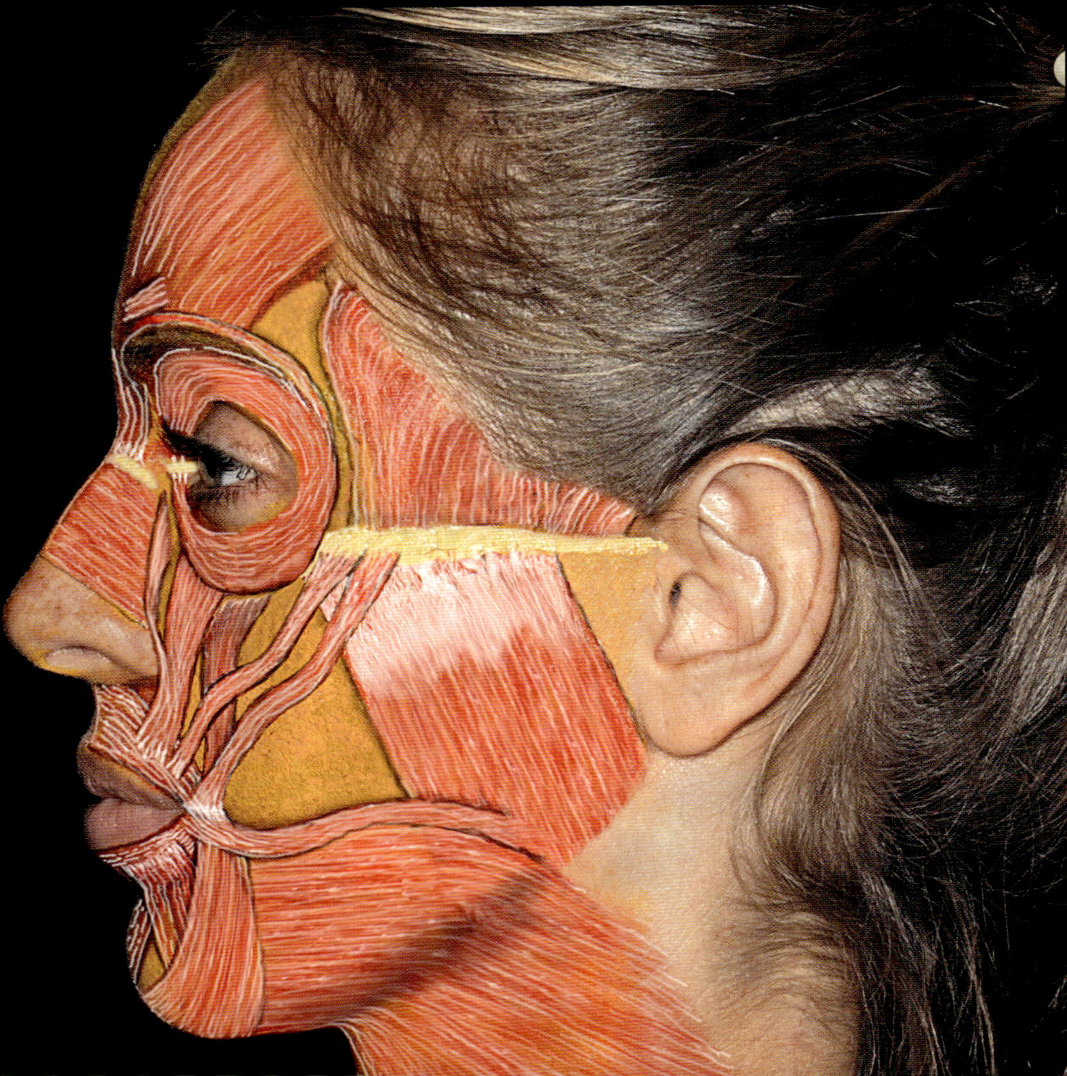

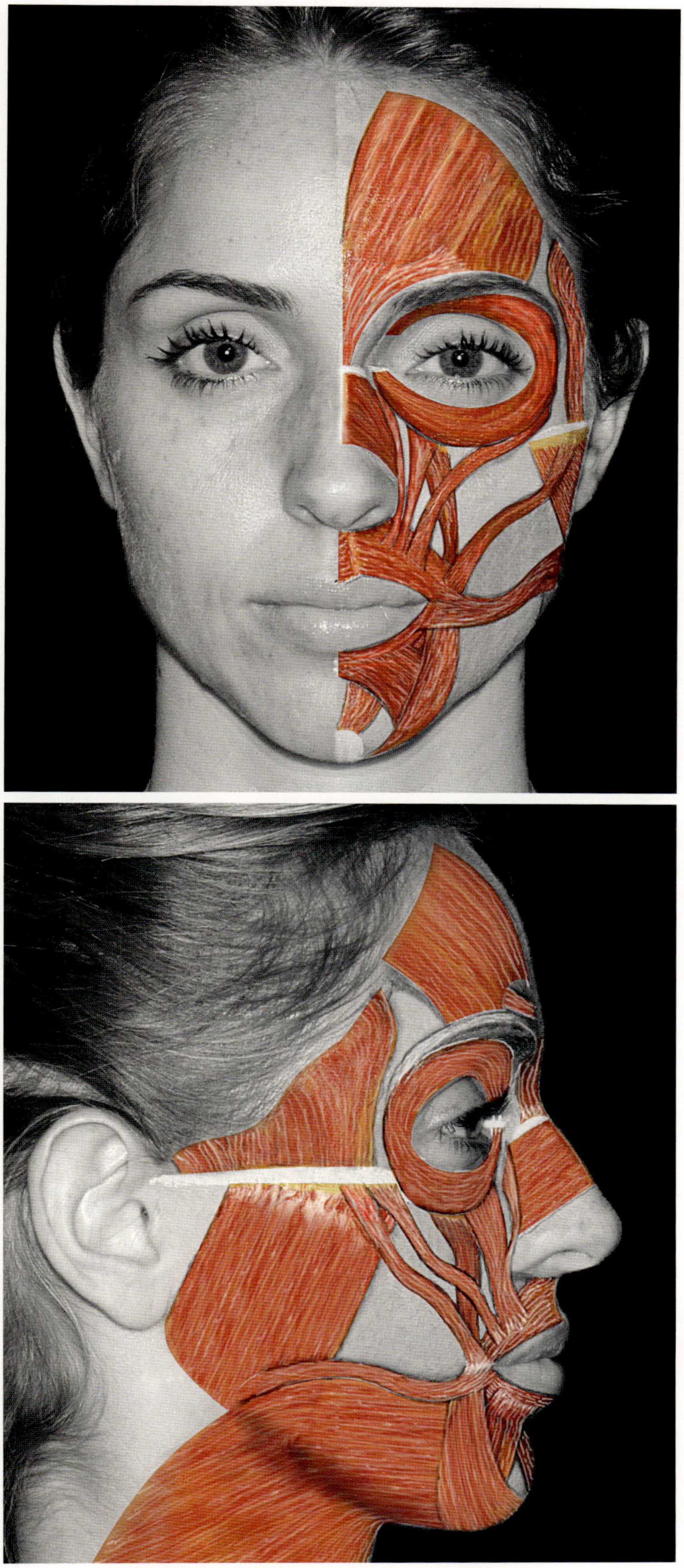

Fig 3-1 Muscles drawn on the face.

Because the insertion plane of botulinum toxin (BTX) is intramuscular, it is fundamental that clinicians know the location and depth of each facial muscle. Once this information has been studied, the muscles can be drawn on the face of a volunteer as an exercise to help the clinician "own the knowledge" (Fig 3-1). The correct position of muscles can be found by using facial expressions, palpation, and facial esthetic references (Box 3-1).

Scan this QR code to access videos demonstrating how to mark injection points for all the muscles illustrated in this chapter.

Box 3-1 **Methods of locating the facial muscles**

FACIAL EXPRESSIONS	PALPATION	ESTHETIC REFERENCES
The muscles of facial expression are not covered by a fascia; they originate and/or insert directly into the skin, thereby pulling the skin during muscle contraction. In order to find these muscles, patients are asked to make a specific facial expression that makes their position predictable. **Muscles:** occipitofrontalis, procerus, corrugator supercilii, orbicularis oculi, nasalis, orbicularis oris, depressor anguli oris, platysma	The muscles of mastication are covered by a fascia that isolates them from the skin. Therefore, they do not cause skin wrinkles and/or mimicry. During contraction, their volume is noticeable through palpation. **Muscles:** temporalis, masseter; use palpation as a complementary method to find the depressor anguli oris	Some muscles are not noticeable through palpation or facial expressions. A better way to find them would be to make drawings over the bones and other anatomical structures. Doing so will create esthetic references that will help to locate the muscles. **Muscles**: depressor septi nasi, levator labii superioris alaeque nasi, levator labii superioris, levator anguli oris, zygomaticus major and minor, mentalis

How Does BTX Affect Facial Muscles?

Some muscles are named for their function. Therefore, an easy way to comprehend the effect of BTX on a muscle is to understand that BTX creates the action opposite to the muscle name. For example, after BTX injection, the action force of the depressor labii inferioris muscle will be reduced so that the muscle will depress to a lesser extent. The final result will be an increased horizontal position of the lower lip from its actual position. Figure 3-2 shows another example.

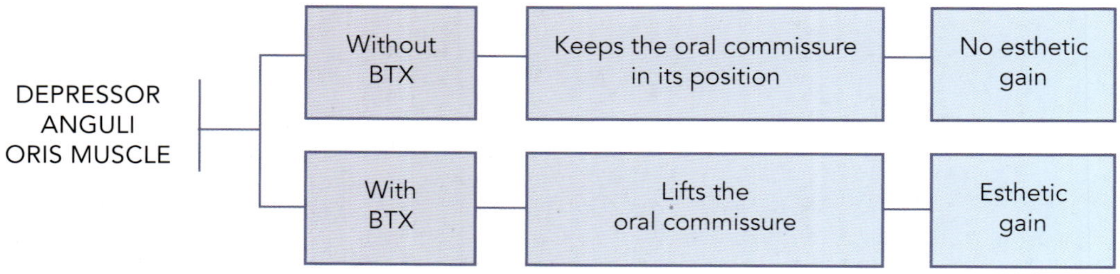

Fig 3-2 Action of BTX on the depressor anguli oris muscle.

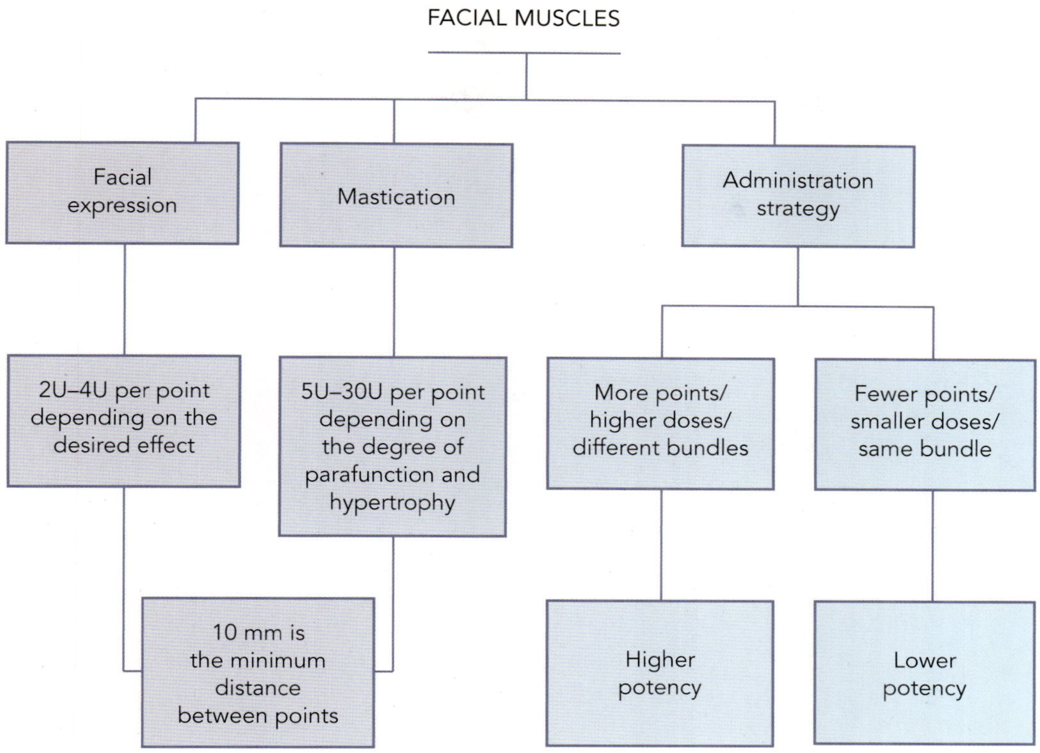

Fig 3-3 General strategy for Botox treatments for the facial muscles.

Dosing by Muscle

A common doubt among novices is the appropriate amount of toxin to inject in each facial muscle. A helpful way to organize these dosages is to separate them by type of muscle. There are two different types of facial muscles: the muscles responsible for mastication and the muscles responsible for facial expression. Because the masticatory muscles are larger, longer, and stronger due to their function, they require larger doses of toxin. On the other hand, the muscles of facial expression are thinner, shorter, and weaker because their only function is to contract the skin. Thus, they require smaller doses of toxin.

There is no such thing as an exact number of units to be injected in each case. Instead, there is an average number of units. The decision as to the number of units to be injected in a specific patient will depend on the diagnosis. For instance, in a patient with a large-volume procerus muscle with static wrinkles, the injection of 4U of BTX may be appropriate. However, in another patient with a smaller procerus muscle and only dynamic wrinkles, 2U may be sufficient.

Another strategy for BTX injection involves administration of the toxin into muscle bundles. For example, the masseter muscle is composed of three different bands: anterior, middle, and posterior. One possible therapy for this muscle is to inject 20U in the whole muscle. It is not advisable to inject two points of 10U only in the middle band because it would result in the decrease of muscle power only in one part of the muscle. To increase the efficacy of the treatment using the same doses and numbers of injections, the best therapy would be to inject 10U in the middle band and 10U in the posterior band.

Figure 3-3 summarizes dosing by muscle group and illustrates the different strategies to adjust the effects.

Occipitofrontalis Muscle (Frontal Belly)

Anatomy and location

Function: It raises the eyebrows and is in part responsible for the "surprised" facial expression.

Location: Forehead.

Origin: Skin of the eyebrows; the fibers are blended with the procerus, corrugator, and orbicularis oculi muscles.

Insertion: Galea aponeurotica.

Fibers: Vertical with an inclination of approximately 30 degrees.

Wrinkles: Horizontal, parallel to the forehead.

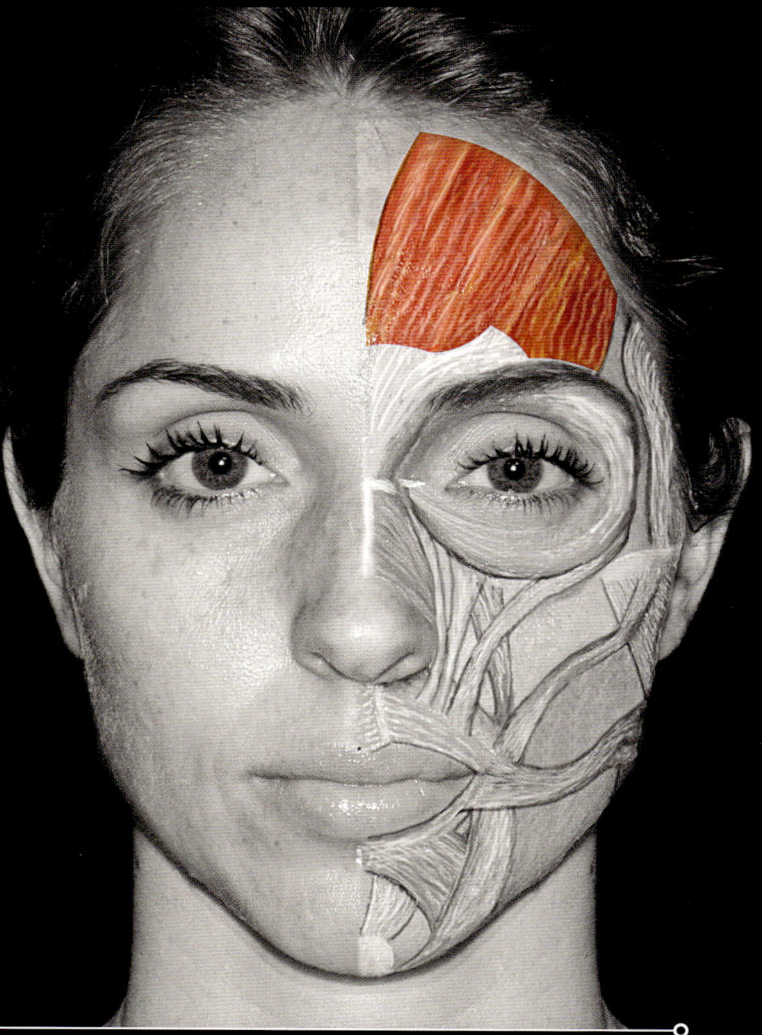

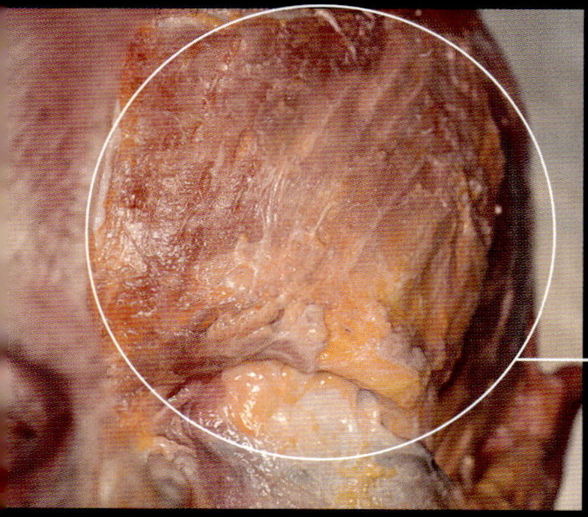

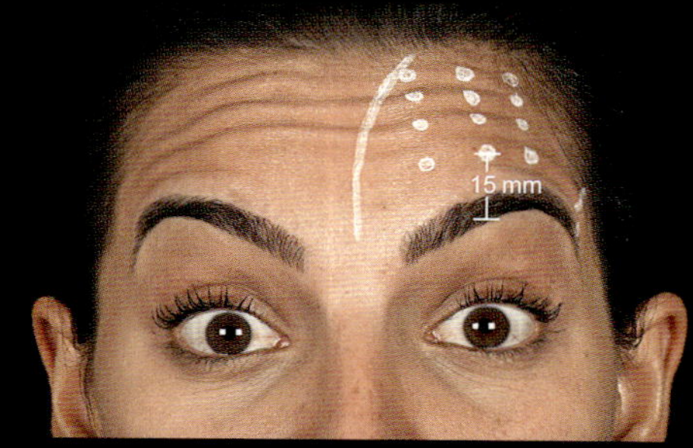

Treatment to smooth wrinkles without lifting the eyebrows

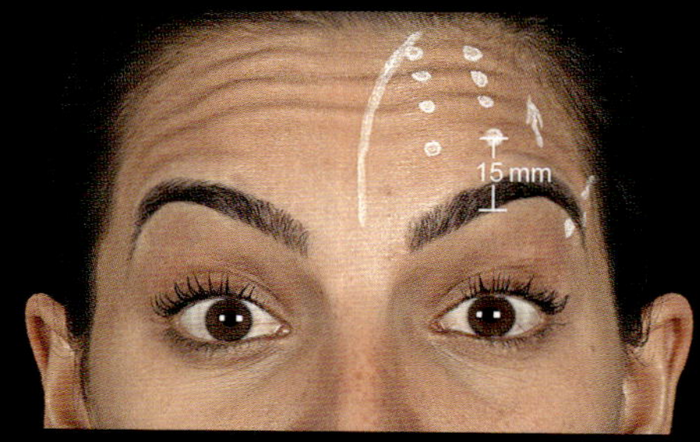

Treatment to smooth wrinkles and lift the eyebrows

Locating and marking the muscle

Markings made when lifting the eyebrows is not an option:

1. Ask the patient to make a surprised facial expression.
2. Mark three points at the highest part of the wrinkle considering three vertical lines: the medial canthus, pupil, and lateral canthus.

Markings made when lifting the eyebrows is the goal: Follow the same procedure as described above but do not mark the line corresponding to the external canthus, because after the injection the muscle in this region will still elevate the eyebrow tail.

Markings made when the goal is intense eyebrow lifting: Follow the same procedure as described above and add one point below the eyebrow tail to relax the orbicularis oculi muscle. After BTX-A injection, the antagonistic effect of this muscle over the occipitofrontalis muscle will be reduced, which will increase the eyebrow lifting.

⚠ A safety distance of 15 mm above the orbital ridge was kept to decrease the chance of diffusion to the levator palpebrae superioris, which could cause an eyebrow ptosis.

BTX injection protocol

OCCIPITOFRONTALIS MUSCLE

Indications	• To smooth wrinkles in the forehead. • To position the eyebrow (different lifting degrees). • When esthetically indicated, the eyebrow lifting accentuates the triangular shape of the face and also makes it look longer (dolichofacial). • Blepharoptosis might be reduced by an eyebrow lift. • Correction of asymmetries might be performed by marking the eyebrow to lift it on one side and not on the other side.		
Contraindications	• Extremely triangular faces will become even more triangular. • Insecure patients might not easily accept brow arching. • Contraindications listed by the manufacturer on the packaging.		
Attention	This muscle does not have fibers in its medial line, eliminating the need to inject toxin at this region.		
Recommended doses (per point)	**Botox** 2U, 3U, or 4U	**Dysport** 6U, 9U, or 12U	**Xeomin** 2U, 3U, or 4U
Injection site	Frontal belly of each wrinkle at its highest point.		
Needle	**Size** 8 mm	**Position** *(in relation to the skin)* 45 degrees	**Insertion** 1/3 of the needle

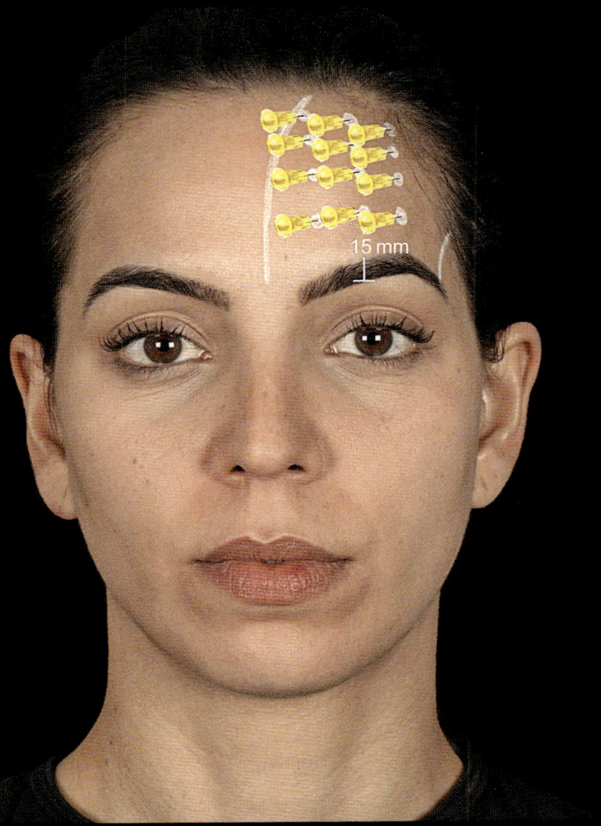

Smoothing wrinkles without lifting the eyebrows

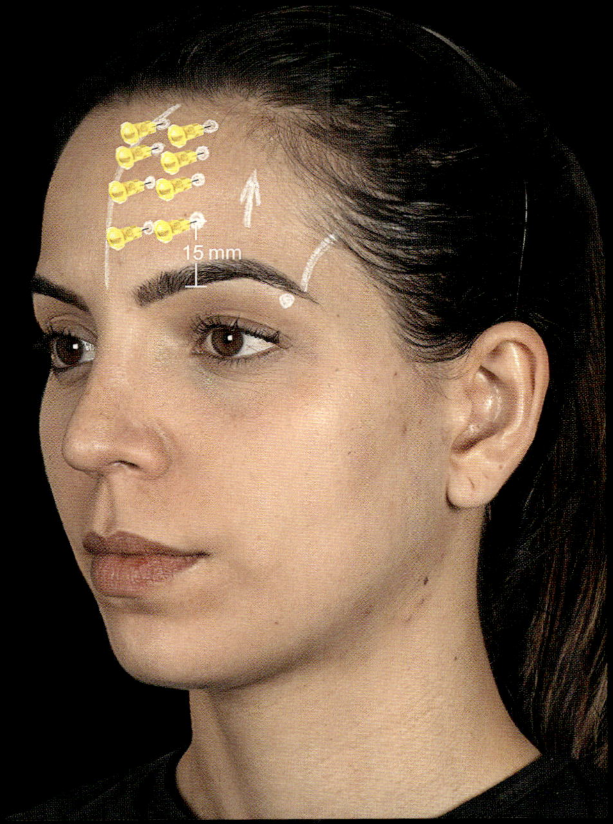

Smoothing wrinkles and lifting the eyebrows

Temporalis Muscle

Anatomy and location

Function: It moves the mandible during mastication and speech. It also helps to elevate the mandible but using less force than the masseter muscle. Its expertise is to move the mandible and not only lift it.

Location: Temples.

Origin: Temporal fossa.

Insertion: Coronoid process of the mandible.

Fibers: Anterior fibers (vertical) elevate the mandible, and posterior (oblique) fibers retract the mandible.

Wrinkles: It is not involved in the formation of wrinkles because it has no fascia.

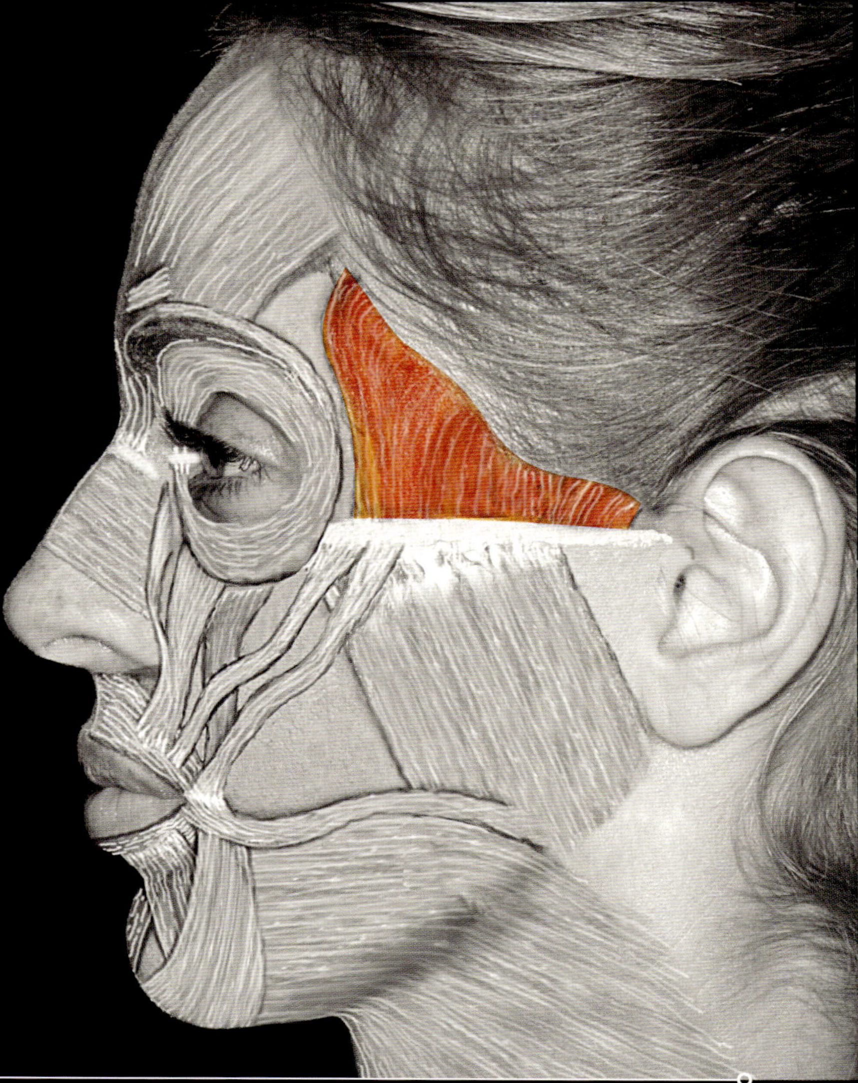

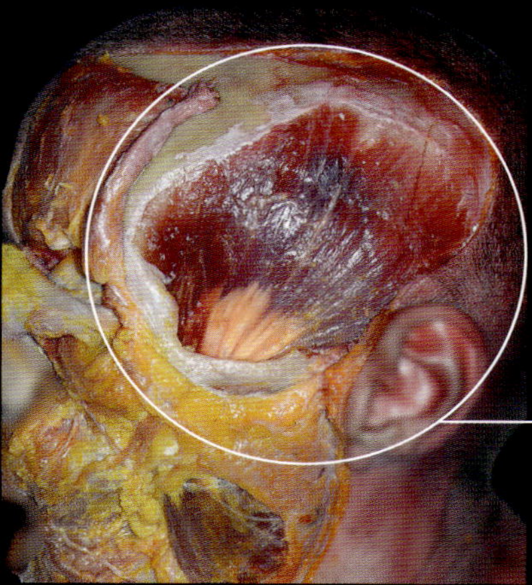

BTX injection protocol

TEMPORALIS MUSCLE			
Indications	• During the mixed dentition phase when the patient presents a severe parafunctional habit. • Coadjuvant treatment in cases of centric, eccentric, diurnal, nocturnal, moderate, and severe bruxism.		
Contraindications	• Patients with no parafunctional habits. • Children younger than 12 years old with light or moderate parafunctional habits can be treated with injections only at the masseter, which is the most potent masticatory muscle. • Contraindications listed by the manufacturer on the packaging.		
Attention	When the BTX is injected in this muscle over skin where there is no hair, it might result in small bruises due to its proximity to parietal branches of the superficial temporal artery. Therefore, injections in areas with hair are beneficial because they hide possible bruises.		
Recommended doses (per point)	**Botox** 5U	**Dysport** 15U	**Xeomin** 5U
Injection site	At the temple, inside and/or outside of areas with hair, always in places where the volume of the fibers is higher during occlusion.		
Needle	**Size** 8 mm	**Position** *(in relation to the skin)* Perpendicular to the side of the face	**Insertion** 1/2 of the needle

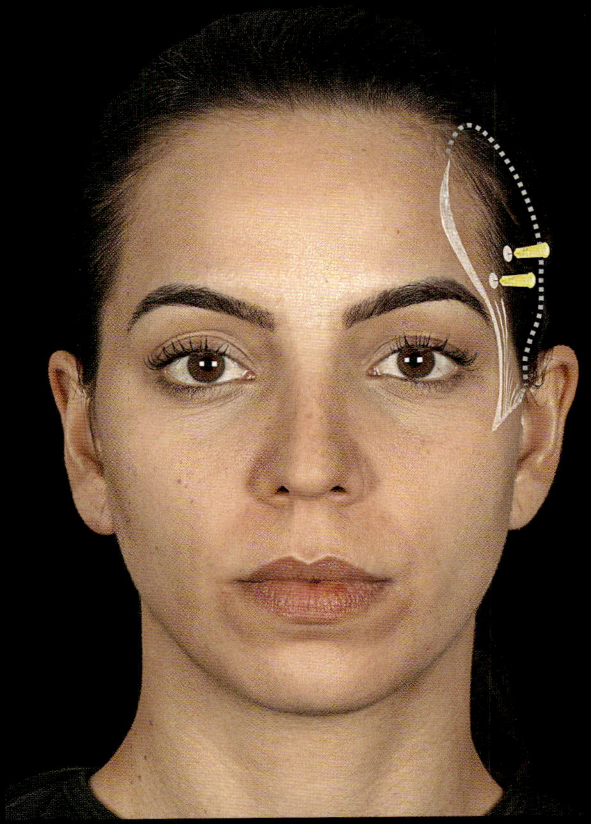

Injection for bruxism: Frontal view

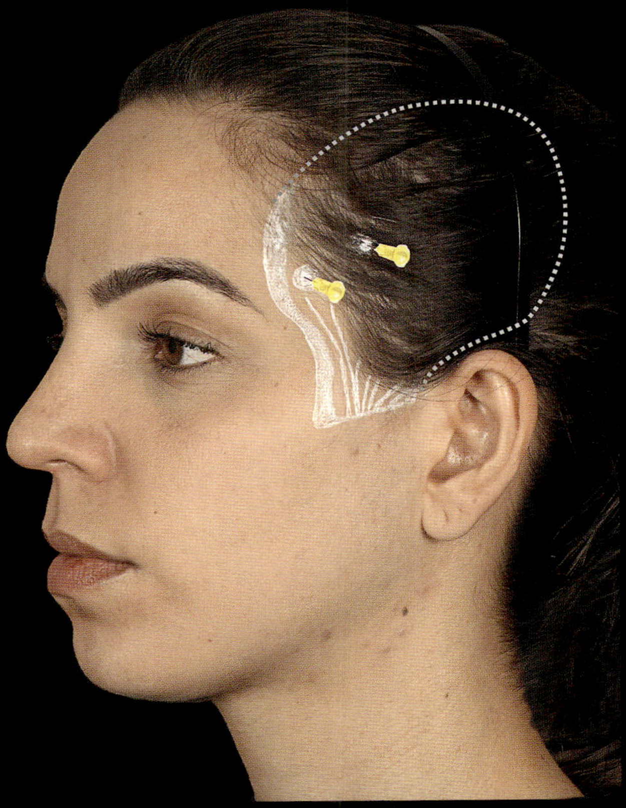

Injection for bruxism: Profile view

Procerus Muscle

Anatomy and location

Function: To lower the medial portion of the eyebrows. It is part of the muscles responsible for the expression of concern.

Location: Glabella.

Origin: Lower part of the nasal bone and upper part of the lateral nasal cartilage.

Insertion: Skin between the forehead and eyebrows.

Fibers: Longitudinal and opening in a fan shape as they bond to the occipitofrontalis muscle.

Wrinkles: Horizontal over the nasal root.

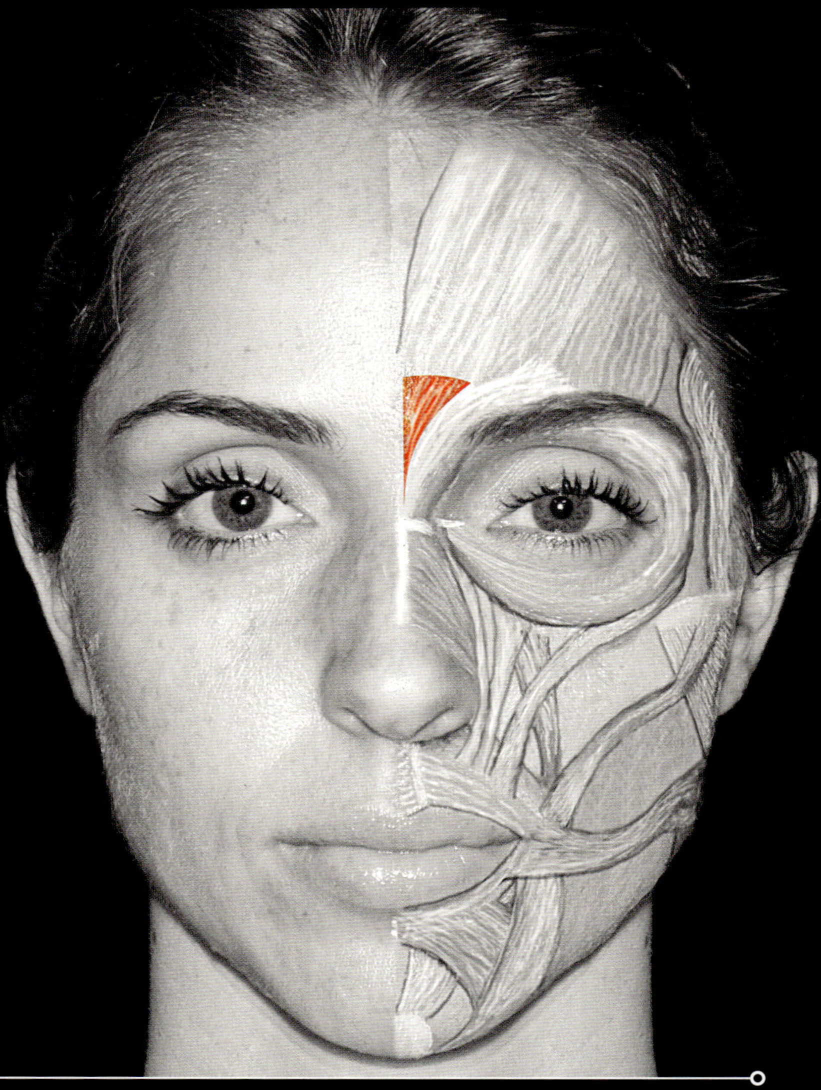

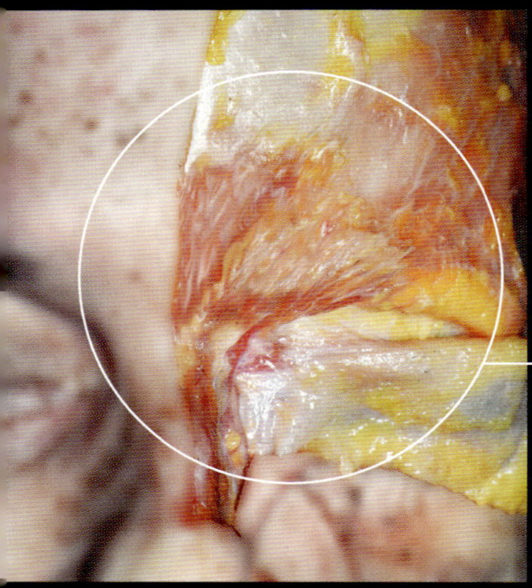

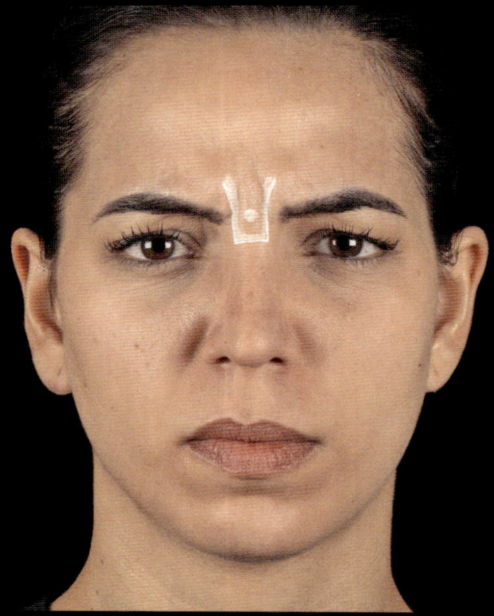

Locating and marking the muscle

1. Ask the patient to make an angry face, lowering the medial portion of the eyebrows and bringing them closer to the nose.
2. Draw a horizontal line corresponding to the deepest part of the nasal root skin, coinciding with the horizontal wrinkle when this groove (wrinkle) is present. This is the lower visible limit of this muscle.
3. The lateral limits correspond to two vertical wrinkles between the eyebrows that correspond to corrugator supercilii muscle. The corrugator generally contracts along with the procerus.
4. The point should be marked at the highest elevation in the skin.

⚠ When injecting the toxin, the needle should penetrate a layer of fat over this muscle called the *glabella fat pad*; otherwise the substance will be diffused in the fat and not in the muscle. The needle should be 4 mm deep.

BTX injection protocol

PROCERUS MUSCLE

Indications	• To smooth horizontal wrinkles at the nasal glabella. • To smooth the wrinkles associated with an angry facial expression. • To control the positioning of the medial eyebrow.		
Contraindications	• Patients whose eyebrows reflect a pity expression (ie, the medial part is higher than the lateral part). • Contraindications listed by the manufacturer on the packaging.		
Attention	The treatment of glabellar wrinkles involves not only this muscle but also the corrugator supercilii.		
Recommended doses	**Botox** 4U, or 2U at two points	**Dysport** 10U, or 5U at two points	**Xeomin** 4U, or 2U at two points
Injection site	One point in the belly of the muscle that coincides with the facial midline. In rare cases, this muscle has no fiber at the midline, instead presenting a depression. In these cases, inject one point in each side of the midline.		
Needle	**Size** 8 mm	**Position** *(in relation to the skin)* Perpendicular to the glabella	**Insertion** 1/2 of the needle

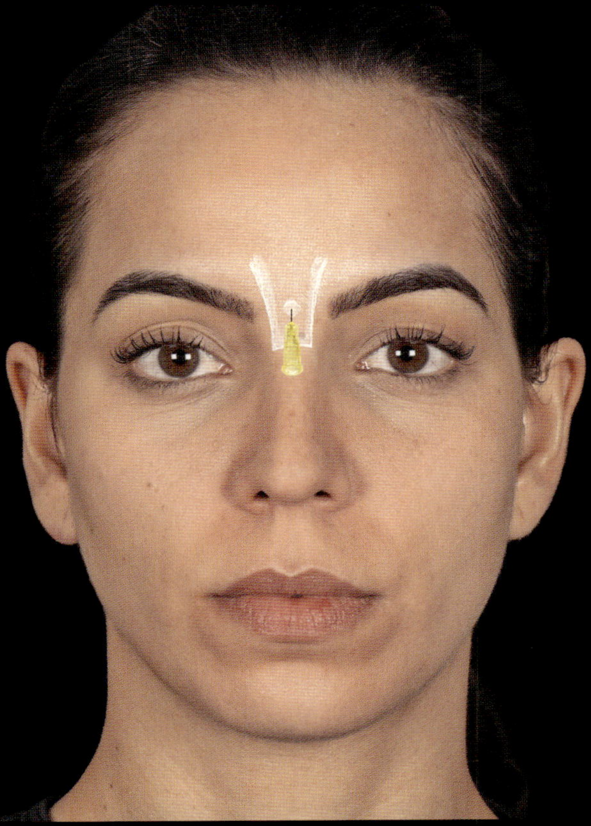

Injection: Frontal view

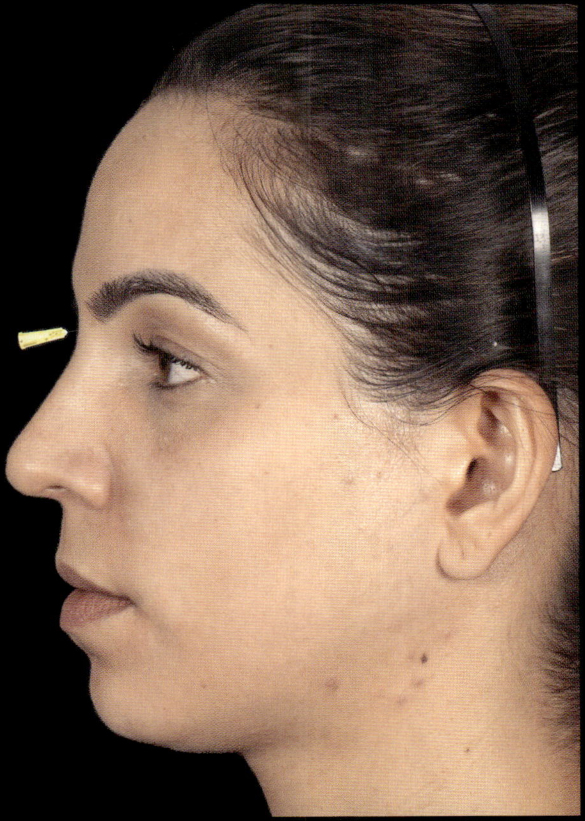

Injection: Profile view

Corrugator Supercilii Muscle

Anatomy and location

Function: To bring the medial part of the eyebrow inward toward the other, slightly depressing it. It is the muscle responsible for the expression of concern. It also assists the procerus and orbicularis oculi when forcefully closing the eyes.

Location: It is located at the medial end of the eyebrow, above the area with hair, inserted into the deep surface of the occipitofrontalis and orbicularis oculi.

Origin: Nasal part of the frontalis at the medial end of the superciliary arch.

Insertion: Superciliary skin at the deep surface of the skin and epicranial aponeurosis.

Fibers: Oblique, ascending in the lateral direction.

Wrinkles: Vertical at the glabellar region and upper internal orbit quadrant. Its action over the procerus muscle results in glabellar longitudinal lines when corrugated. They are known as the "11s."

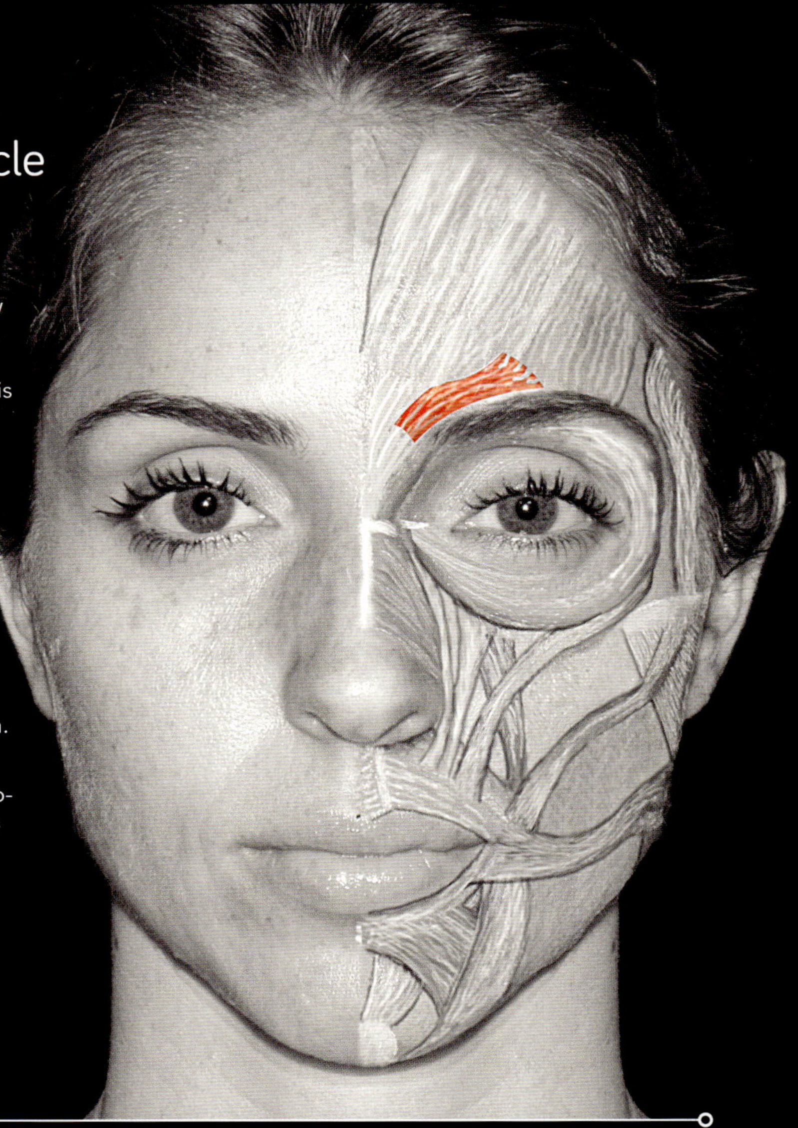

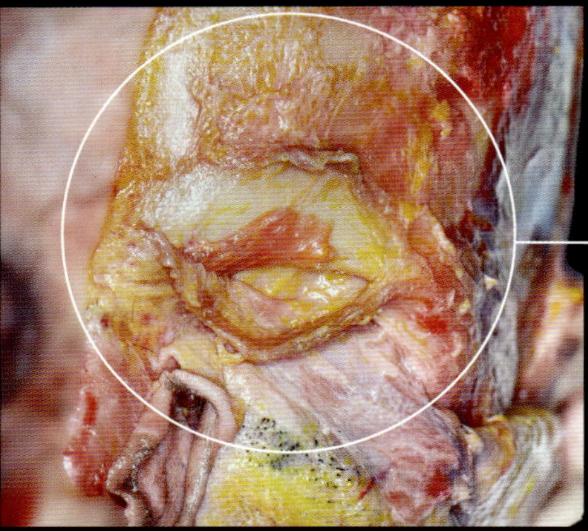

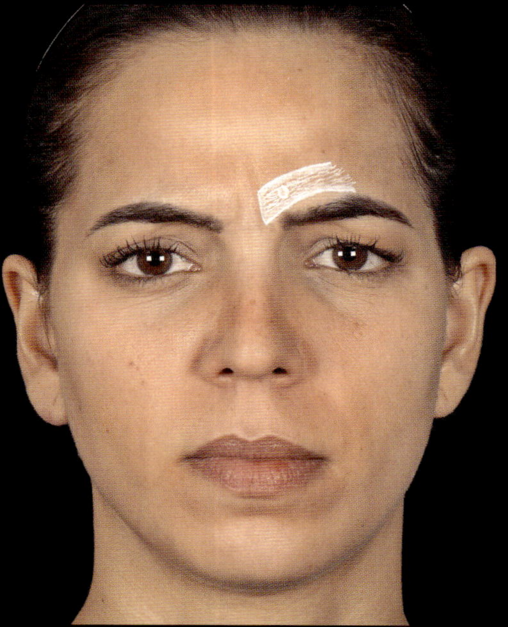

Locating and marking the muscle

1. Ask the patient to make an angry face, bringing the medial portions of the eyebrows together.
2. Draw a vertical line inside the vertical wrinkle that will correspond to the medial limit of the muscle.
3. The upper and lower limits do not need to be marked because they are similar to the width of the eyebrow.
4. A point should be drawn lateral to the vertical line at the point of the skin with the highest elevation.

The more lateral the injection point is, the greater will be the proximity with the levator palpebrae superioris muscle, thus increasing the chances of an eyebrow ptosis.

BTX injection protocol

CORRUGATOR SUPERCILII

Indications	• To smooth glabella vertical wrinkles of the nasal root. • To smooth anger lines. • To adjust the position of the eyebrow.		
Contraindications	Contraindications listed by the manufacturer on the packaging.		
Attention	This muscle is deeper than the occipitofrontalis and orbicularis oculi. Therefore, the needle should penetrate 4 mm to reach the muscle.		
Recommended doses	**Botox** 3U	**Dysport** 6U	**Xeomin** 3U
Injection site	One point in the part of the skin that is most elevated during facial expression, immediately lateral to the vertical glabella wrinkles.		
Needle	**Size** 8 mm	**Position** *(in relation to the skin)* 45 degrees	**Insertion** 1/2 of the needle

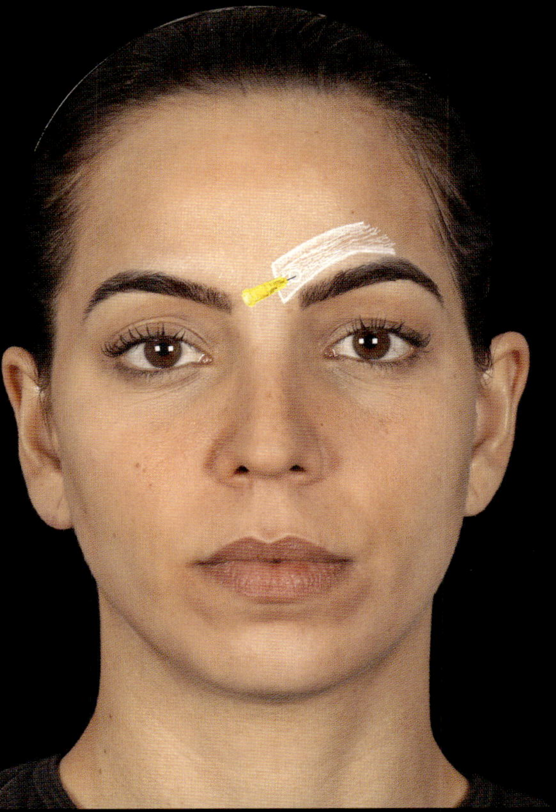

Injection: Frontal view

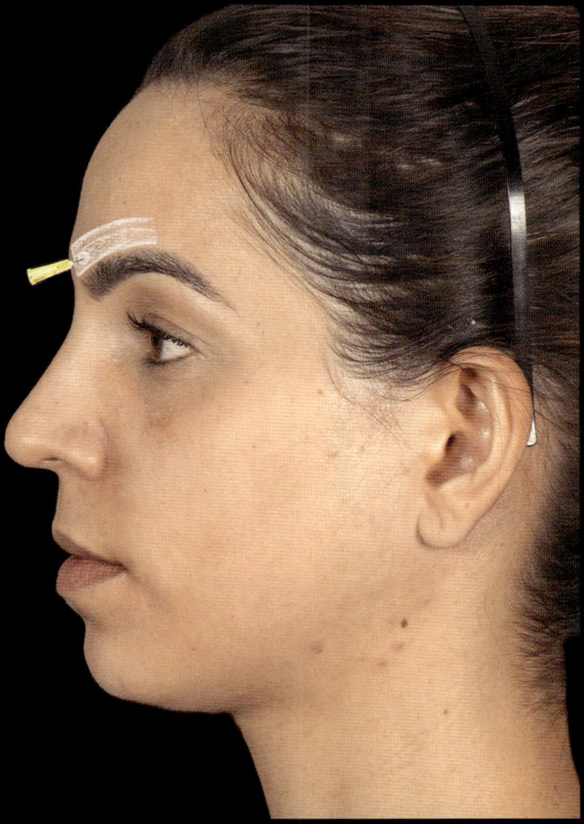

Injection: Profile view

Orbicularis Oculi Muscle

Anatomy and location

Function: To close the eyes in a sphincter action (orbital and palpebral portions), blink (palpebral portion), and drain the lacrimal sac (lacrimal portion).

Location: It encircles the eyes.

Origin: Orbital portion—nasal part of the frontal process of the maxilla, in the medial eye angle and medial palpebral ligament. Palpebral portion—medial palpebral ligament. Lacrimal portion—posterior lateral crest.

Insertion: Orbital portion—skin around the eye, forehead, and cheeks. Palpebral portion—lateral palpebral raphe and lateral palpebral ligament. Lacrimal portion—around the lacrimal canaliculi and lacrimal sac, frontalis bone, glabella skin, and lacrimal gland.

Fibers: Elliptical.

Wrinkles: Lateral canthus lines, or periorbital wrinkles or "crow's feet."

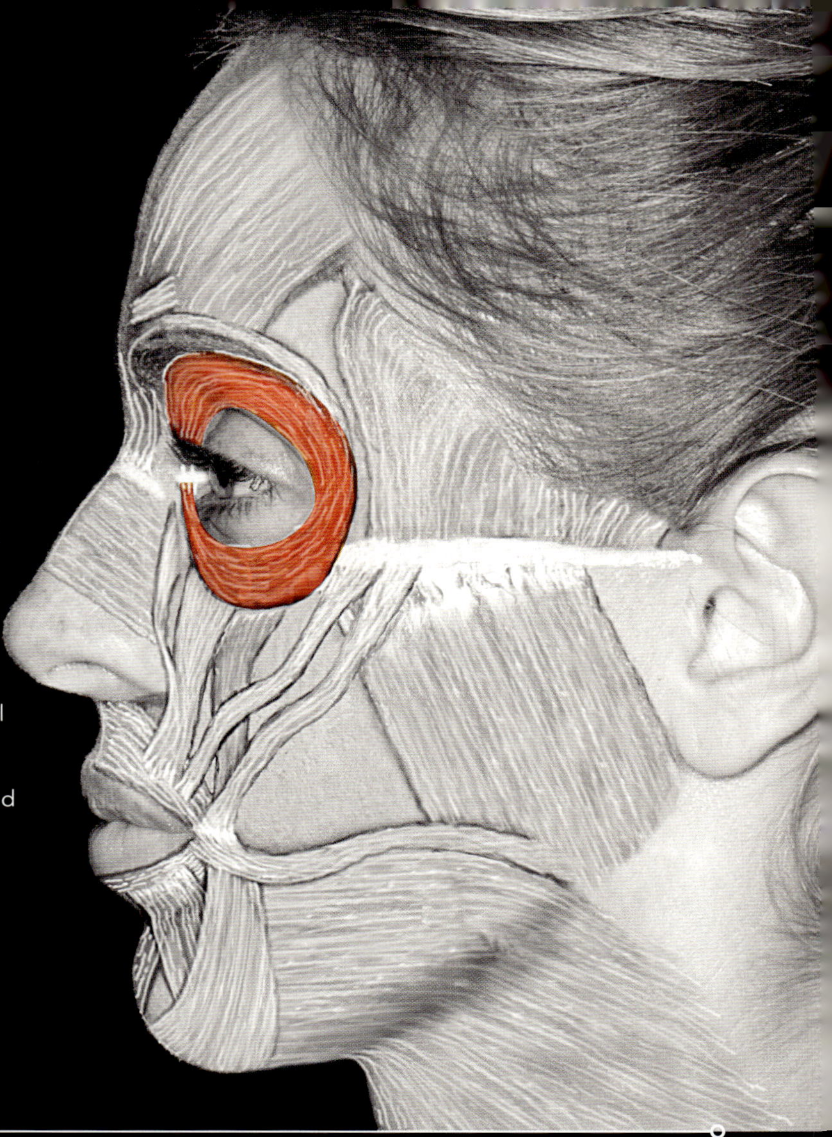

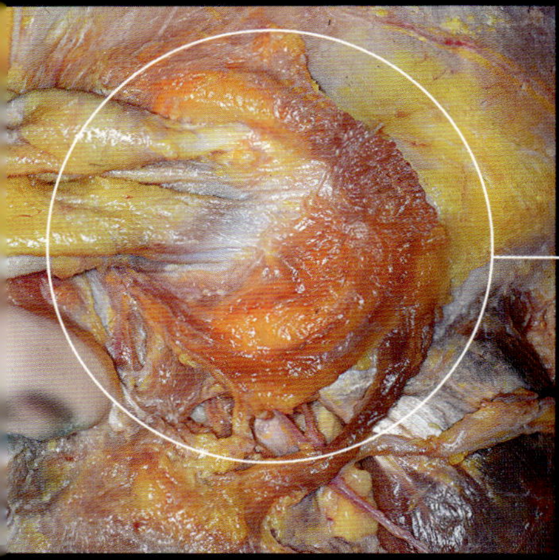

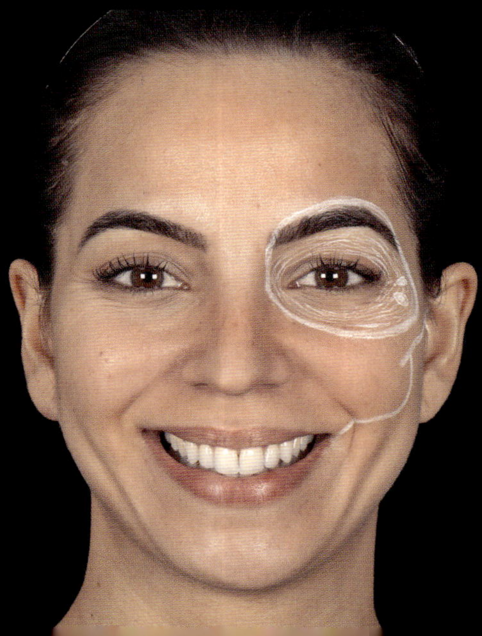

Locating and marking the muscle

1. Ask the patient to smile and to keep smiling.
2. Mark one or more points at the highest parts of the wrinkles around the eye. The number of points to be established depends on the size of the wrinkled area. The points should be marked by following a semicircle lateral to the orbit. Keep a distance of 10 mm between each of the points, because at this distance toxin diffusion will effectively treat the muscle. Also keep a distance of 10 mm from each of the points up to the orbital ridge to avoid possible diffusions to the muscles that move the eyes (lateral rectus muscle and superior and inferior oblique muscles).
3. Draw the horizontal zygomatic bone ridge via palpation and keep a distance of 10 mm from the lowest mark. This prevents possible diffusion to the zygomaticus major muscle.

Injections at the lower eyelid might cause flaccidity, making it distant from the bulbar conjunctiva and causing an ectropion and consequently persistent eye watering and irritation.

BTX injection protocol

ORBICULARIS OCULI MUSCLE			
Indications	• To smooth lateral canthus or periorbital wrinkles as well as crow's feet. • To adjust the position of the eyebrow.		
Contraindications	Contraindications listed by the manufacturer on the packaging.		
Attention	This region shows a tendency to develop bruises because of its proximity to the zygomatico-orbital artery. The orbicularis oculi muscle has an antagonist action over the movement of the occipitofrontalis muscle. Therefore, the injection at one point in the skin of the eyebrow tail, a little below the area with hair, will relax the orbicularis oculi, facilitating brow arching through the occipitofrontalis muscle.		
Recommended doses (per point)	**Botox** 2U–4U	**Dysport** 6U–12U	**Xeomin** 2U–4U
Injection site	10 mm lateral to the orbital ridge		
Needle	**Size** 8 mm	**Position** *(in relation to the skin)* 45 degrees	**Insertion** 1/3 of the needle

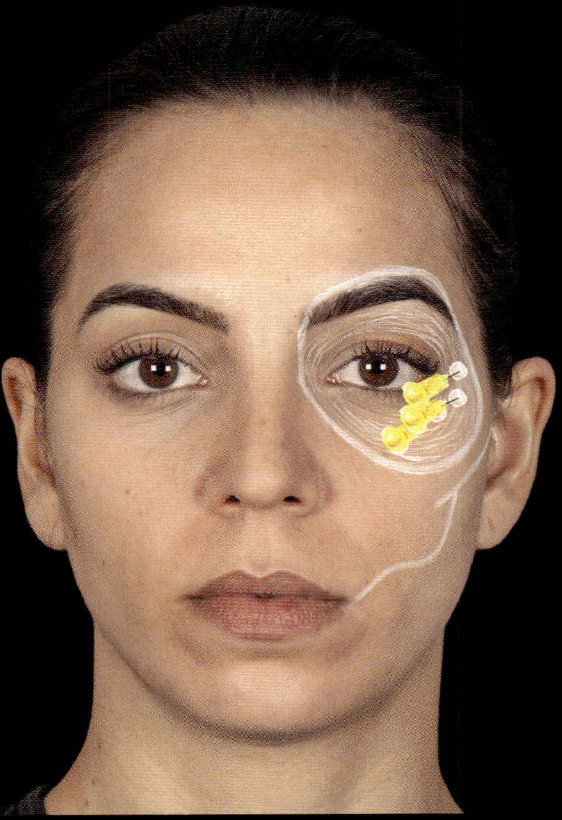
Injection: Frontal view

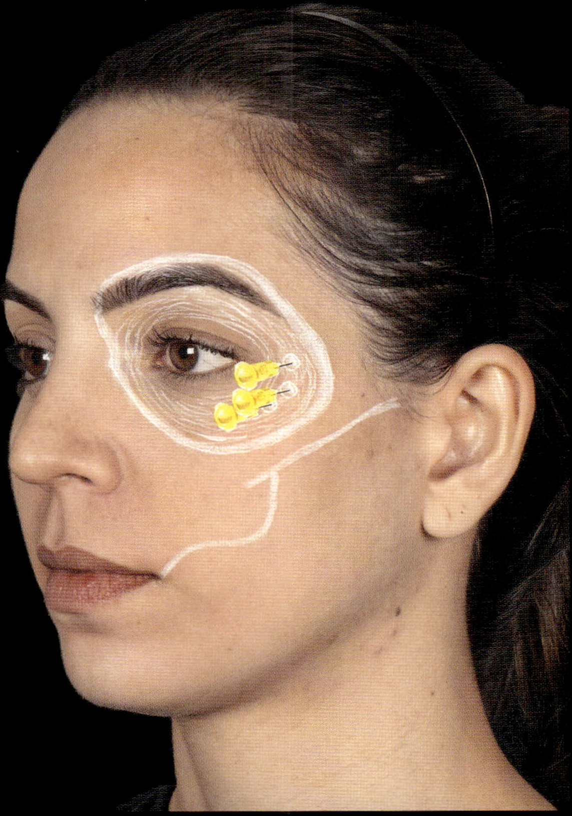
Injection: Oblique view

Nasalis Muscle (Transverse Part)

Anatomy and location

Function: It compresses the nose, slightly lowering the tip.

Location: Nasal dorsum.

Origin: Alveolar eminence of the canines and maxillary lateral incisors.

Insertion: Tendinous lamina of the nasal dorsum.

Fibers: Transverse, descendent and lateral to the midline.

Wrinkles: Perpendicular to the direction of the muscle fibers. They are known as *bunny lines*. The levator labii superioris alaeque nasi muscle is also in part responsible for producing this wrinkle.

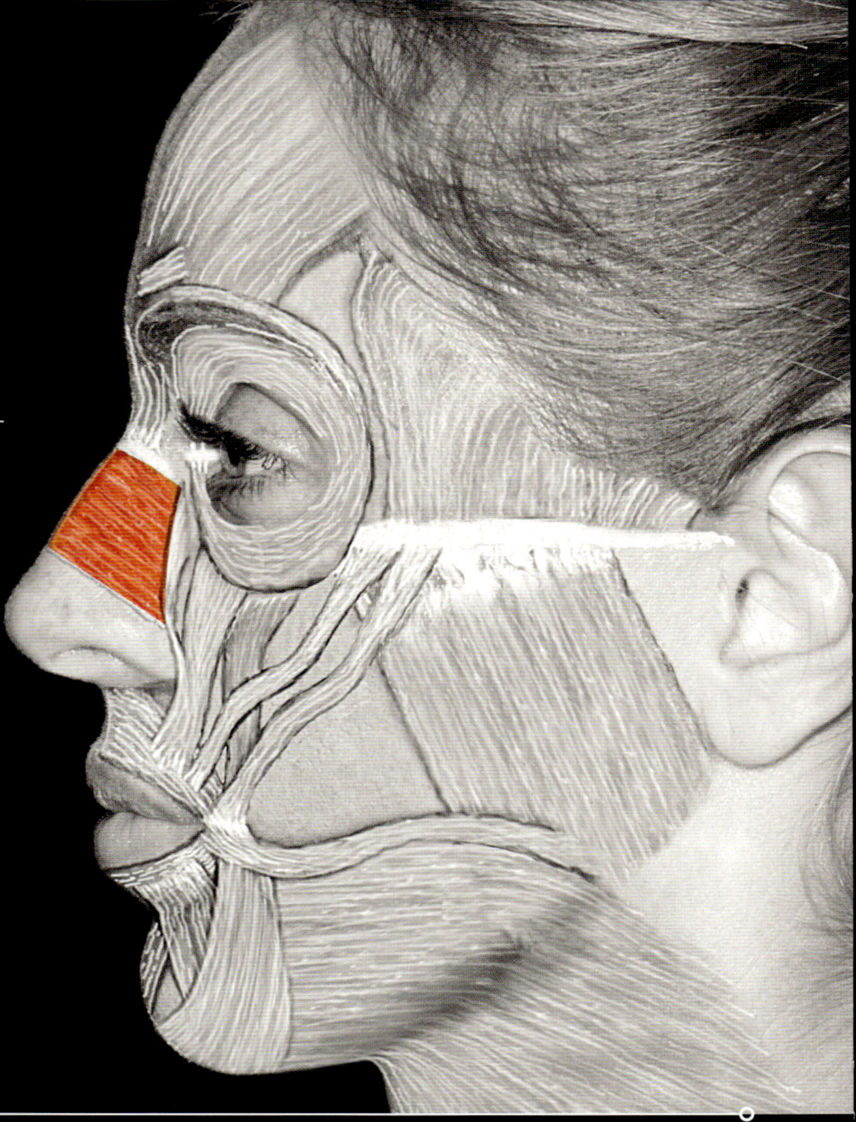

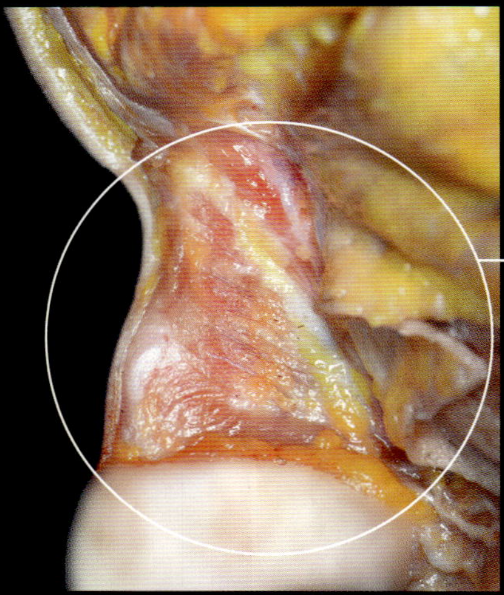

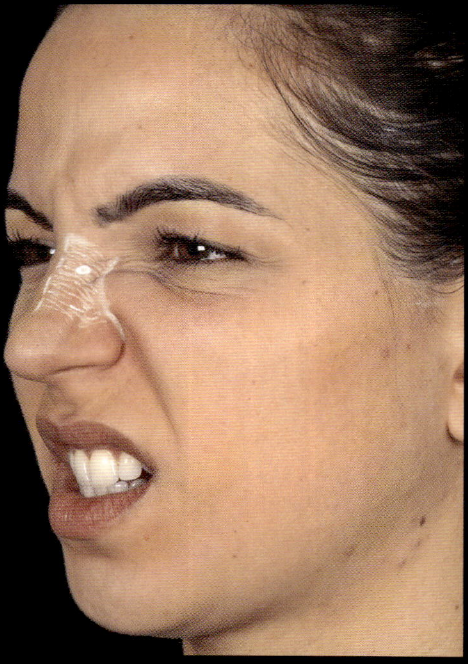

Locating and marking the muscle

1. Draw a midline over the nasal dorsum.
2. Ask the patient to smile and make wrinkles in the nose and then hold that expression.
3. Mark the point that shows the highest elevation of the skin corresponding to each wrinkle. Mark one point in each wrinkle, in case there is more than one. Even when the highest volumes of these wrinkles are distant from the midline, the risk of injections close to the levator labii superioris alaeque nasi muscle should be considered. Injections close to the midline prevent undesired diffusion to this muscle.

Injections too close to the levator labii superioris alaeque nasi muscle should be avoided to prevent diffusion to this muscle. This diffusion would compromise the elevation of the upper lip during a smile.

BTX injection protocol

NASALIS MUSCLE (TRANSVERSE PART)			
Indications	• To smooth dynamic wrinkles of bunny lines showing during the smile. • To smooth static wrinkles of bunny lines showing at rest. • In cases where BTX-A will be used to control the gummy smile.		
Contraindications	Contraindications listed by the manufacturer on the packaging.		
Attention	Patients who had toxin injected in the upper third of the face and/or who were treated for gummy smile and did not have injections in this muscle might show more wrinkled skin in this site due to a "compensatory activation." This can clearly show that the patient was treated with BTX-A. Therefore, this muscle should also be injected with toxin in case the patient already shows wrinkles in the nose while smiling.		
Recommended doses (per point)	**Botox** 1U	**Dysport** 3U	**Xeomin** 1U
Injection site	Belly of the muscle, one to two points on each side, at the highest elevation of the skin.		
Needle	**Size** 8 mm	**Position** *(in relation to the skin)* Parallel	**Insertion** Only the bevel should penetrate the skin

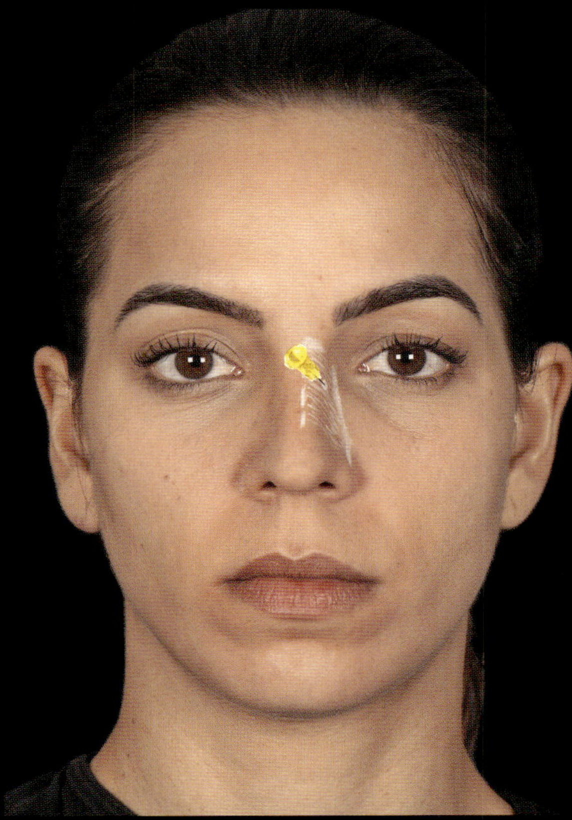

Injection: Frontal view

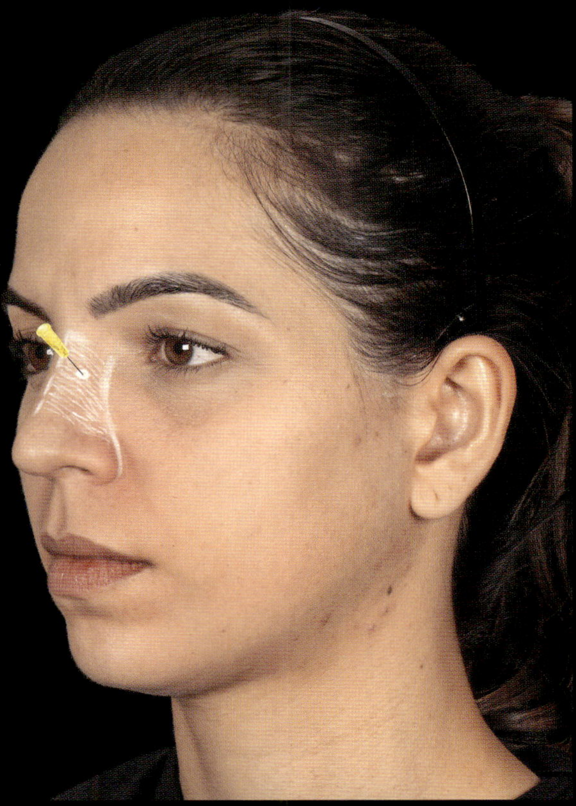

Injection: Oblique view

Depressor Septi Nasi Muscle

Anatomy and location

Function: It depresses the nasal septum and narrows the nostrils.

Location: Below the columella insertion.

Origin: Incisive fossa of the maxilla.

Insertion: Nasal septum cartilage and dorsal portion of the ala of the nose.

Fibers: Longitudinal.

Wrinkles: Horizontal, at the upper lip skin. Next to the nasal septum base.

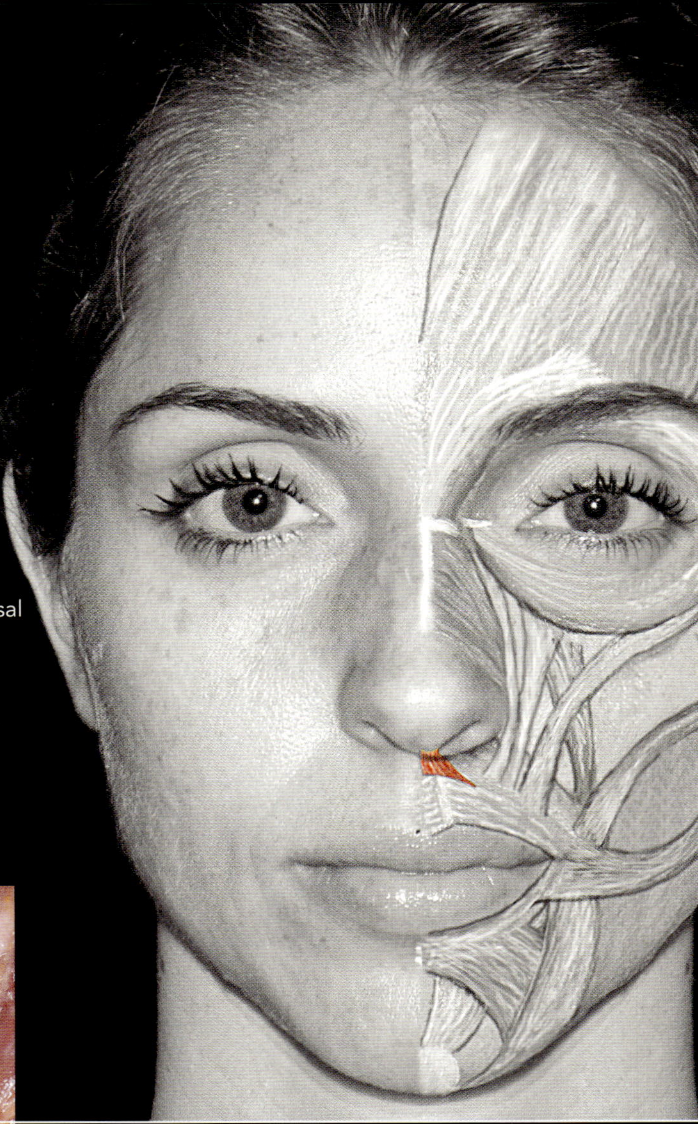

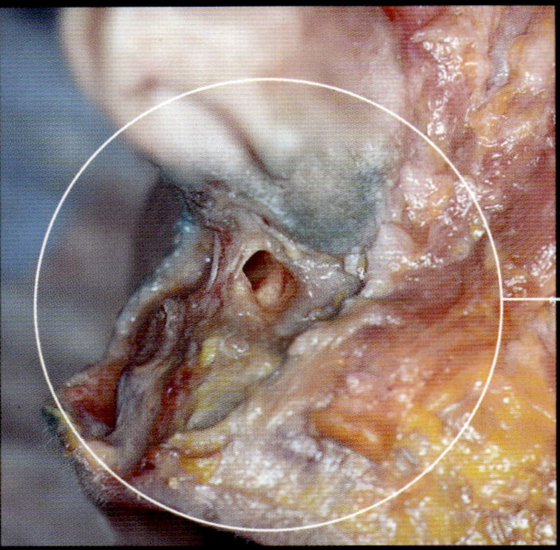

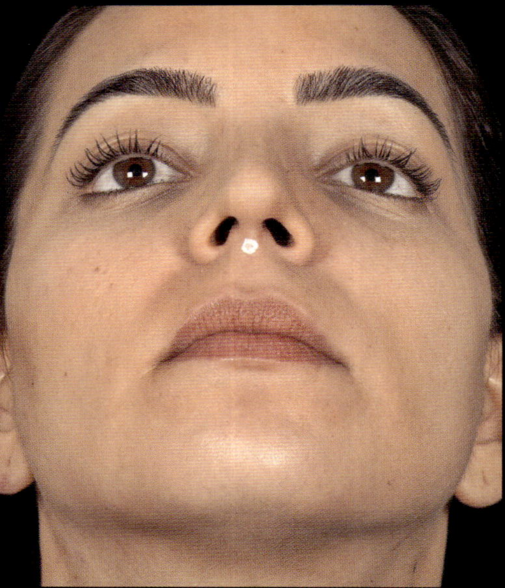

Locating and marking the muscle

- It cannot be identified through facial expressions or via palpation. It should be located through facial esthetic references.
- A point in the facial midline should be marked at th level of the nasolabial angle, that is, at the insertion of the nasal columella with the upper lip skin.

Although the BTX-A injection in this muscle wi result in a pleasant elevation of the nasal tip, the horizontal level of the upper lip will be lowered, covering part of the anterosuperior crown length, which is very unesthetic. This injection can only be used in cases associated with an upper gummy smile.

BTX injection protocol

DEPRESSOR SEPTI NASI MUSCLE

Indications	• Patients who move the tip of the nose during speech. • To move the nose tip up and at the same time to lower the horizontal level of the anterior part of the upper lip. • Patients with a gummy smile showing more than 3 mm of gingival tissue around the maxillary central incisors. • To smooth the horizontal fold at the upper lip produced during a smile. • Patients with a gummy smile whose upper lip stomion is horizontally higher than the oral commissures during the smile.		
Contraindications	• Patients not showing a gummy smile. • Contraindications listed by the manufacturer on the packaging.		
Attention	This is the most painful injection in the face. If possible, it should be the last injection to be administered to avoid scaring the patient at the beginning of the appointment. Injection in the middle of the cartilage is very painful and does not work.		
Recommended doses	**Botox** 2U, 3U, or 4U	**Dysport** 6U, 9U, or 12U	**Xeomin** 2U, 3U, or 4U
Injection site	Nasolabial angle.		
Needle	**Size** 8 mm	**Position** *(in relation to the skin)* 70 degrees	**Insertion** The whole needle

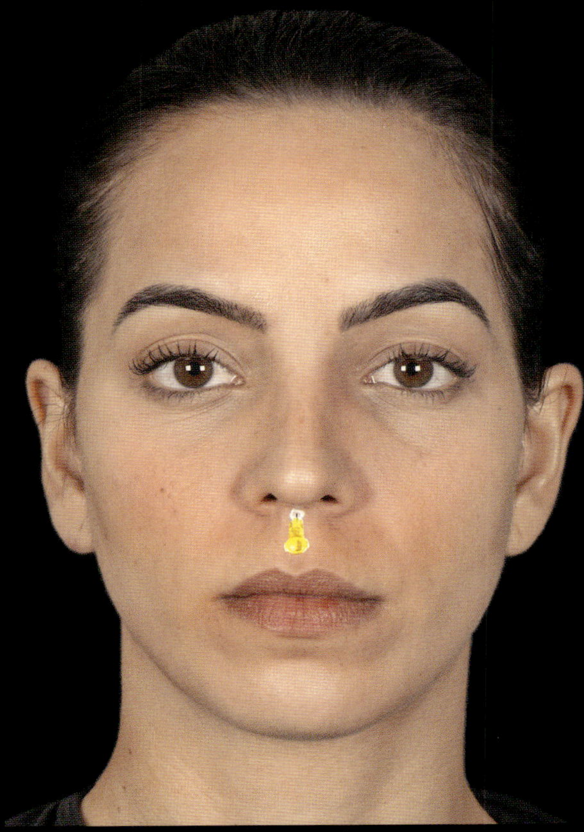

Injection: Frontal view

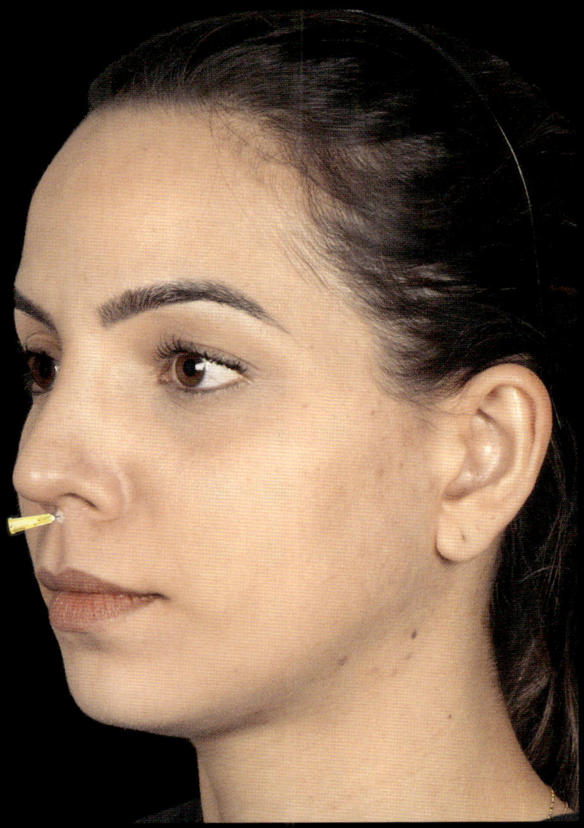

Injection: Oblique view

Levator Labii Superioris Alaeque Nasi and Levator Labii Superioris Muscles

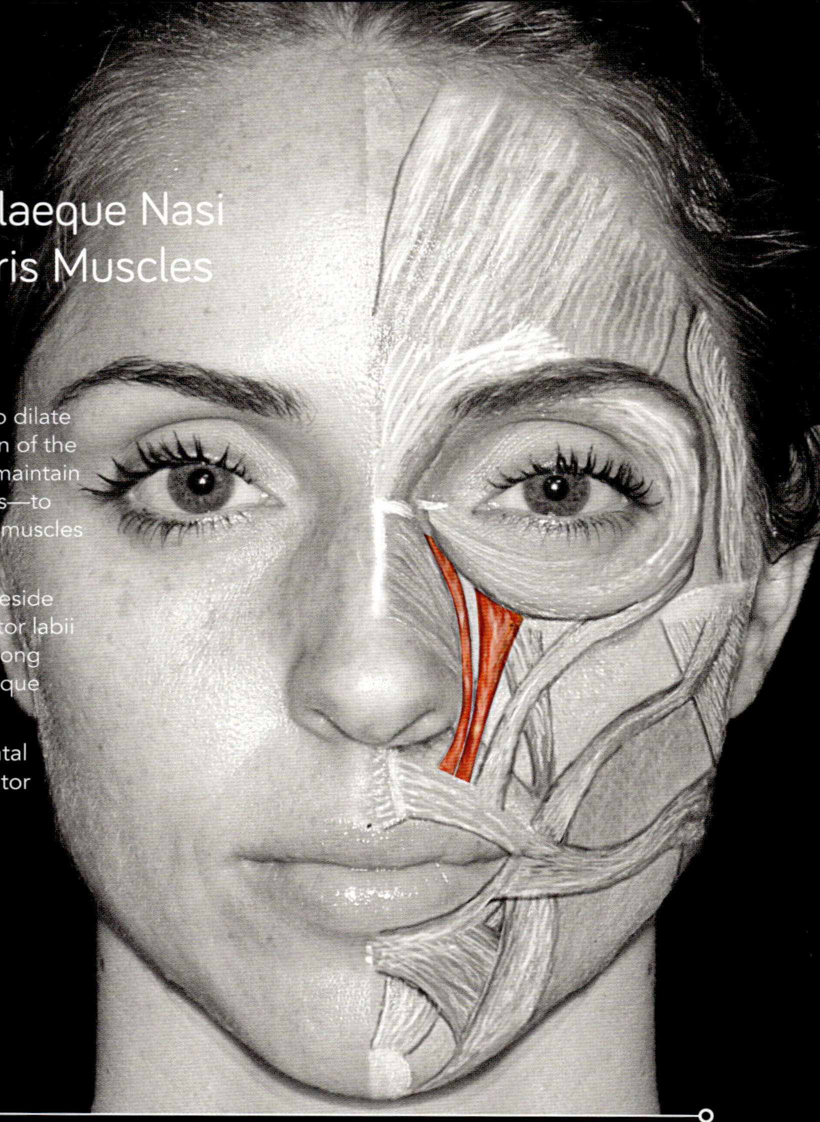

Anatomy and location

Function: Levator labii superioris alaeque nasi—to dilate the nostrils and lift and elevate the middle portion of the upper lip. When the muscle is at rest, it helps to maintain the position of the nostrils. Levator labii superioris—to elevate the medial portion of the upper lip. Both muscles work through eversion of the upper lip.

Location: Levator labii superioris alaeque nasi—beside and along the nose between the nasalis and levator labii superioris. Levator labii superioris—beside and along the nose between the levator labii superioris alaeque nasi and zygomaticus minor.

Origin: Levator labii superioris alaeque nasi—frontal process of the maxilla and infraorbital edge. Levator labii superioris—infraorbital edge at the maxilla above the infraorbital foramen.

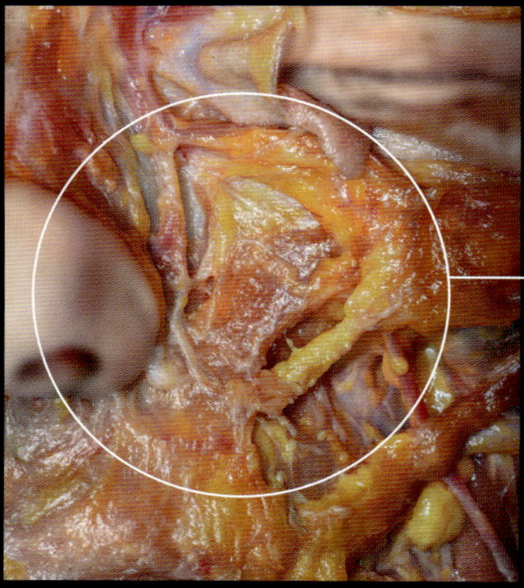

Insertion: Levator labii superioris alaeque nasi—greater alar cartilage, wing of the nose, and upper lip skin. Levator labii superioris—upper lip skin and fibers blending with the orbicularis oculi muscle.

Fibers: Vertical direction.

Wrinkles: Help to produce wrinkles lateral to the nose at the internal canthus of the eyes. Also causes the initial process of the nasolabial sulcus near the nose.

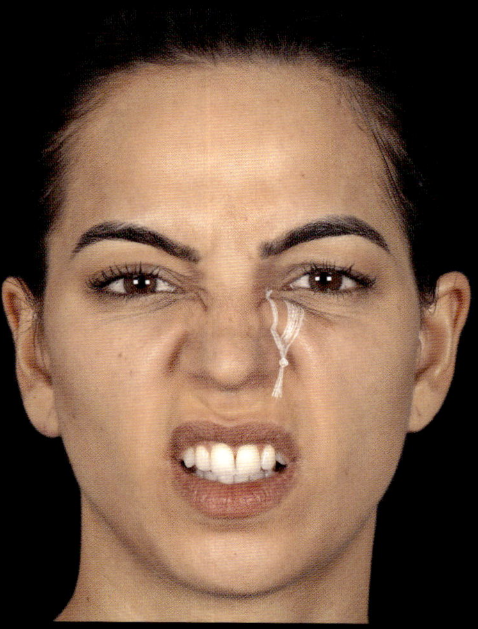

Locating and marking the muscle

- These two muscles cannot be perceived through facial expression or via palpation. They are found through facial esthetic references.
- A 3-mm-wide line should be drawn along the side of the nose. A second drawing is made lateral to the first and further from the nose, approximately 9 mm wide.
- The ideal injection point to affect both muscles at the same time is a point lateral to the wing of the nose and at the middle of the nasolabial end.
- These two muscles have separate origins, but they are near the insertion. Therefore, only one injection is enough to treat both muscles at the same time.

⚠ Individual injections in each of these two muscles are not recommended because above the wing of the nose its location becomes more difficult. Errors in the injection site might result in bilateral asymmetries.

BTX injection protocol

LEVATOR LABII SUPERIORIS ALAEQUE NASI AND LEVATOR LABII SUPERIORIS MUSCLES			
Indications	• Posterior gummy smile (when there is an excessive, esthetically unpleasant gingival exposure at the maxillary canines). It is a very successful approach in cases where muscle hyperactivity is the cause of the gummy smile. • It can be used as a palliative approach in cases of nonoperable vertical maxillary excess. • Asymmetries at the horizontal level of the upper lip.		
Contraindications	• This technique does not fully work in patients whose gummy smile is caused by a short upper lip. • Contraindications listed by the manufacturer on the packaging.		
Attention	If the smile is gummy and the horizontal level of the upper lip stomion is higher than the commissures, the toxin should also be injected in the depressor septi nasi. By reducing the gummy smile, the passive labial seal will be improved, contributing to better nasal breathing.		
Recommended doses (per point)	**Botox** 2U, 3U, or 4U	**Dysport** 6U, 9U, or 12U	**Xeomin** 2U, 3U, or 4U
Injection site	Inject the toxin at the same height in both sides using the same inclination and depth of the needle, immediately beside the wing of the nose and medial to the nasolabial groove.		
Needle	**Size** 8 mm	**Position** *(in relation to the skin)* Perpendicular to the face	**Insertion** 1/2 of the needle

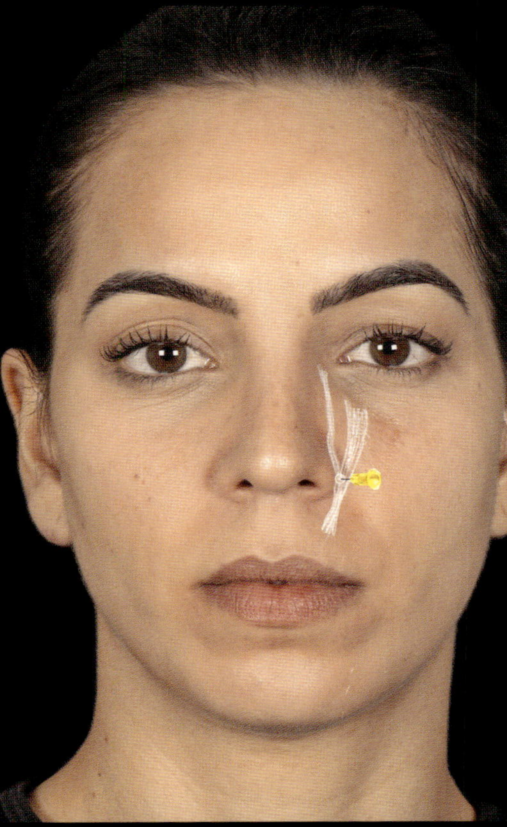

Injection: Frontal view

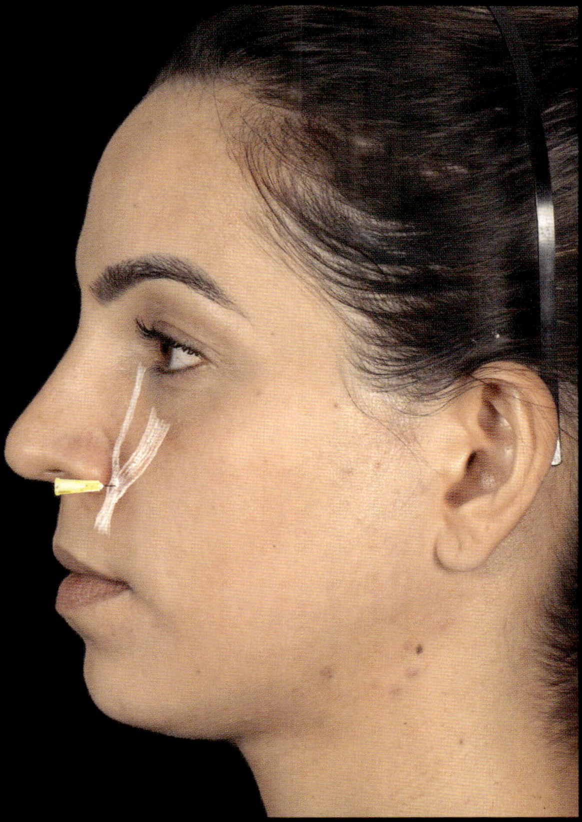

Injection: Profile view

Levator Anguli Oris Muscle

Anatomy and location

Function: To elevate the angle of the mouth. It is one of the muscles involved in the smile.

Location: It ascends from the modiolus in the direction of the eye.

Origin: Canine fossa of the maxilla.

Insertion: Angle of the mouth.

Fibers: Vertical.

Wrinkles: Helps in the formation of the nasolabial sulcus.

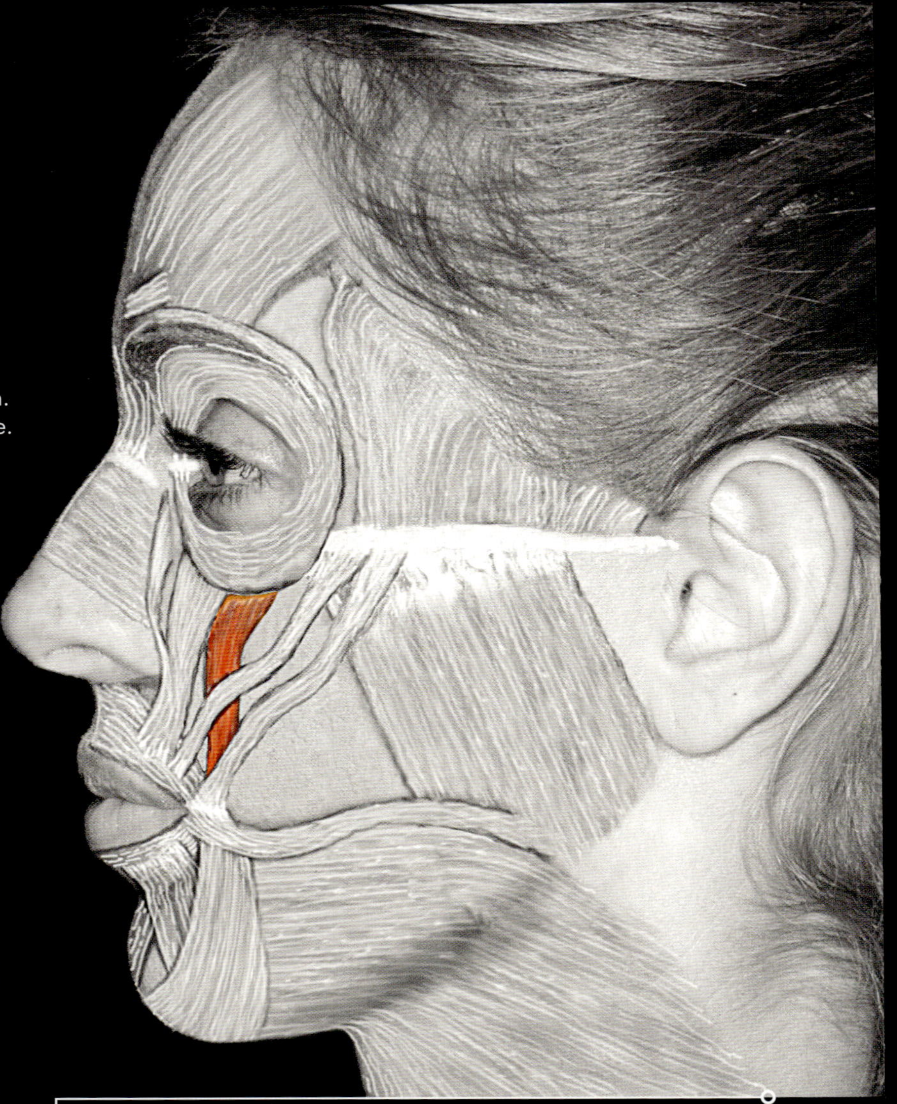

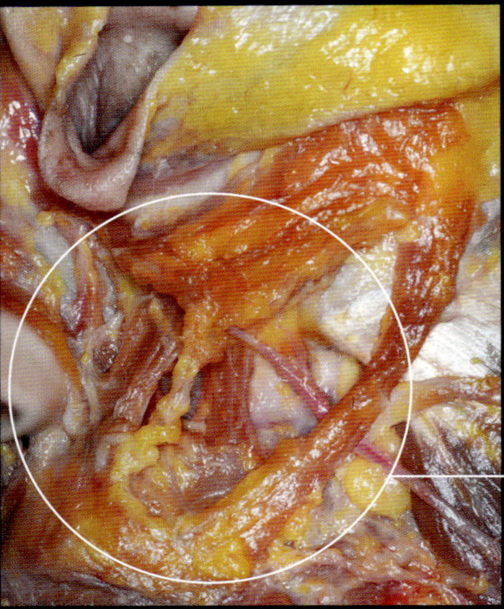

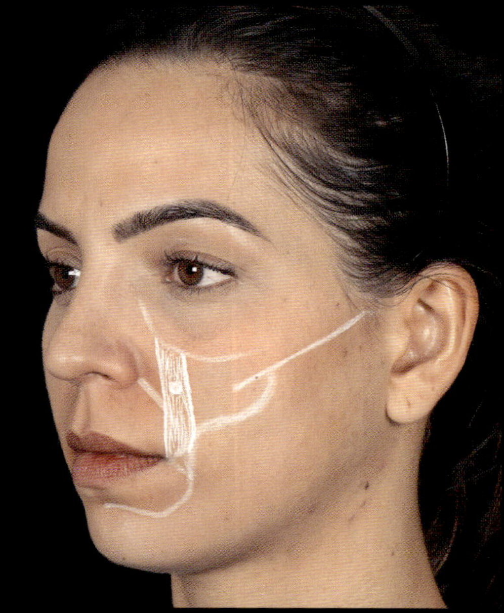

Locating and marking the muscle

- This muscle cannot be found through facial expression or via palpation. It should be located through facial esthetic references.
- The superior limit of the drawing is the inferior limit of the orbicular oculi that is located approximately 10 mm below the lower orbital ridge.
- Its lower limit is the modiolus; that is, the middle portion of this muscle coincides with the oral commissure, laterally extending approximately 5 mm.
- Draw the orbicularis oris muscle to exclude it from the injection area.
- The injection point should be equidistant from the orbicularis oculi and orbicularis oris muscle.

Draw the orbicularis oculi, orbicularis oris, and zygomaticus major muscles to exclude them from the injection area, thereby avoiding undesired effects. Do not inject the toxin too close to the modiolus, as there are fibers from different muscles inserted in this region.

BTX injection protocol

LEVATOR ANGULI ORIS MUSCLE

Indications	• Asymmetries caused by hyperkinesia or facial paralysis where the patient predominantly elevates one of the oral commissures. • Patients with asymmetries at the horizontal level of the commissures and also posterior gummy smile. • Patients whose smiles present excessive elevation of both oral commissures ("joker face"), exposing excessive gingiva above the clinical crowns of posterior teeth.		
Contraindications	• Patients with a good horizontal level of the gingival tissue not showing a posterior gummy smile. When the toxin is injected in these patients, the oral commissures might be low during the smile, hiding the clinical crowns of the maxillary premolars. • Contraindications listed by the manufacturer on the packaging.		
Attention	In the case of horizontal asymmetry of the commissures not associated with a gummy smile, the ideal approach is to inject the toxin into the depressor anguli oris muscle on the side that is less elevated. This will stop the muscle from lowering this commissure and result in horizontal symmetry.		
Recommended doses	**Botox** 2U, 3U, or 4U	**Dysport** 6U, 9U, or 12U	**Xeomin** 2U, 3U, or 4U
Injection site	An equidistant point between the orbicularis oculi and orbicularis oris muscles following an imaginary vertical ascending line from the middle of the modiolus.		
Needle	**Size** 8 mm	**Position** *(in relation to the skin)* Perpendicular	**Insertion** The whole needle

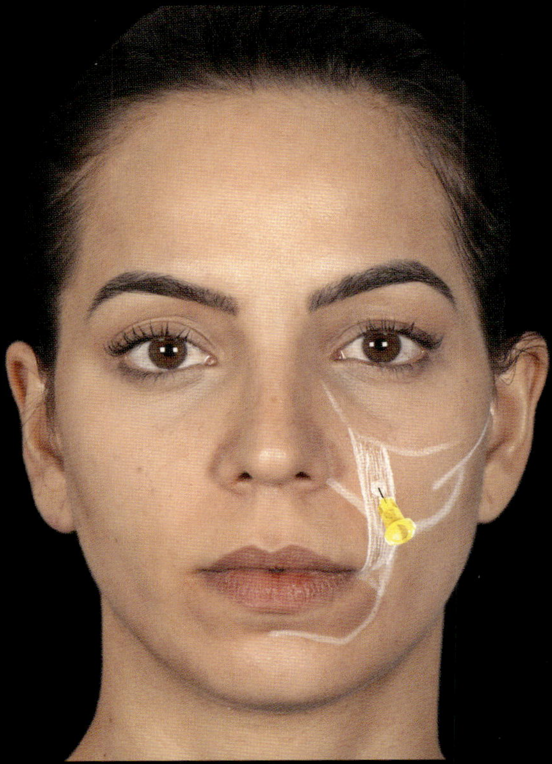

Injection: Frontal view

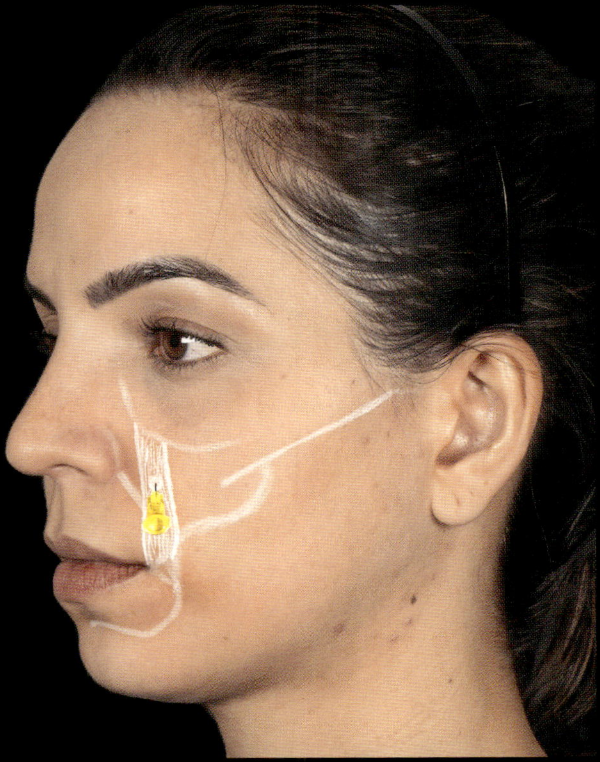

Injection: Oblique view

Zygomaticus Major Muscle

Anatomy and location

Function: To lift the angle of the mouth superiorly and pull it slightly to the lateral, helping to form a smile. It assists other muscles in mastication.

Location: At the cheek, from the anguli oris to the zygomatic bone in an ascending pathway of approximately 45 degrees, similar to the zygomaticus minor pathway.

Origin: Lateral surface of the zygomatic bone.

Insertion: Skin of the angle of the mouth and fibers blending with the orbicularis oris and levator anguli muscles.

Fibers: Ascending and with an inclination of approximately 45 degrees.

Wrinkles: Helps in the production of the nasolabial sulcus and wrinkles around the eyes.

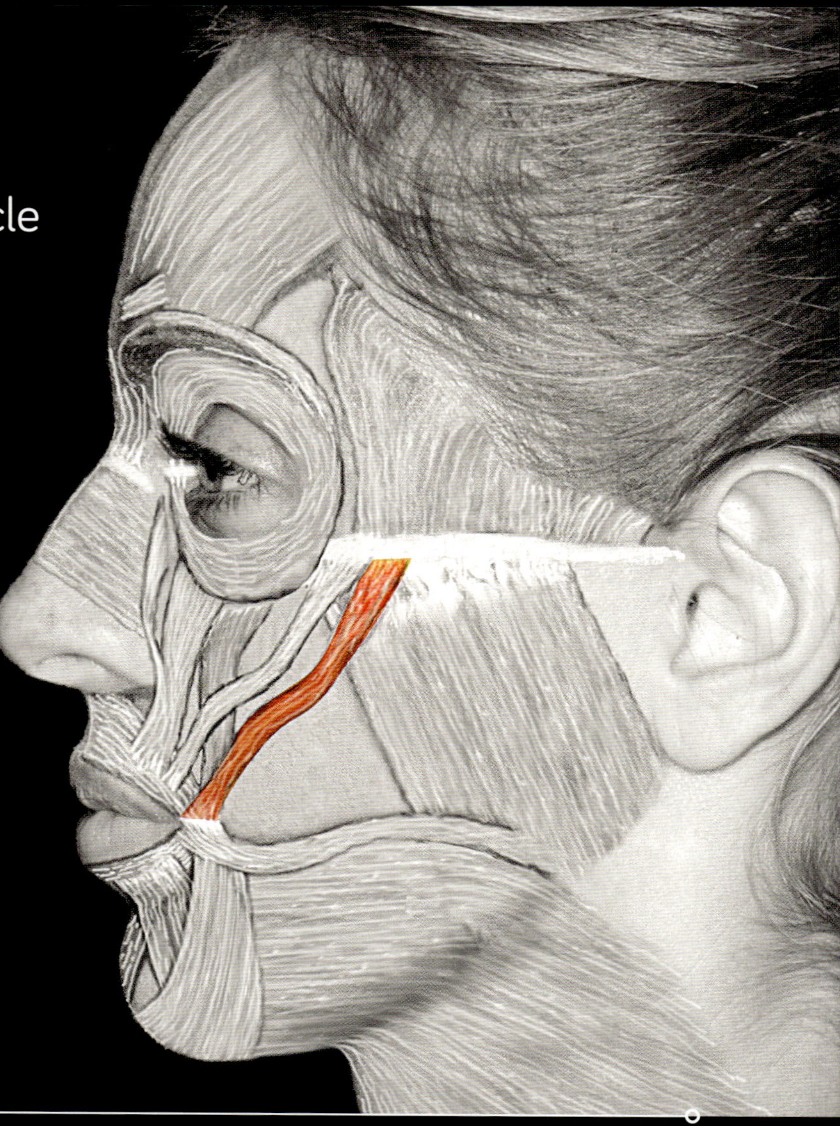

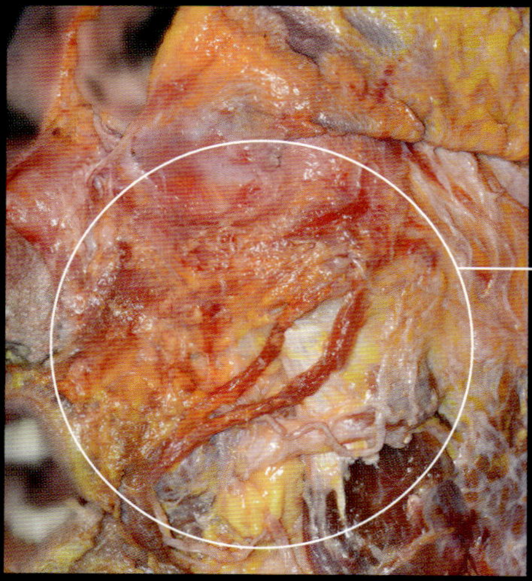

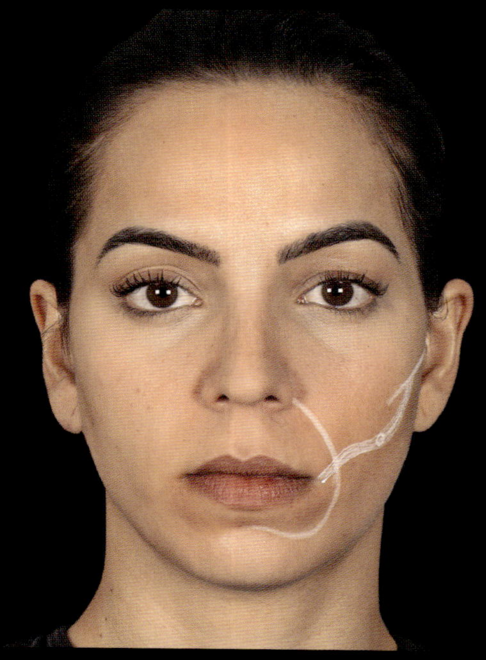

Locating and marking the muscle

Although it helps to produce wrinkles at the side of the eyes and increases the nasolabial sulcus, it cannot be located using facial expressions. In this case, facial esthetic references are used to find the muscle location.

1. Ask the patient to relax all facial musculature. Via palpation, draw the zygomatic bone.
2. Start the drawing from the anguli oris going upward in the direction of the lateral surface of the zygomatic bone.
3. Ask the patient to strongly close the mouth (without smiling), biting and relaxing several times, and draw the anterior masseter ridge via palpation.

The fixation of this muscle in the zygomatic bone is 15 mm lateral to the anterior border of the masseter muscle. The zygomaticus major is superficial to the masseter muscle. The injection site is an equidistant point between the origin and insertion.

! It is not advisable to inject BTX in this muscle without a previous drawing.

BTX injection protocol

ZYGOMATICUS MAJOR MUSCLE			
Indications	Asymmetries caused by hyperkinesia or facial paralysis resulting in a smile where patients show a wider oral corridor than their contralateral side.		
Contraindications	• Symmetric smiles where the amplitude of the oral corridor is excessive. • Excessive oral corridor caused by maxillary atresia and/or by the lingual inclination of maxillary posterior teeth. • Contraindications listed by the manufacturer on the packaging.		
Attention	Although the zygomaticus major muscle assists with the elevation of the anguli oris, asymmetries at the horizontal level of the oral commissures ideally should be treated with injections at the levator anguli oris or depressor anguli oris muscle.		
Recommended doses	**Botox** 2U, 3U, or 4U	**Dysport** 6U, 9U, or 12U	**Xeomin** 2U, 3U, or 4U
Injection site	A point equidistant to two extremities of the muscle drawing.		
Needle	**Size** 8 mm	**Position** *(in relation to the skin)* Perpendicular to the skin of the cheek	**Insertion** 1/3 of the needle

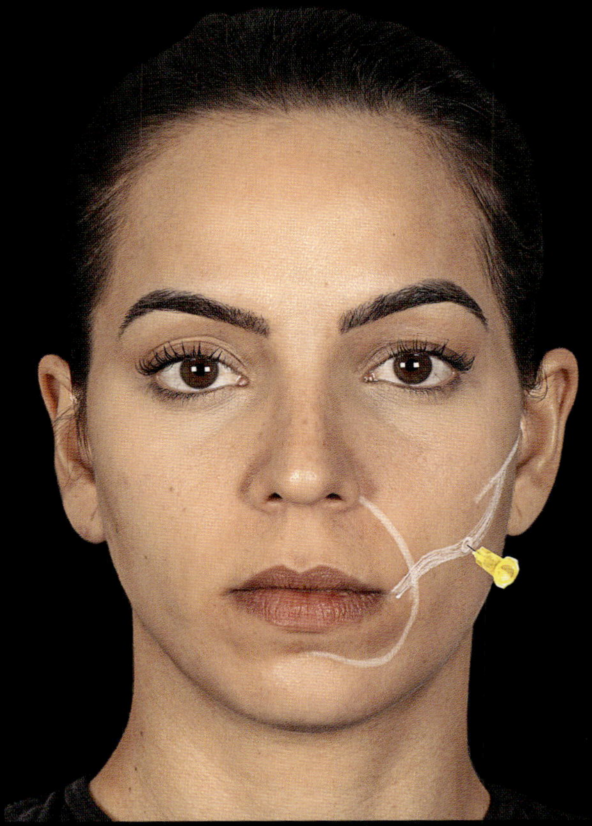

Injection: Frontal view

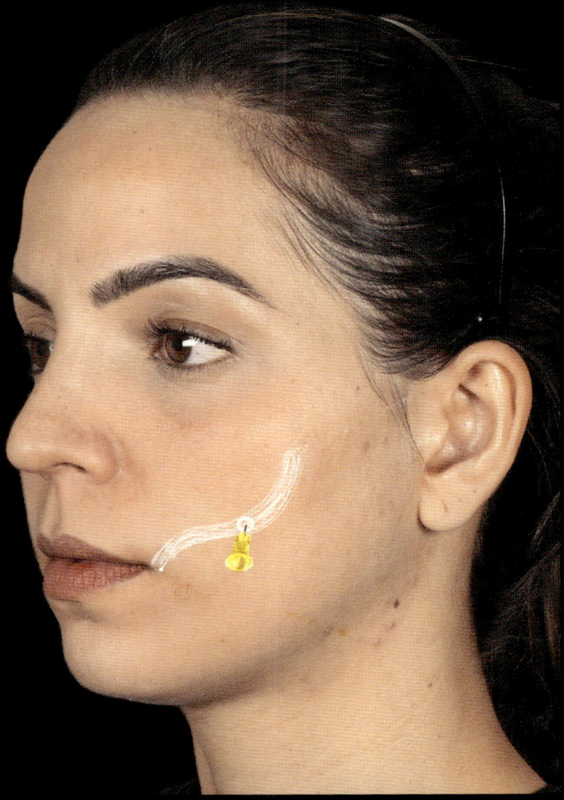

Injection: Oblique view

Masseter Muscle

Anatomy and location

Function: Elevation of the mandible and helps with mastication.

Location: Lateral to the mandibular ramus.

Origin: Zygomatic arch.

Insertion: Masseteric tuberosity located at the lateral lower two-thirds of the face of the mandibular ramus and the gonial angle.

Fibers: Lower posterior direction at approximately 45 degrees.

Wrinkles: It does not cause wrinkles because of its fascia.

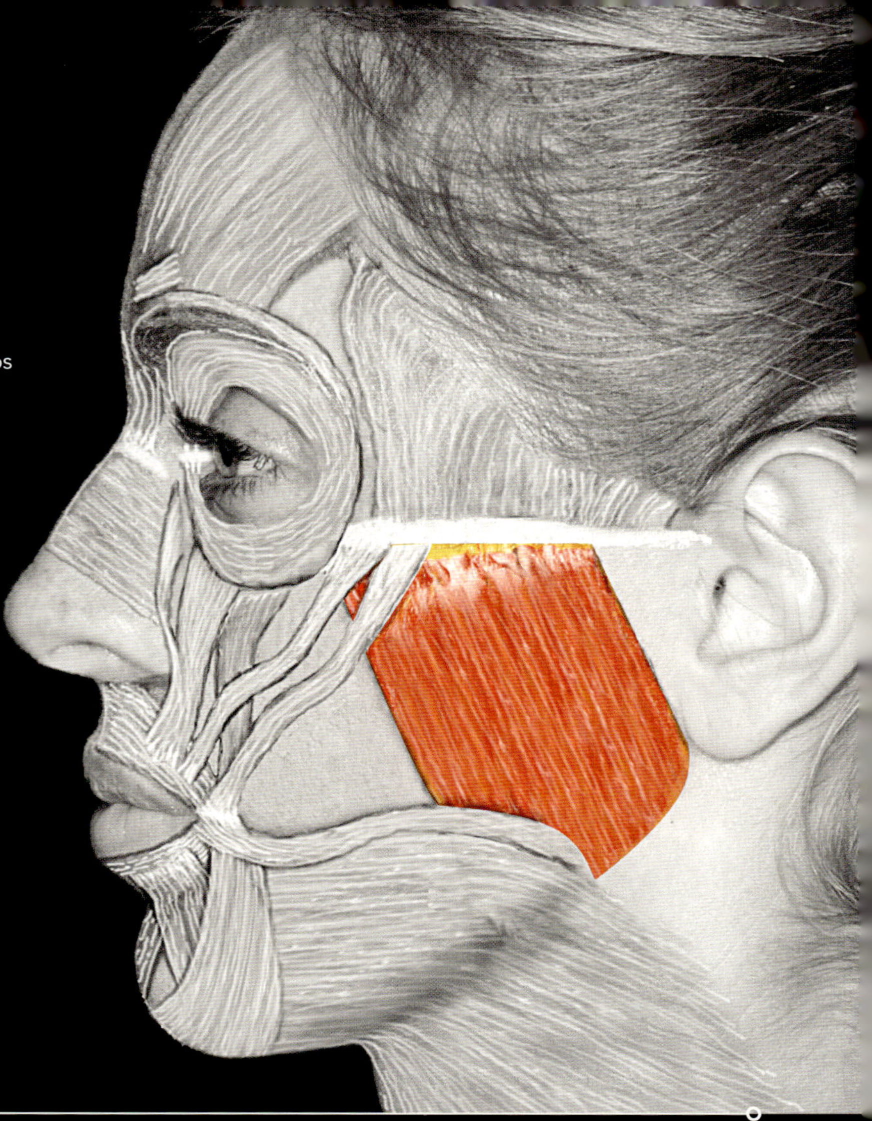

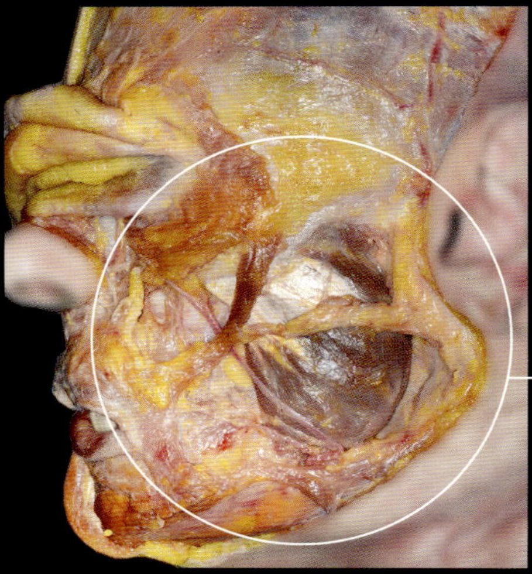

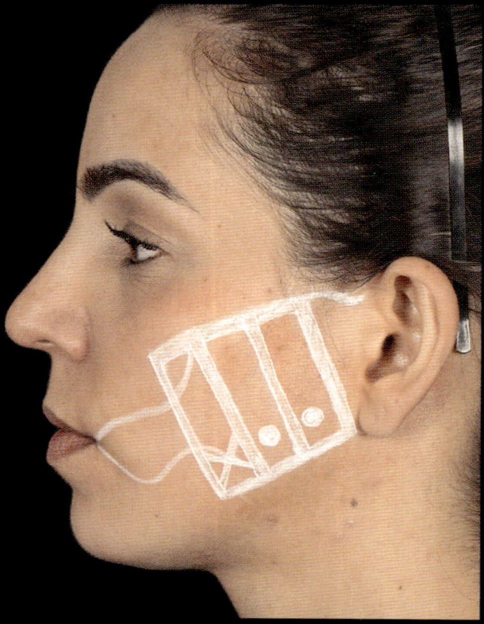

Locating and marking the muscle

1. Draw the zygomatic bone via palpation.
2. Ask the patient to close the mouth (without smiling), biting and relaxing several times, and draw the anterior and posterior limits of this muscle feeling the extension of the fibers that are contracted.
3. Draw two vertically inclined lines to divide this area into three parts.
4. Mark a point below the center corresponding to the medium bundle. Repeat the procedure for the posterior bundle.
5. Place your finger over the medial bundle and ask the patient to close the mouth while biting and relaxing. The finger should be pushed only to the lateral. Do the same at the posterior bundle. This time the finger should be moved to the lateral and posterior.

Observation: Mark the lower injection points where the muscle volume is greater. This muscle does not cover the temporomandibular joint.

The following should be avoided:

- Injections at the anterior bundle of the masseter muscle because of its proximity to the risorius muscle that originates at the masseteric fascia (at the anterior third of the masseter muscle).
- Injections toward the top of the muscle because of its proximity to the origin of the zygomaticus major muscle at the zygomatic arch.

BTX injection protocol

MASSETER MUSCLE			
Indications	• During the mixed dentition when the patient presents with severe parafunction. • Coadjuvant in cases of centric, eccentric, diurnal, nocturnal, moderate, and severe bruxism. • Preoperatively in dental rehabilitations to restore the vertical dimension of occlusion. • Masseter hypertrophy.		
Contraindications	• Patients who do not show bruxism. • Contraindications listed by the manufacturer on the packaging.		
Attention	Half of the dose should be administered in children younger than 12 years old. BTX injections at the masseter might cause a width reduction in the lower third of the face. As a result, the face will be more triangular.		
Recommended doses	**Botox** 10U–20U	**Dysport** 30U–60U	**Xeomin** 10U–20U
Injection site	A lower point at the middle bundle and another at the posterior bundle as shown in the photographs. In order to obtain symmetric points, use a ruler to measure from the tragus to the points on one side, and make corresponding marks on the other side.		
Needle	**Size** 13 mm	**Position** *(in relation to the skin)* Perpendicular to the lateral side of the face	**Insertion** The whole needle

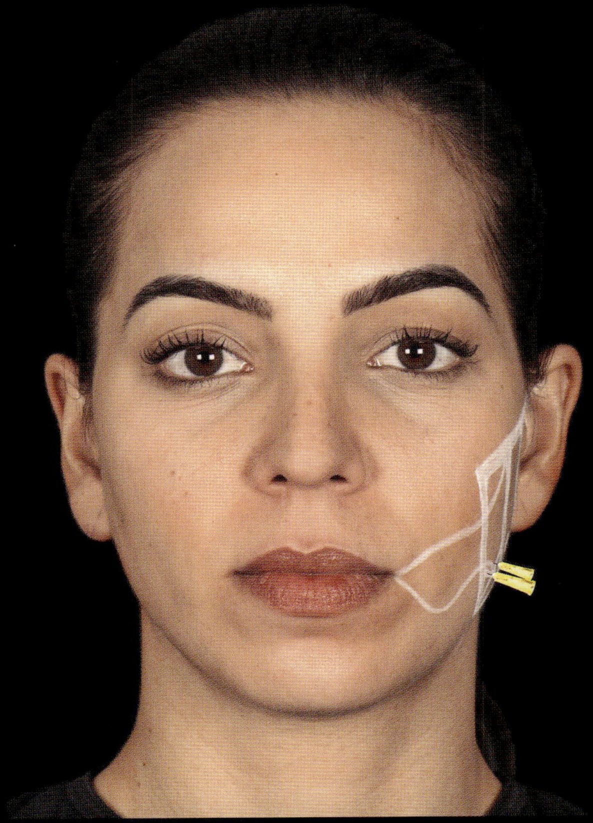

Injection: Frontal view

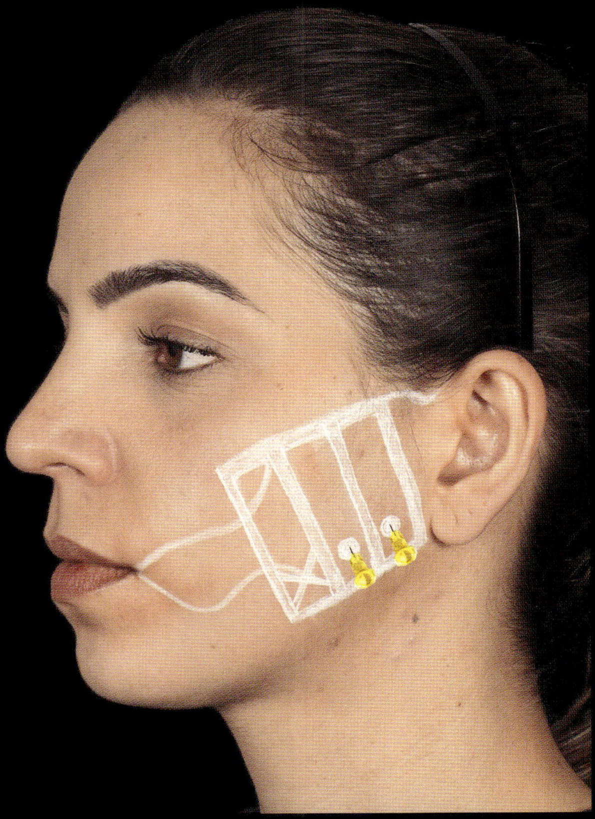

Injection: Profile view

Orbicularis Oris Muscle

Anatomy and location

Function: Responsible for closing the lips and compressing them against the teeth. It also participates in the eversion of the lips.

Location: Encircles the lips.

Origin: At the alveolar ridges of the maxilla and mandible, next to the midline and modiolus.

Insertion: Fascia and skin around the lips and bundles with fibers from the buccinator.

Fibers: Circular around the mouth.

Wrinkles: Vertical lines around the mouth or "radial lip lines."

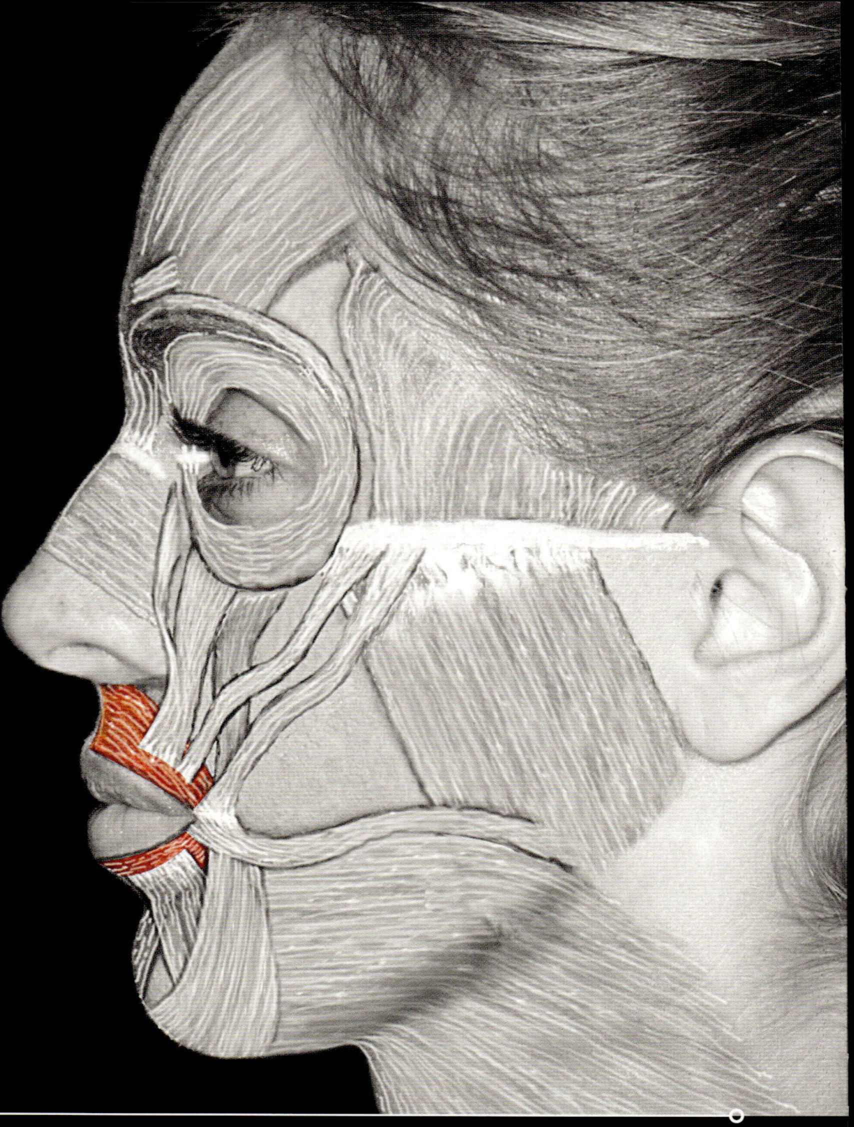

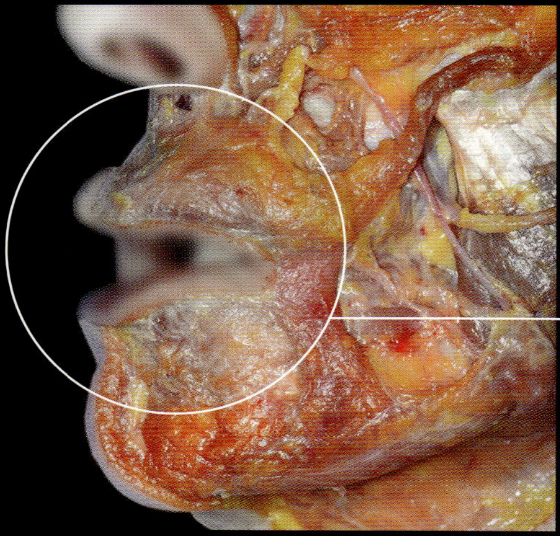

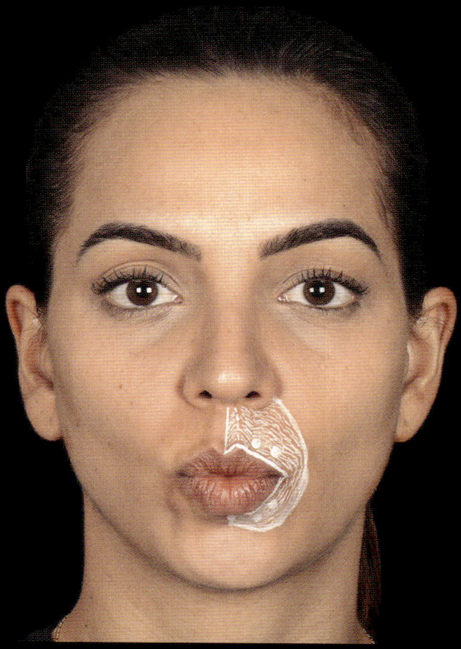

Locating and marking the muscle

1. Ask the patient to squeeze the upper lip against the lower lip but not narrow the distance between the commissures. Mark the first curved wrinkle that shows in the lateral side of the commissures; this will be its lateral limit.
2. Continue this line to the superior aspect of the muscle, following the nasolabial sulcus. The nasolabial angle will be its upper limit.
3. Mark the mentolabial sulcus, which divides the chin and lower lip. This will be its lower limit.
4. The internal limit is the vermilion of the lips. That is, inside the vermilion of the lips there are no muscle fibers.

Marking injection points: Ask the patient to make a "throwing a kiss" facial expression and to keep it. Mark the highest points.

At first, a loss of sphincter power might occur for up to 2 weeks. The function will then return to normal and be stable for months. This effect should be discussed with the patient. The use of high doses might damage the function.

BTX injection protocol

ORBICULARIS ORIS MUSCLE

Indications	• To smooth vertical wrinkles around the mouth. • Patients with a habit of frowning the lips due to tension. • Smokers with the habit of grabbing the cigarette with their lips tend to show premature wrinkles in the skin of the lips. • Patients without a passive lip seal as in cases of vertical maxillary excess or Class II malocclusions who activate this muscle to seal the lips. This generates a muscle hypertrophy noticeable under the skin, which decreases the perception of the vermilion of the lips.		
Contraindications	• Patients who are not emotionally stable enough to withstand a temporary decrease of the sphincter competence at this muscle. • Contraindications listed by the manufacturer on the packaging.		
Attention	Do not inject the toxin near the philtrum to avoid its flattening. Maintain a distance of 5 mm. Do not inject near the commissure because it causes saliva to accumulate there. Maintain a distance of 5 mm. Do not inject near the eversion line of the lips to avoid the flattening of this line. Maintain a distance of 5 mm.		
Recommended doses (per point)	**Botox** 1U	**Dysport** 3U	**Xeomin** 1U
Injection site	One point in each high part of the skin that is produced during the "kiss" facial expression.		
Needle	**Size** 8 mm	**Position** *(in relation to the skin)* Almost parallel to the skin	**Insertion** Only the bevel

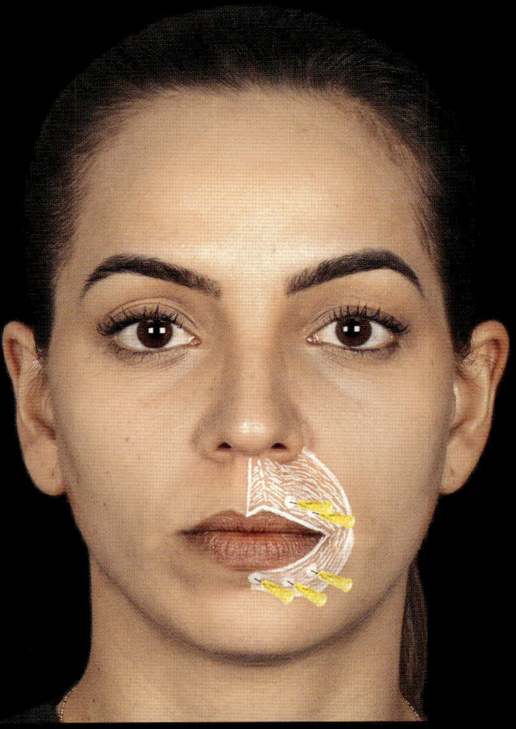

Injection: Frontal view

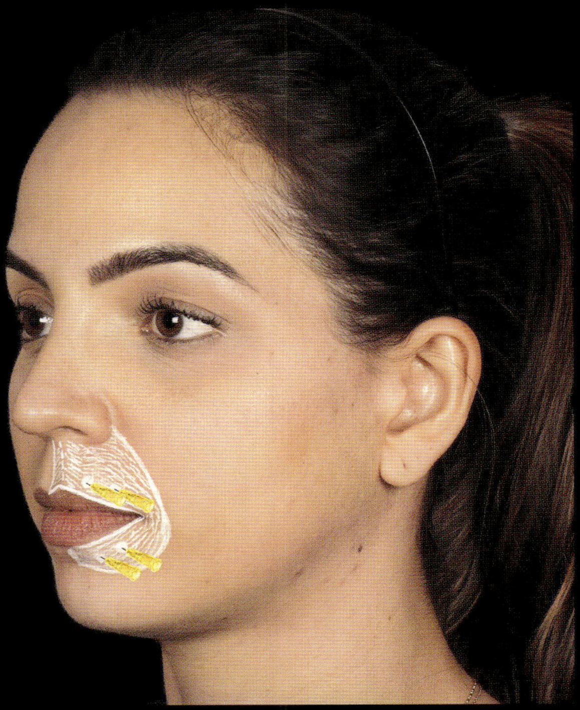

Injection: Oblique view

Depressor Anguli Oris Muscle

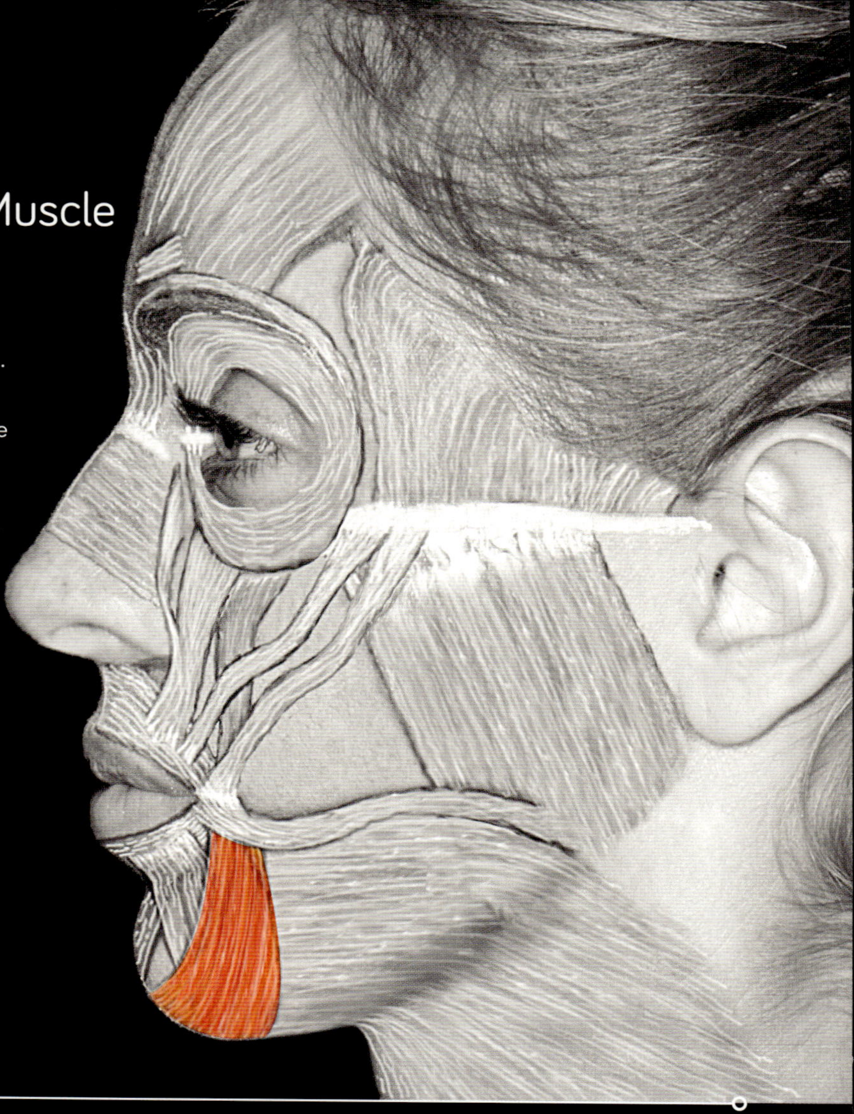

Anatomy and location

Function: It depresses the angle of the mouth.

Location: Lateral part of the chin. From the oral commissure, it goes downward and to the medial. It is superficial to the depressor labii inferioris muscle.

Origin: Oblique line in the base of the mandible at the inferior limit of the mandible.

Insertion: Angle of the mouth (modiolus) and fibers blending with the platysma muscle.

Fibers: Opened in a fan shape toward the maxillary ridge in a medial direction.

Wrinkles: Helps form the sulcus in the chin or "marionette" lines.

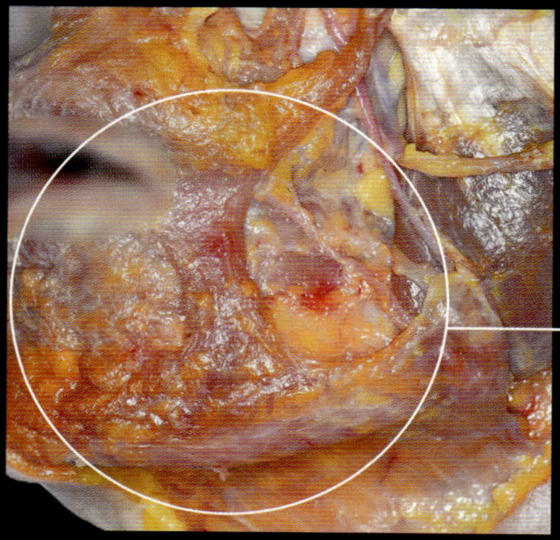

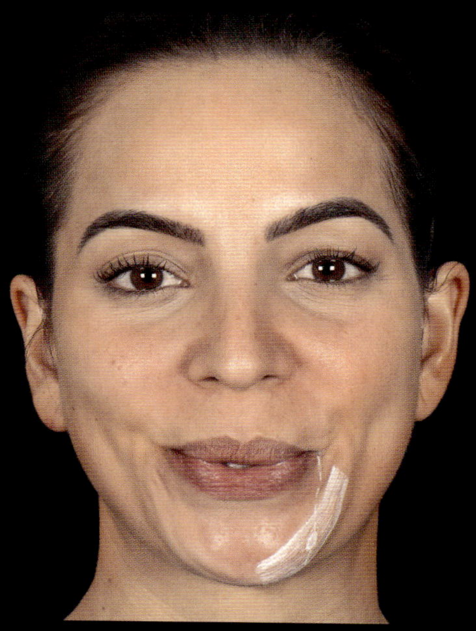

Locating and marking the muscle

This muscle may be found through facial expression and palpation:

1. Ask the patient to squeeze the upper lip against the lower lip without shortening the distance between the commissures. This will emphasize the skin over the muscle.
2. Palpate the volume created by the facial expression, outlining the anterior and posterior limit of this muscle. The final drawing has the shape of a comma.

Marking injection points: Find the most voluminous and most equidistant point between the anterior and posterior border of the muscle. This will decrease the chance of error. Keep distance from the modiolus so that it will not affect other muscles.

In case the muscle is not found by palpation and/or during facial expression, ask the patient to keep a resting posture and then draw a line descending from the oral commissure; mark a point 10 mm from the inferior limit of the mandible.

Among all BTX injection sites in the face, this is the site with the highest risk for asymmetries. Asymmetries will occur when the clinician injects the toxin in one side of the target muscle but makes a mistake concerning the position and/or depth of the muscle on the other side. Patients should be warned that in case of asymmetries, the muscle that was not injected will be highlighted during facial expression. This can be corrected with a new injection containing the same units as in the initial treatment.

BTX injection protocol

DEPRESSOR ANGULI ORIS MUSCLE			
Indications	• Patients with low commissures at rest, giving the patient a sad or bored appearance. • When during the smile the oral commissure is low, preventing the complete visualization of the maxillary premolar crown. • In case of smile asymmetries where one of the oral commissures is elevated more than the other and when the clinical crowns of the premolars are not visualized at the lowest oral commissure. In such cases, inject the toxin on this side to elevate the commissure, leveling it with the other and at the same time enabling the visualization of the maxillary premolar crowns.		
Contraindications	• Patients with posterior gummy smile. Injections of BTX in this muscle of such patients will make the problem worse because the commissures will be more elevated, increasing the gingival exposure at the maxillary premolars. • Contraindications listed by the manufacturer on the packaging.		
Attention	Older patients with ptosis at the superficial muscular aponeurotic system who want to improve marionette lines should also be treated with fillers and/or rhytidoplasties.		
Recommended doses	**Botox** 2U, 3U, or 4U	**Dysport** 6U, 9U, or 12U	**Xeomin** 2U, 3U, or 4U
Injection site	Lateral side of the chin in the thickest part of the muscle shown during contraction.		
Needle	**Size** 8 mm	**Position** *(in relation to the skin)* 90 degrees	**Insertion** 1/3 of the needle

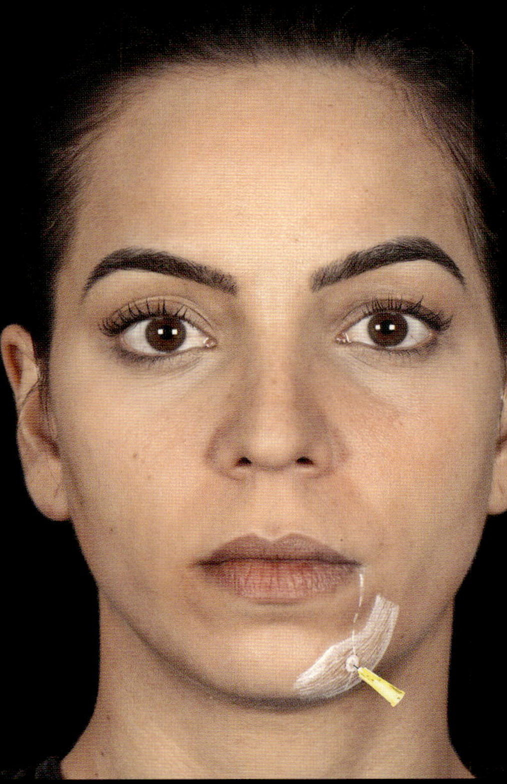

Injection: Frontal view

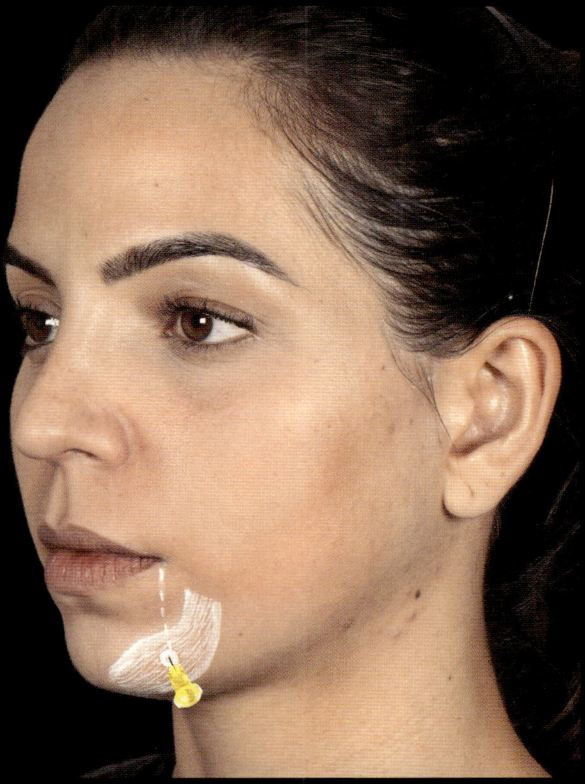

Injection: Oblique view

Depressor Labii nferioris Muscle

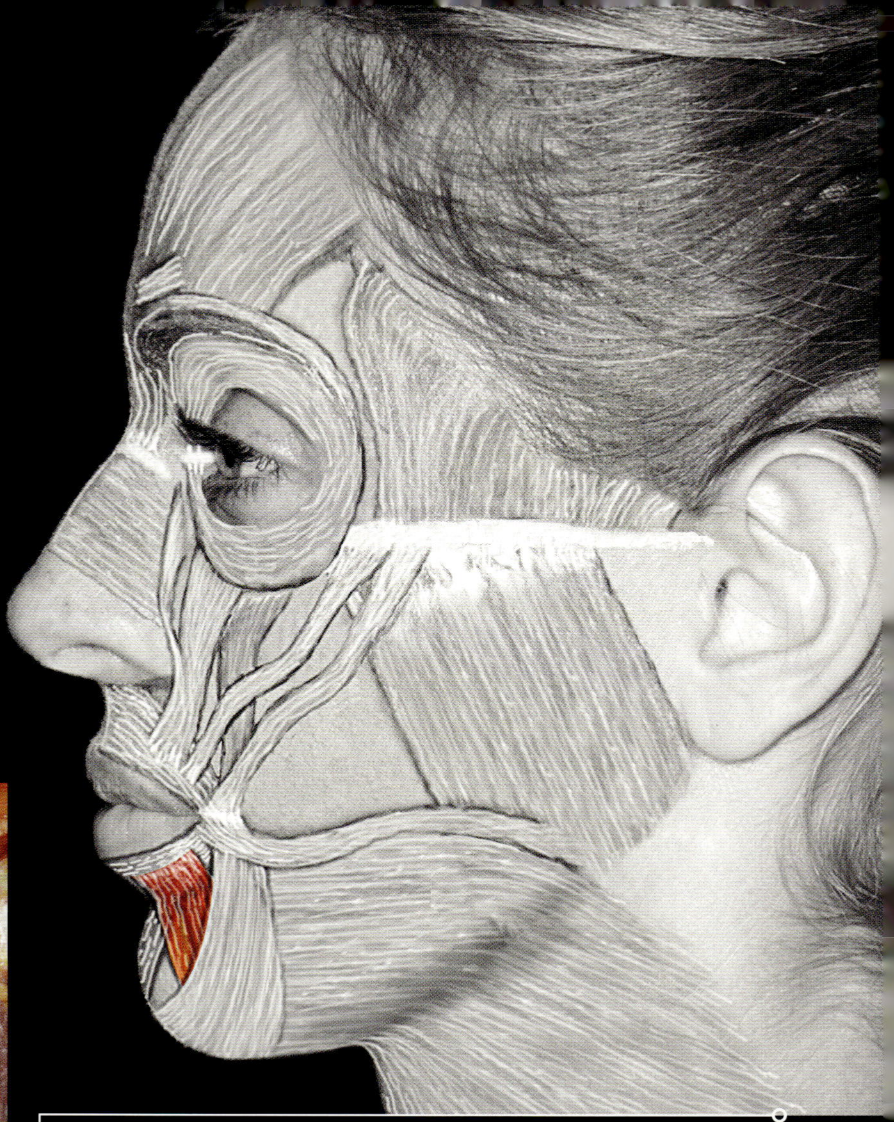

Anatomy and location

Function: It lowers the lower lip, helping ts eversion.

Location: Chin.

Origin: Anterior portion of the mandible following the oblique line.

nsertion: Skin of the lower lip.

Fibers: Descending from the midline and aterally inclined.

Wrinkles: It does not produce wrinkles.

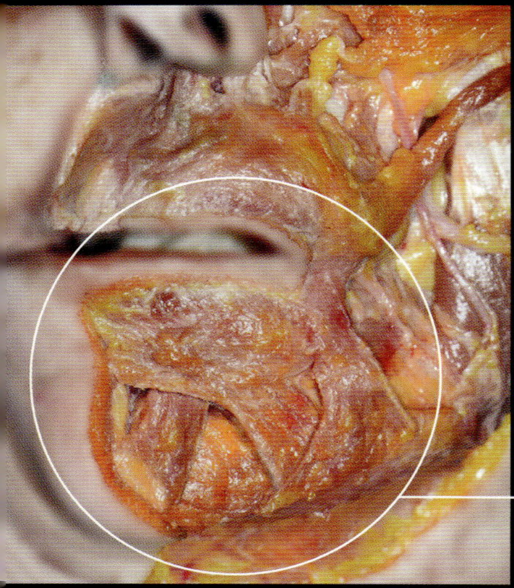

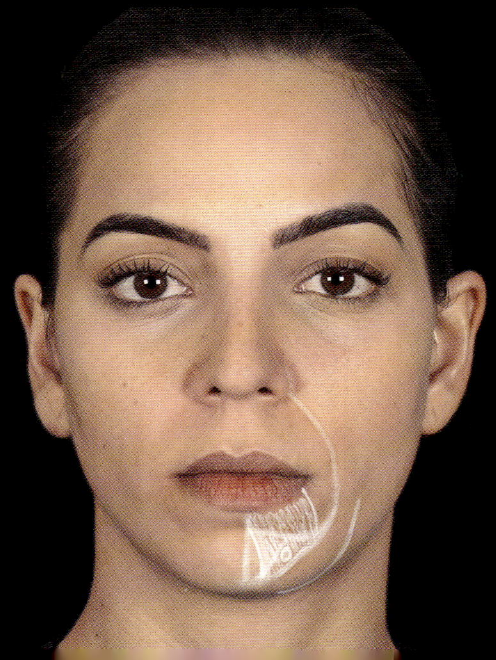

Locating and marking the muscle

This muscle does not cause wrinkles, nor does it become palpable during facial expressions. Therefore, it should be located using facial esthetic references.

Draw the muscles that will not be injected to help locate the other targeted muscles:

- Orbicularis oris
- Depressor anguli oris
- Mentalis

There will only be a small triangular area left between the drawings of these three muscles. The marking should be made in the center of the triangle to prevent the diffusion to other muscles.

Use small doses because BTX injections in this muscle will cause an excessive elevation of the lower lip.

BTX injection protocol

DEPRESSOR LABII INFERIORIS MUSCLE

Indications	• Patients with lower gummy smile, that is, gingival exposure in the mandible during spontaneous smile. This is considered unesthetic because it decreases the dominance of the maxillary teeth during the smile. • Asymmetric smiles where one side of the lower lip is more depressed than the other side. The injection should be on the side that is lower. If the injection is unilateral for asymmetry, use only 1U. • To help promote the passive seal of lips in patients with vertically maxillary excess. The ideal treatment in these cases is orthognathic surgery. However, the toxin might be used when surgery is not possible.
Contraindications	• Patients who do not display the mandibular gingiva when smiling. • Contraindications listed by the manufacturer on the packaging.
Attention	When the toxin is injected in patients without gingival exposure when smiling, an excessive elevation of the lower lip will occur, pressing it to the incisal of the maxillary teeth during the smile and also interposing it between the anterior teeth during mastication. This might be very uncomfortable for the patient.
Recommended doses	**Botox** 1U–2U; **Dysport** 3U–6U; **Xeomin** 1U–2U
Injection site	Chin, below the inferior limit of the orbicularis oris, lateral to the mentalis muscle, and medial to the depressor anguli oris muscle.
Needle	**Size** 8 mm; **Position** *(in relation to the skin)* 90 degrees; **Insertion** 1/2 of the needle

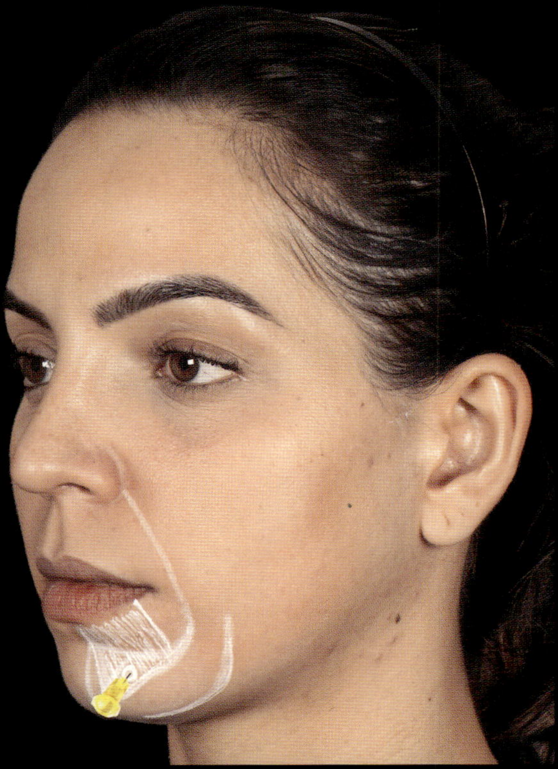

Injection: Frontal view

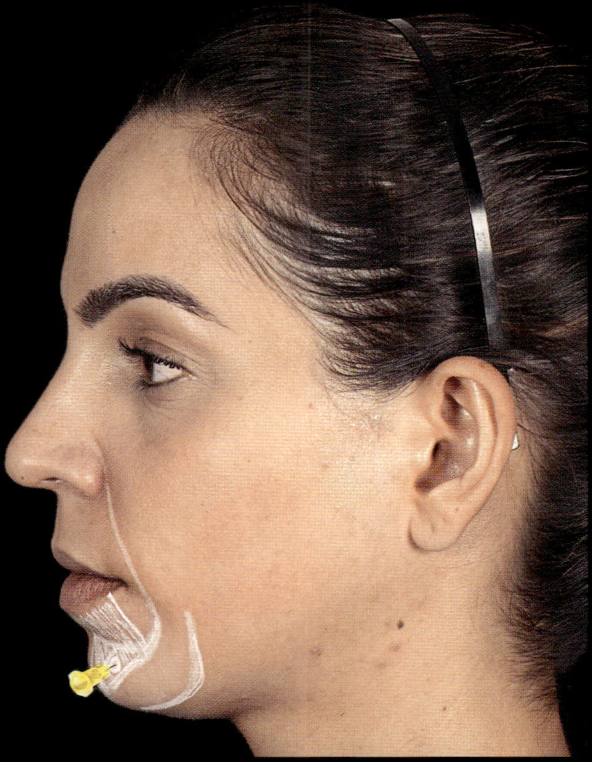

Injection: Oblique view

Mentalis Muscle

Anatomy and location

Function: To elevate the medial part of the lower lip and skin of the chin. In its maximum action, it projects the lower lip forward.

Location: Chin.

Origin: Alveolar eminence of the mandibular lateral incisor.

Insertion: Skin of the chin.

Fibers: Oblique ascending fibers that open in a fan shape in the superior and lateral direction.

Wrinkles: Results in several wrinkles in the skin of the chin, leading to a "golf ball" appearance.

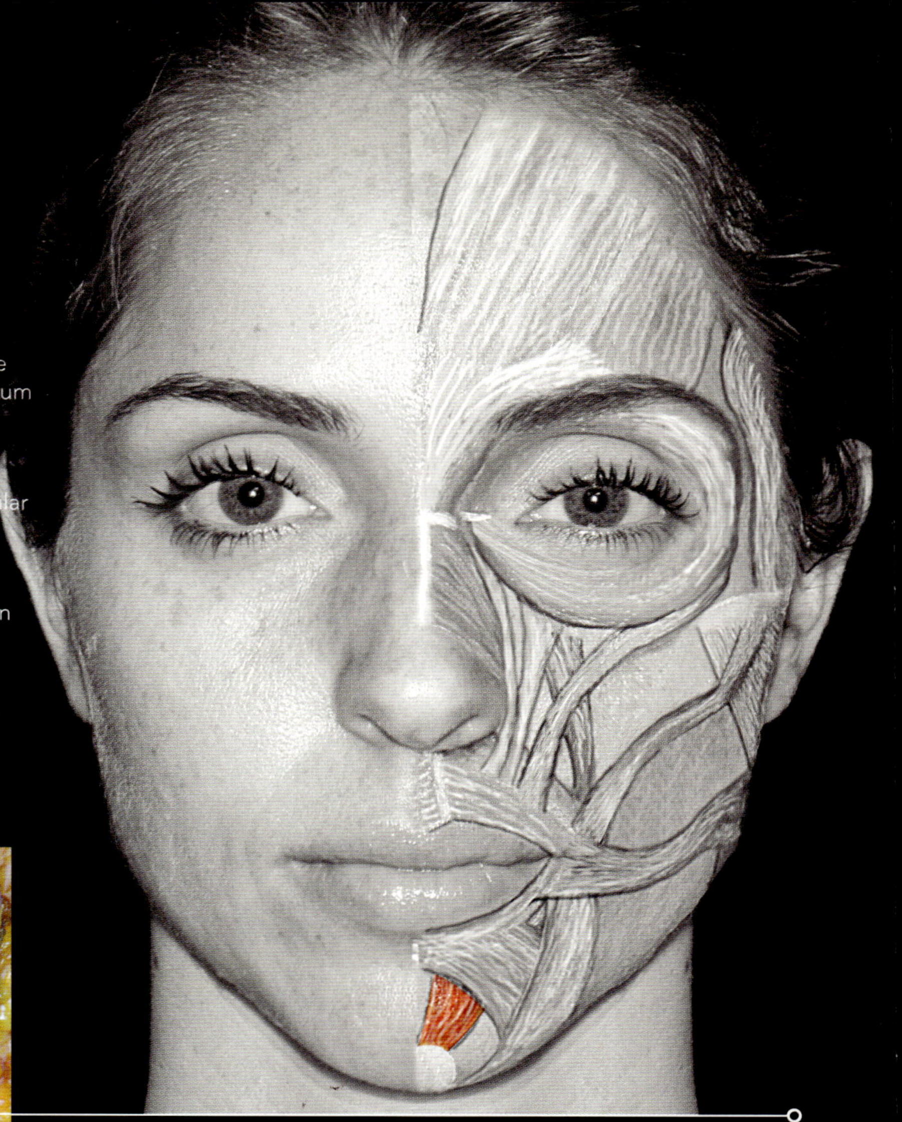

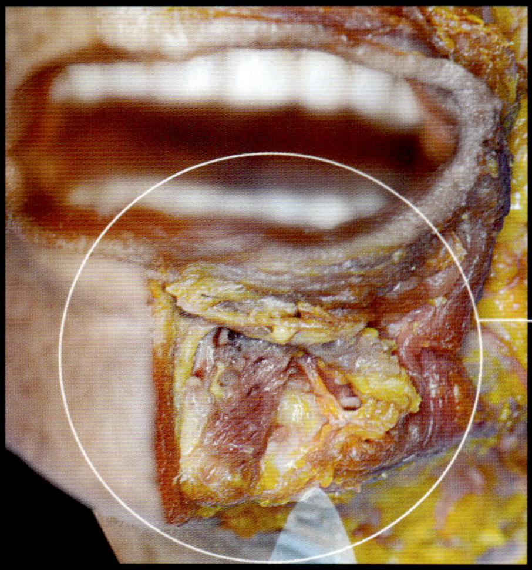

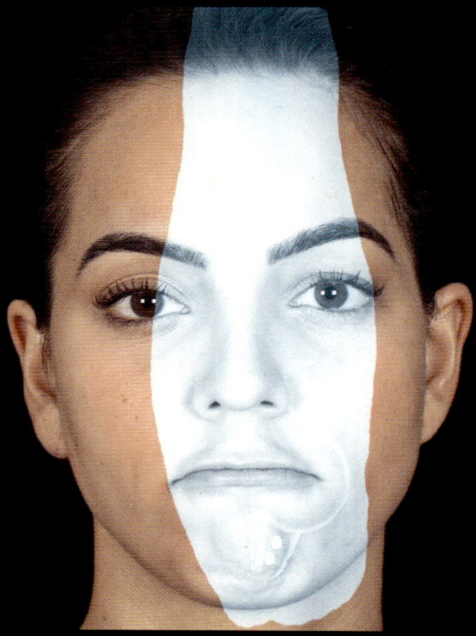

Locating and marking the muscle

Although it is a muscle with a deep origin, its insertion is in the skin of the chin. Therefore, facial expressions might help to outline its lateral limit.

1. Draw the midline.
2. Draw the orbicularis oris muscle to exclude it from the application.
3. Ask the patient to elevate the medial portion of the lower lip, making an "upset" facial expression, and hold it.
4. First draw the medial limit along with the midline; as it approaches the orbicularis oris, it will be distant from the midline, which will result in a line inclined to the lateral.
5. Draw its lateral limit inside the depression lateral to the volume of wrinkles created by the facial expression. The distance between the two lines ranges from 10 to 16 mm, corresponding to the muscle width.

Marking injection points: Two vertical points should be marked.

In case the toxin is injected in only one point, the fibers that did not receive the injection might be highlighted. To prevent this, inject two points in each side of the muscle. To correct highlighted fibers, reinject the same dosage in the highlighted points.

BTX injection protocol

MENTALIS MUSCLE

Indications	• Patients with no passive seal of the lips might use the mentalis muscle to elevate the medial portion of the lower lip to obtain labial seal. In these cases, the mentalis muscle might become hyperkinetic, turning the skin of the chin constantly wrinkled, with the dimpled appearance of a golf ball. BTX-A can soften this aspect. • Patients with paralysis or hemifacial spasms, where this muscle is contributing to the asymmetries.		
Contraindications	Contraindications listed by the manufacturer on the packaging.		
Attention	Toxin should not be injected in the mentalis and levator labii inferioris muscles at the same treatment, because it would highly decrease the patient's lip seal. If necessary, these muscles can be treated at different periods of time.		
Recommended doses (per point)	**Botox** 2U, 3U, or 4U	**Dysport** 6U, 9U, or 12U	**Xeomin** 2U, 3U, or 4U
Injection site	Two points in the belly of the muscle (highest part during facial expression).		
Needle	**Size** 8 mm	**Position** *(in relation to the skin)* 90 degrees	**Insertion** The whole needle

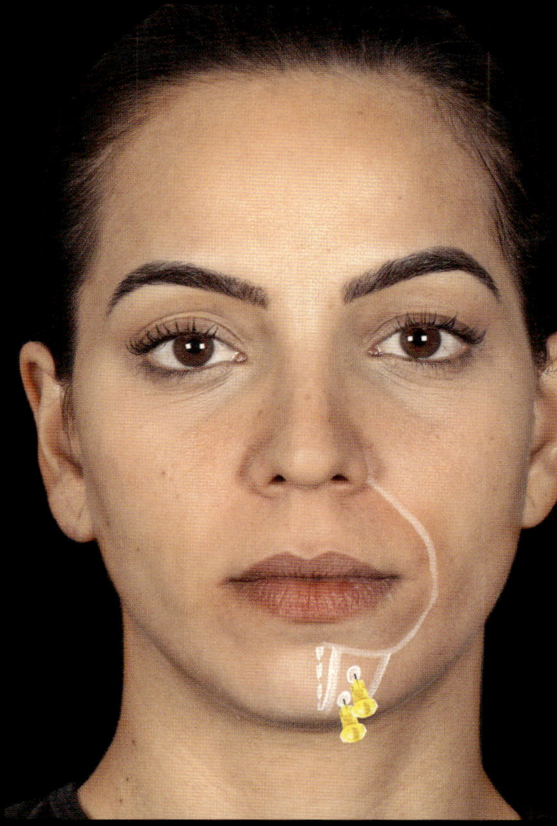

Injection: Frontal view

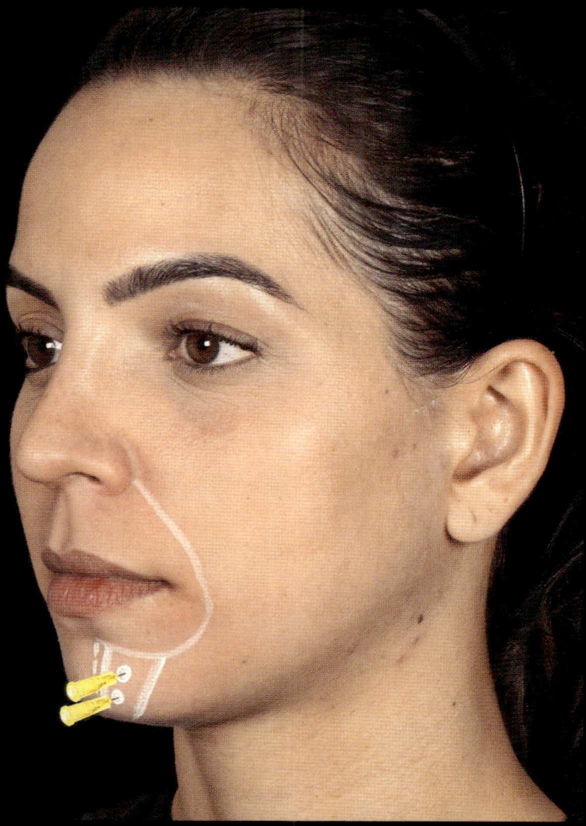

Injection: Oblique view

Platysma Muscle

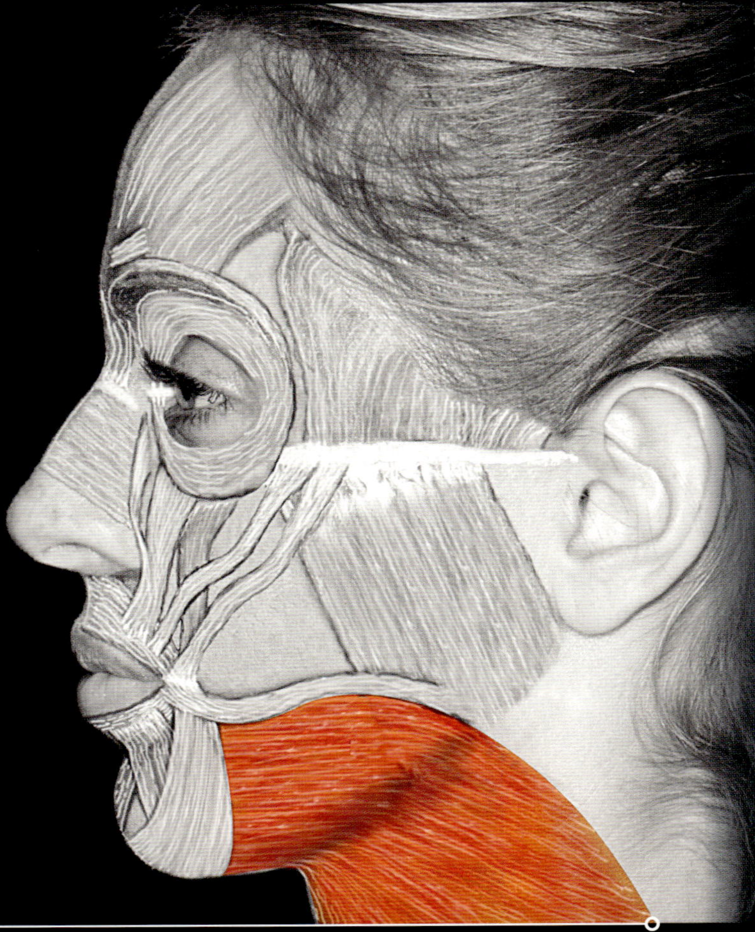

Anatomy and location

Function: It acts by tightening up the neck skin and helps to pull down the mandible, lower lip, and angle of the mouth.

Location: Neck.

Origin: Lower border of the clavicle (over the fascia of the pectoralis major and anterior and middle deltoid muscles).

Insertion: Upper border of the mandible body.

Fibers: Parallel, longitudinal, and inclined fibers along the mandibular border that proceed over the cervical fascia at the neck.

Wrinkles: No wrinkles. When small portions of this muscle are hyperkinetic, platysmal bands are formed in the neck. In this anterior region of the neck, these bands are popularly called "turkey neck." When the muscle is hyperkinetic in more extended areas, it reduces the definition of the jawline.

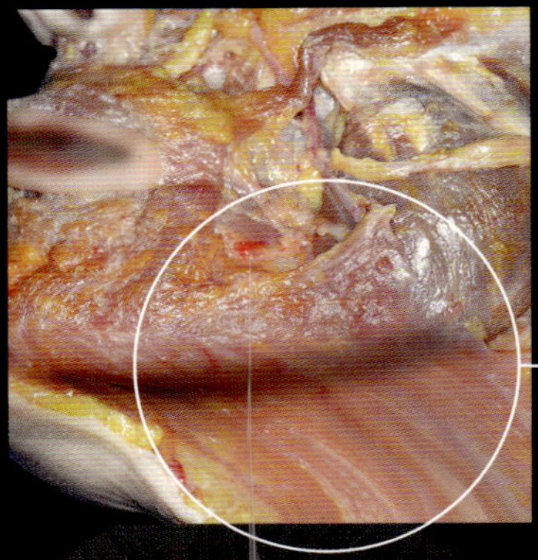

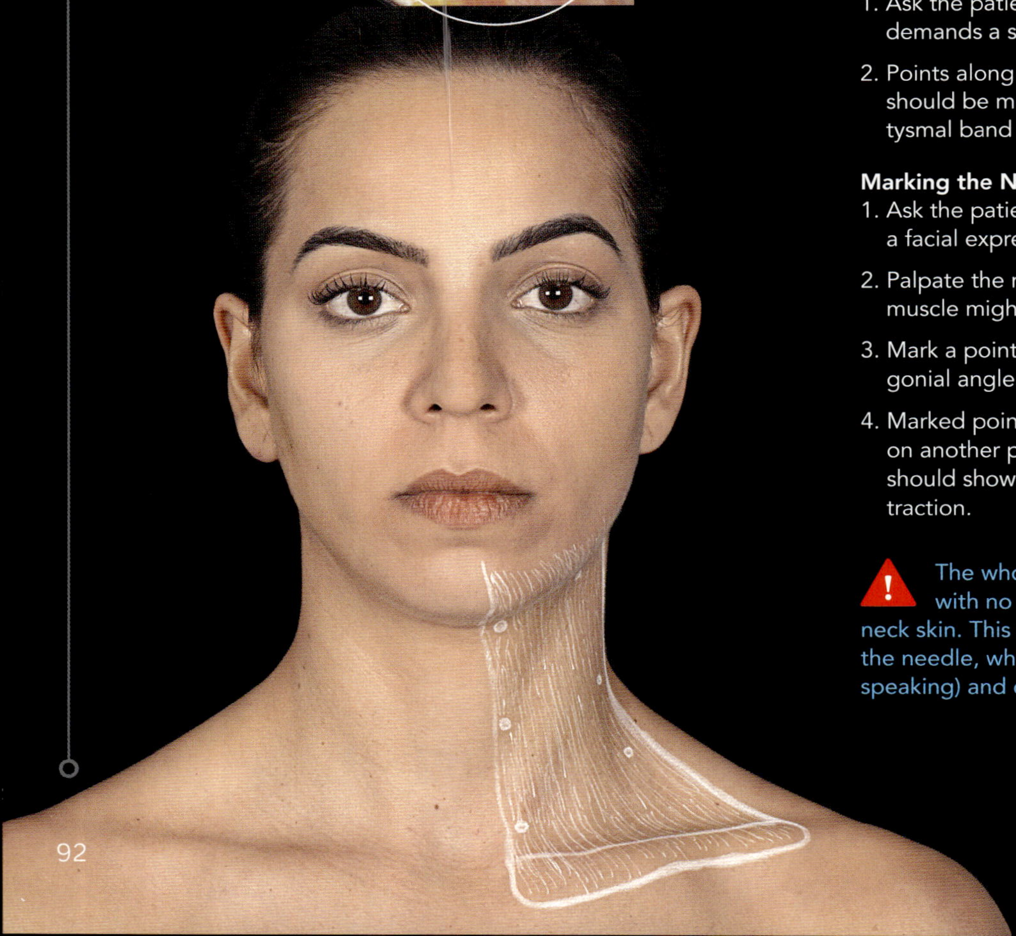

Locating and marking the muscle

Marking the platysmal bands:

1. Ask the patient to make a facial expression that demands a strong neck contraction.
2. Points along the extension of the platysmal bands should be marked. Two to three points in each platysmal band should be marked.

Marking the Nefertiti lift:

1. Ask the patient to strongly contract the neck through a facial expression.
2. Palpate the neck below the mandible to verify if the muscle might be felt.
3. Mark a point lateral to the midline, another at the gonial angle, and two others equidistant to those.
4. Marked points can be modified or deleted based on another palpation; the areas close to the marks should show a greater volume during muscle contraction.

⚠ The whole needle should penetrate the skin but with no pressure on the needle hub against the neck skin. This will avoid an excessive deepening of the needle, which would result in dysphonia (difficulty speaking) and dysphagia (difficulty swallowing).

BTX injection protocol

PLATYSMA MUSCLE

Indications	• In the presence of static or dynamic platysmal bands (observed when talking and/or smiling). • Coadjuvant in the elevation of the horizontal level of the oral commissures when they are low. • To slightly elevate the angles of the mouth when they are low, as the posterior fibers of the platysma muscle blend to the depressor anguli oris muscle. • For better definition of the jawline when it is not noticeable.		
Contraindications	• To smooth horizontal neck lines. Not even fillers are able to smooth these lines. • Contraindications listed by the manufacturer on the packaging.		
Attention	Facial expressions should not be used to verify the indication but only to locate the injection points. The professional should observe the two natural facial expressions—smile and speech—in order to diagnose.		
Recommended doses (per point)	**Botox** 2U, 3U, or 4U	**Dysport** 6U, 9U, or 12U	**Xeomin** 2U, 3U, or 4U
Injection site	Platysmal bands and/or right below the mandible.		
Needle	**Size** 8 mm	**Position** *(in relation to the skin)* Perpendicular to the skin	**Insertion** The whole needle, but avoid depressing deeply the skin of the neck

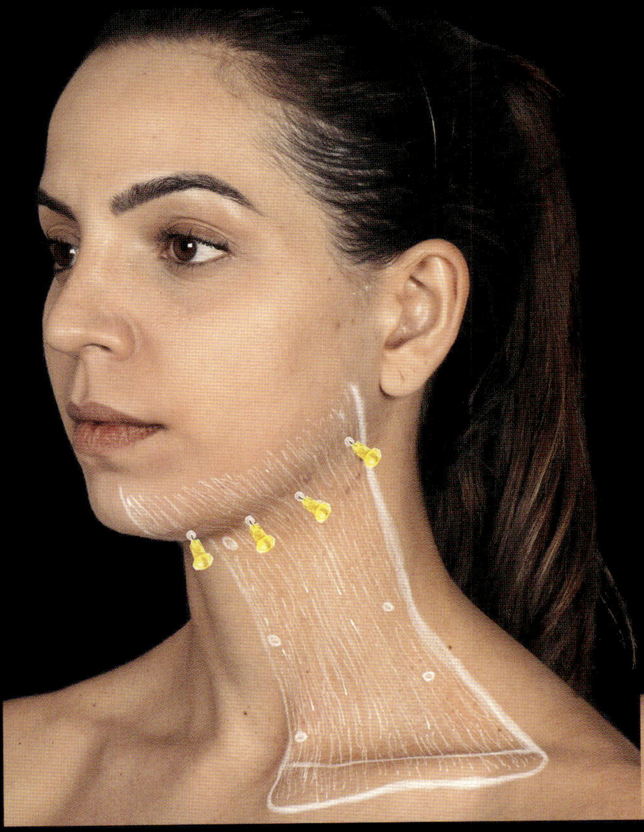

Marking the outline of the mandible

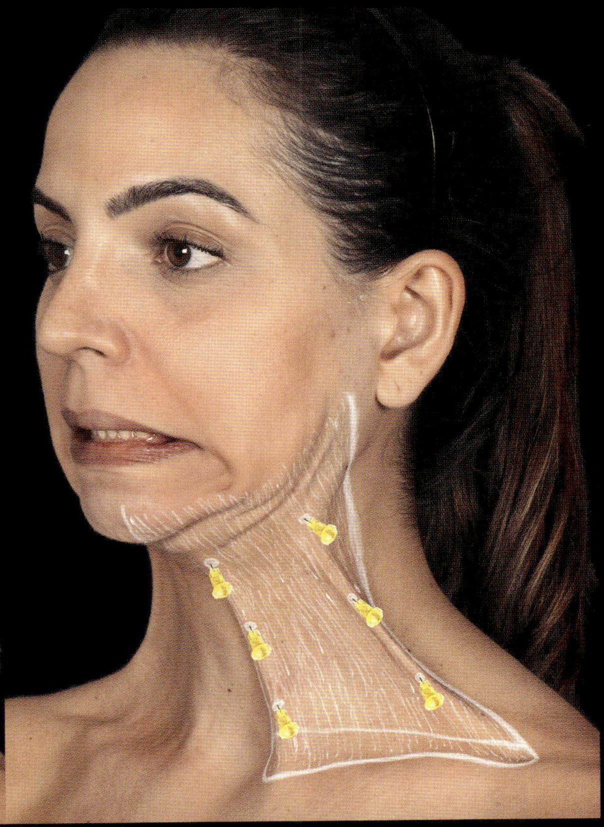

Marking the platysmal bands

Diagram of BTX Injection

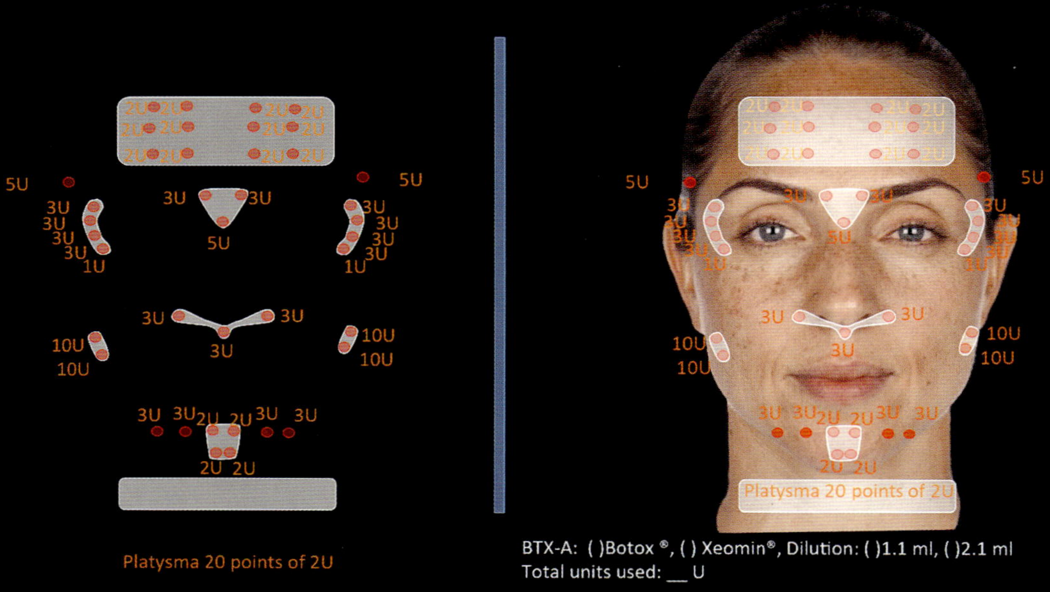

This diagram lists all of the injection points and doses for the various muscles previously described. Available via QR code, it can be used to present the treatment plan by placing the patient's photograph over it and then using the option "Send to back." Delete the points not involved in the treatment.

The Muscles in Fresh Frozen Cadavers

The following images show all of the previously described muscles in fresh frozen cadavers.

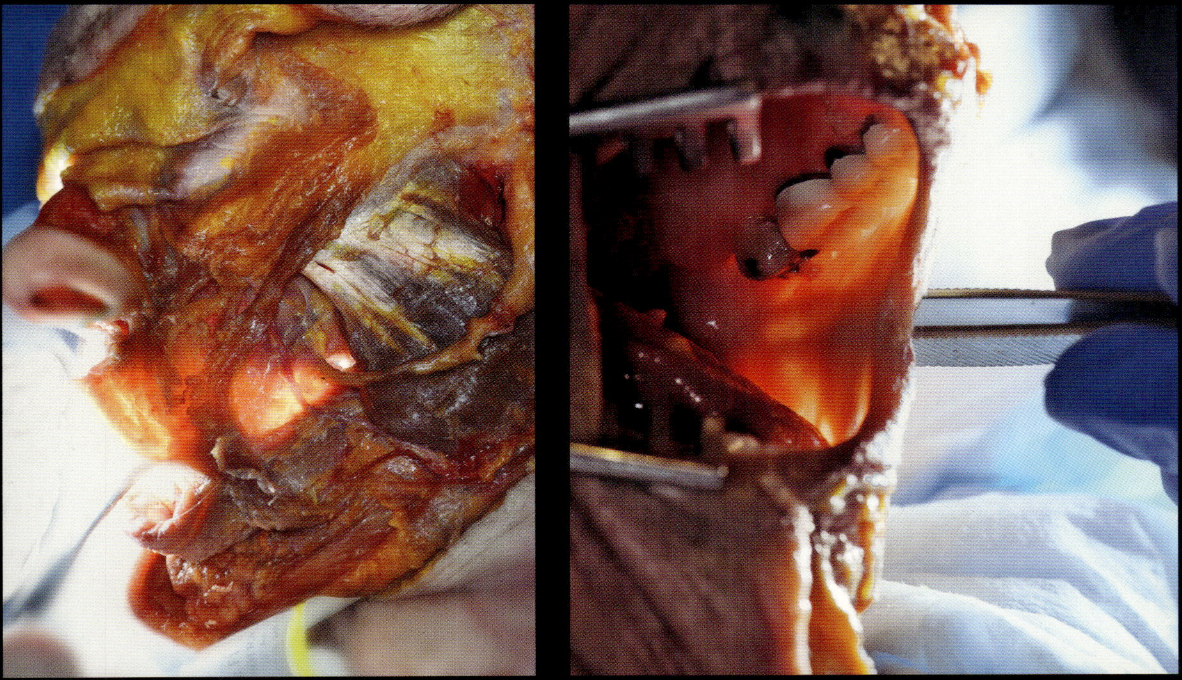

Buccinator transilluminated

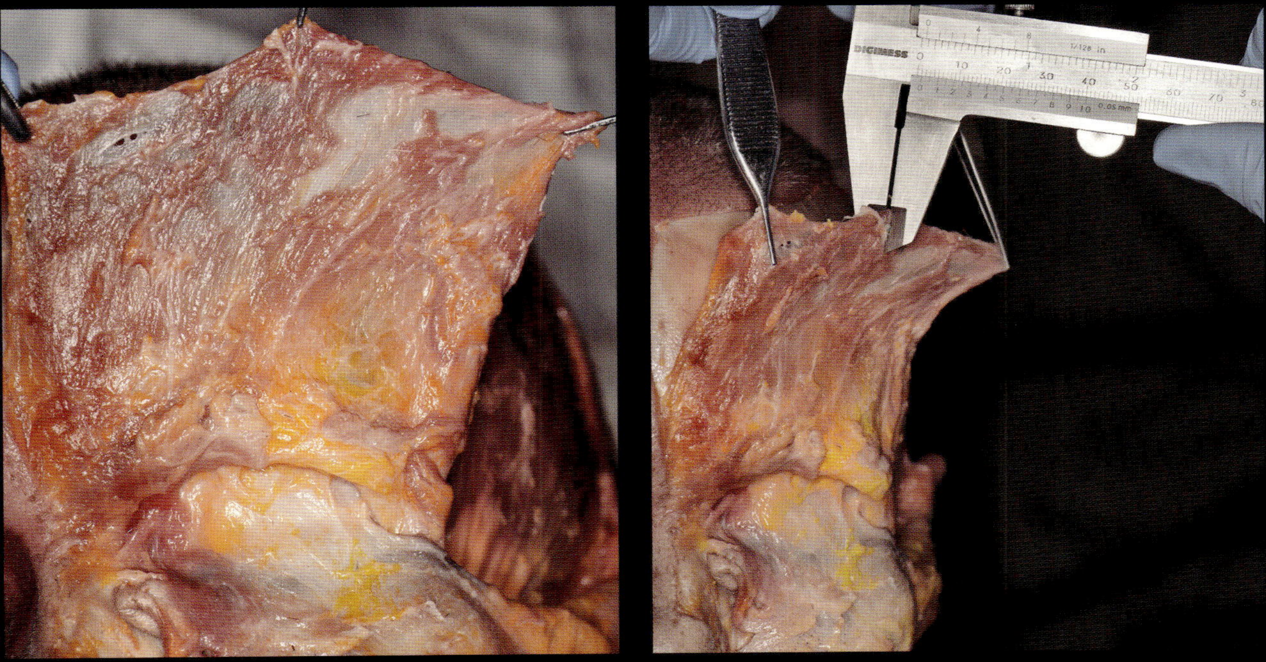

Occipitofrontalis thickness = 1 mm

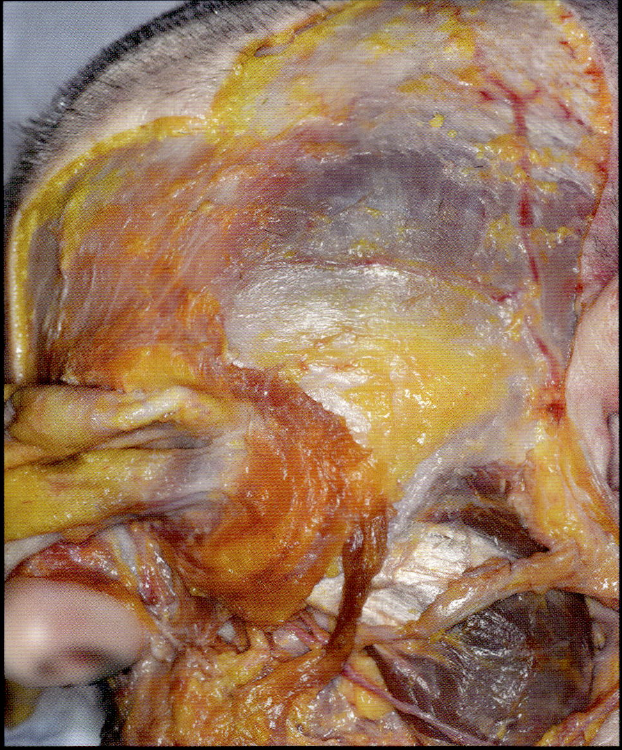

Temporalis covered by its fascia

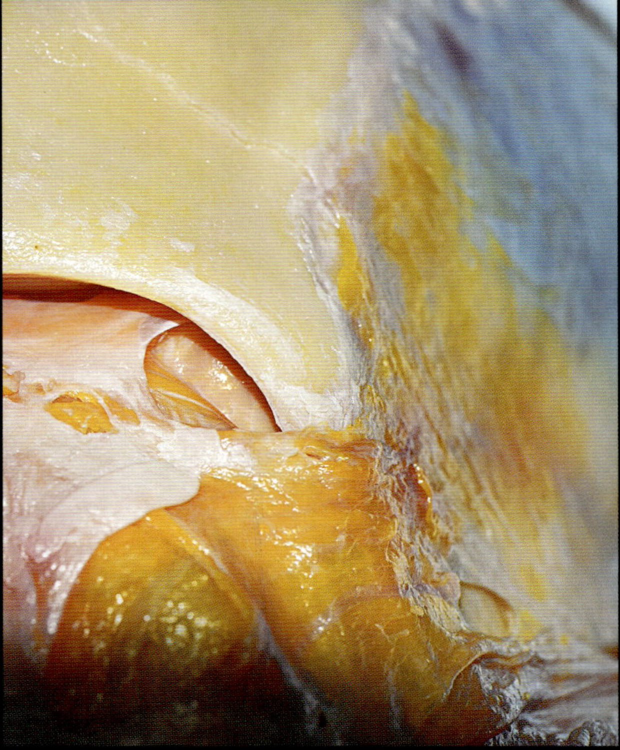

Temporalis inside its fossa

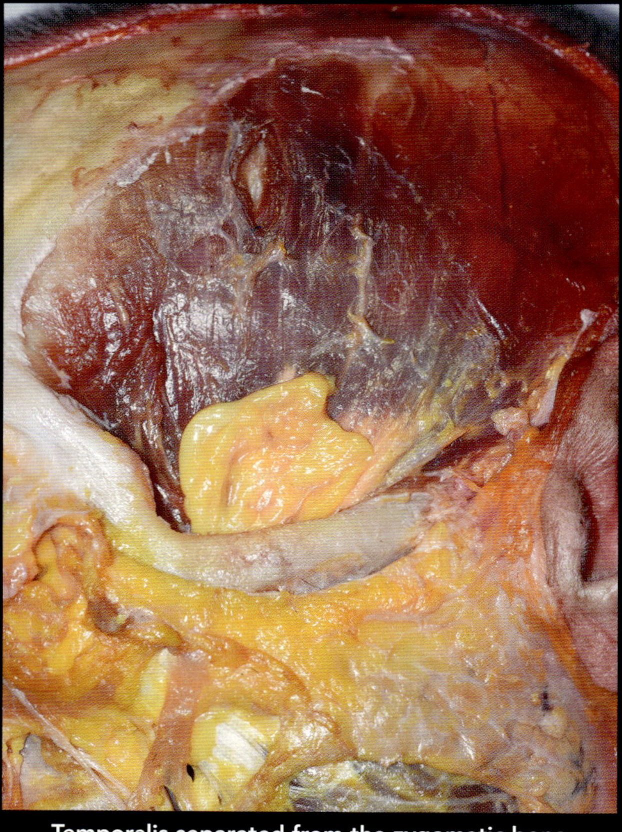

Temporalis separated from the zygomatic bone
by the buccal fat pad

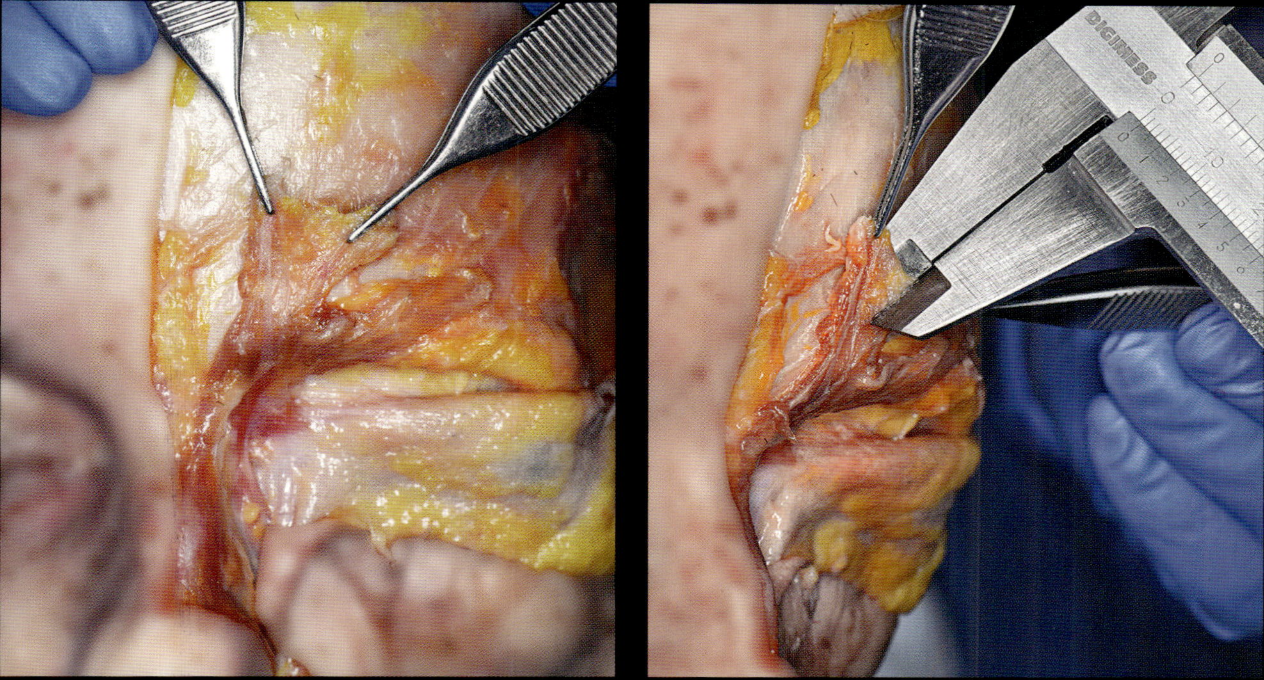

Procerus thickness = 0.4 mm

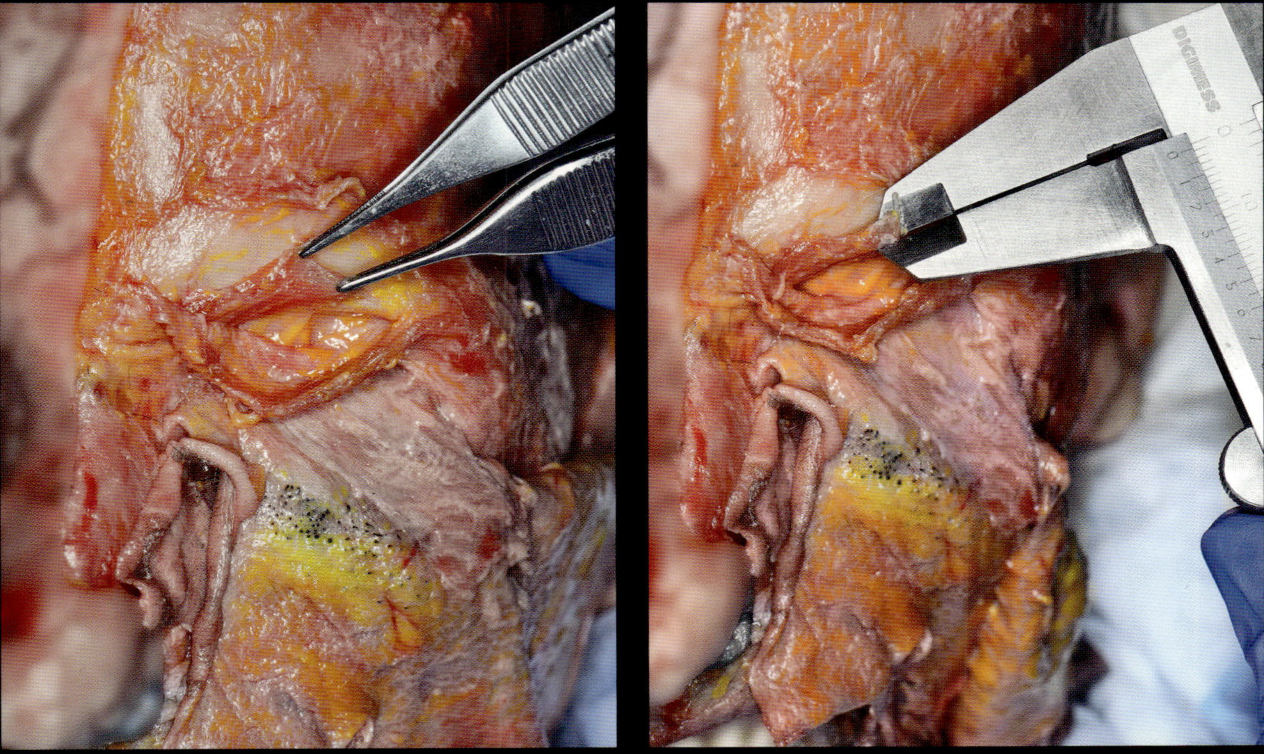

Corrugator supercilii thickness = 0.5 mm

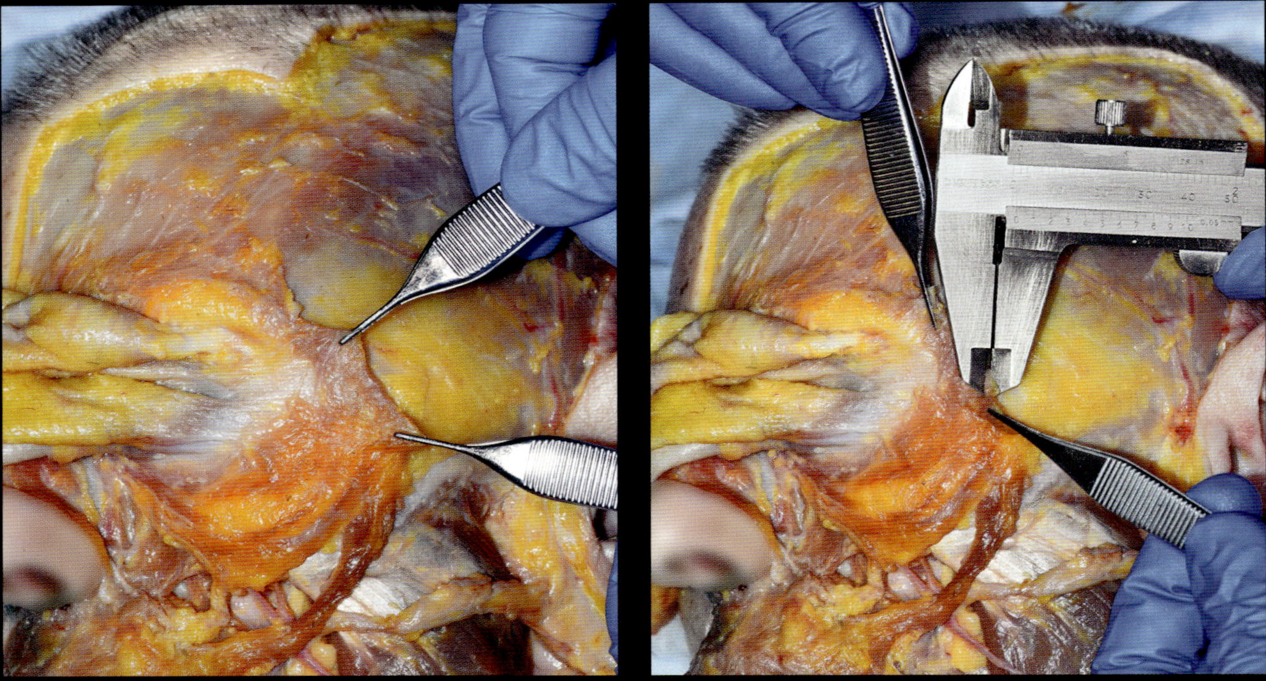

Orbicularis oculi thickness = 1 mm

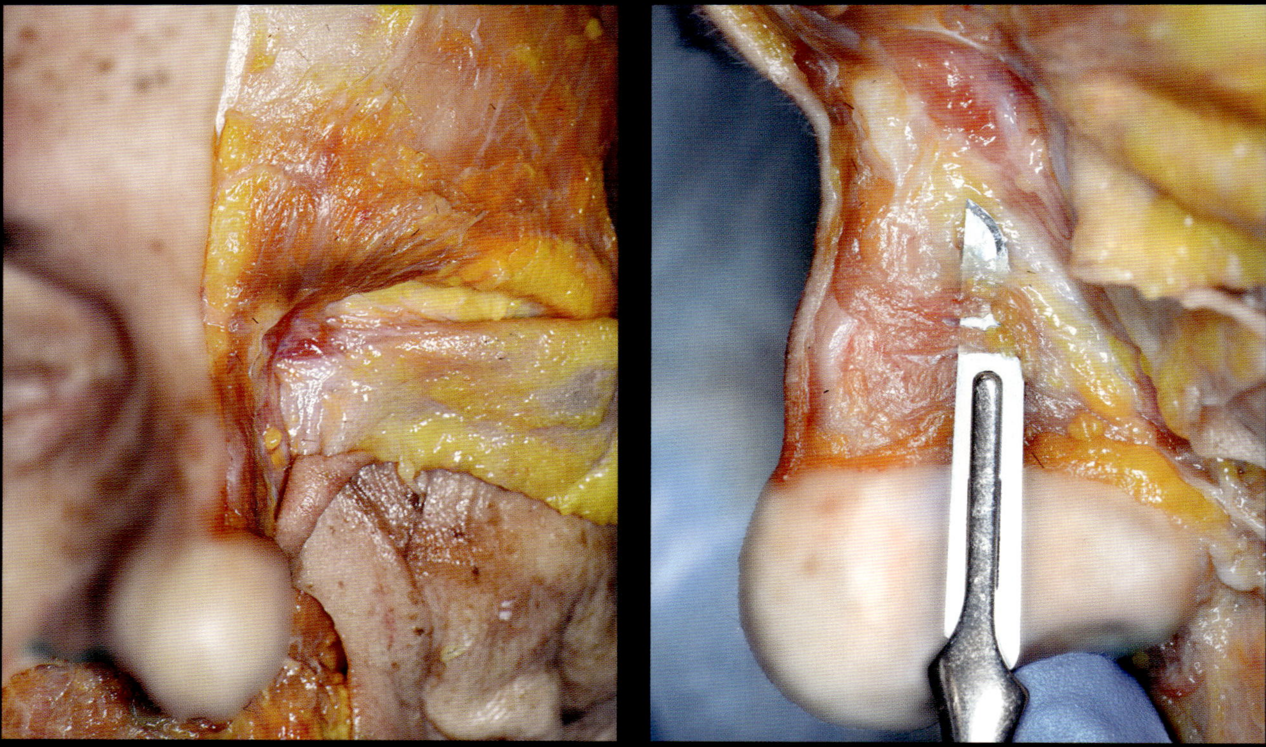

Nasalis thickness

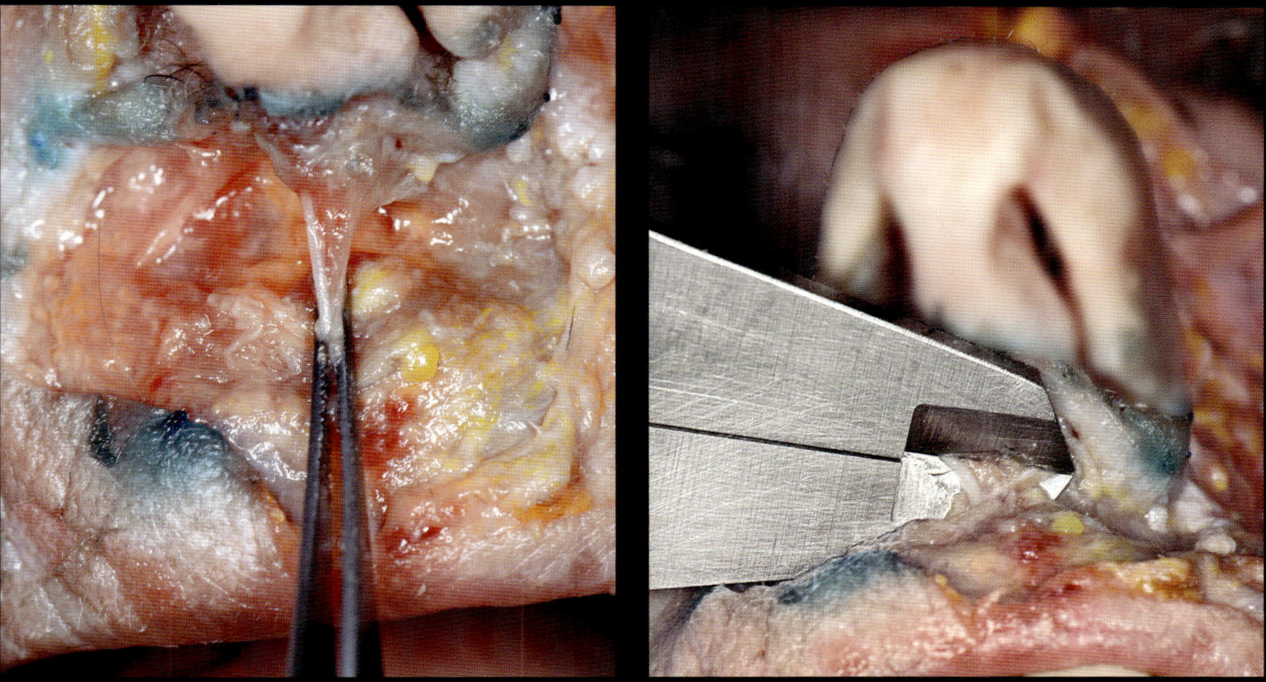

Depressor septi nasi thickness = 0.2 mm

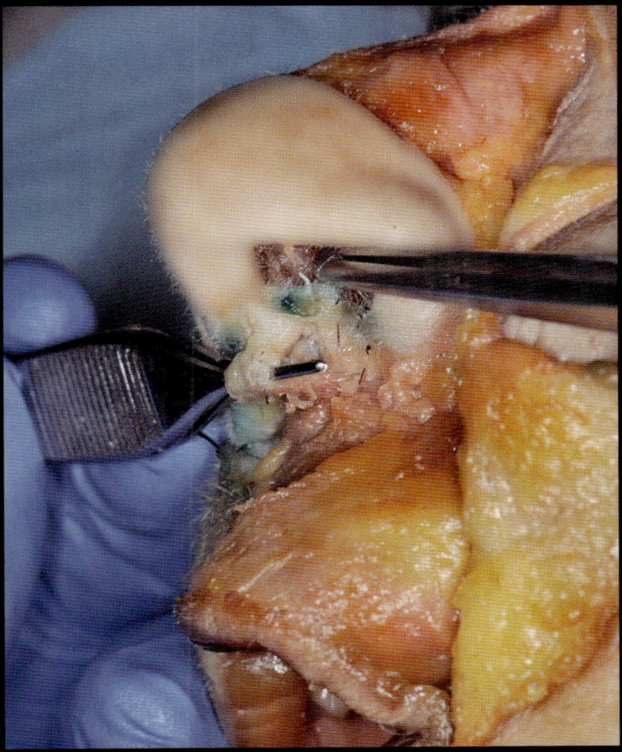

Depressor septi nasi detached from the columella

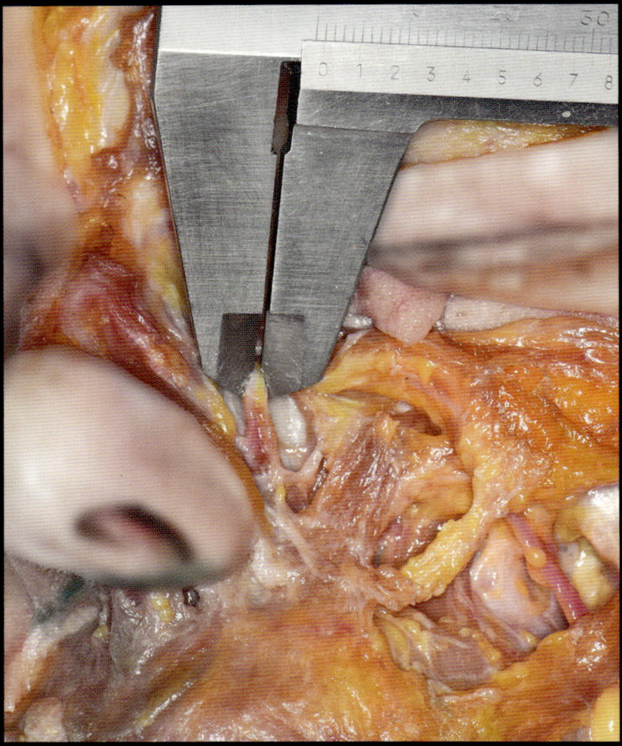

Levator labii superioris alaeque nasi thickness = 0.8 mm

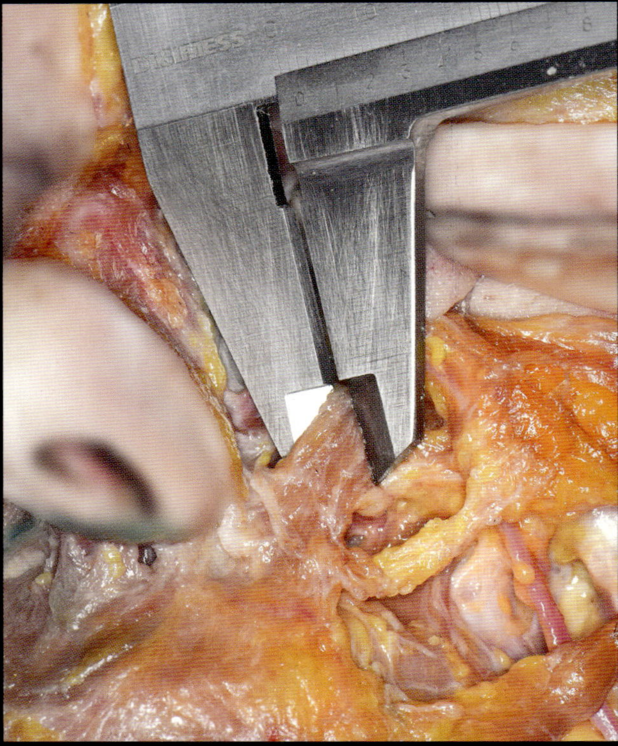

Levator labii superioris thickness = 1.6 mm

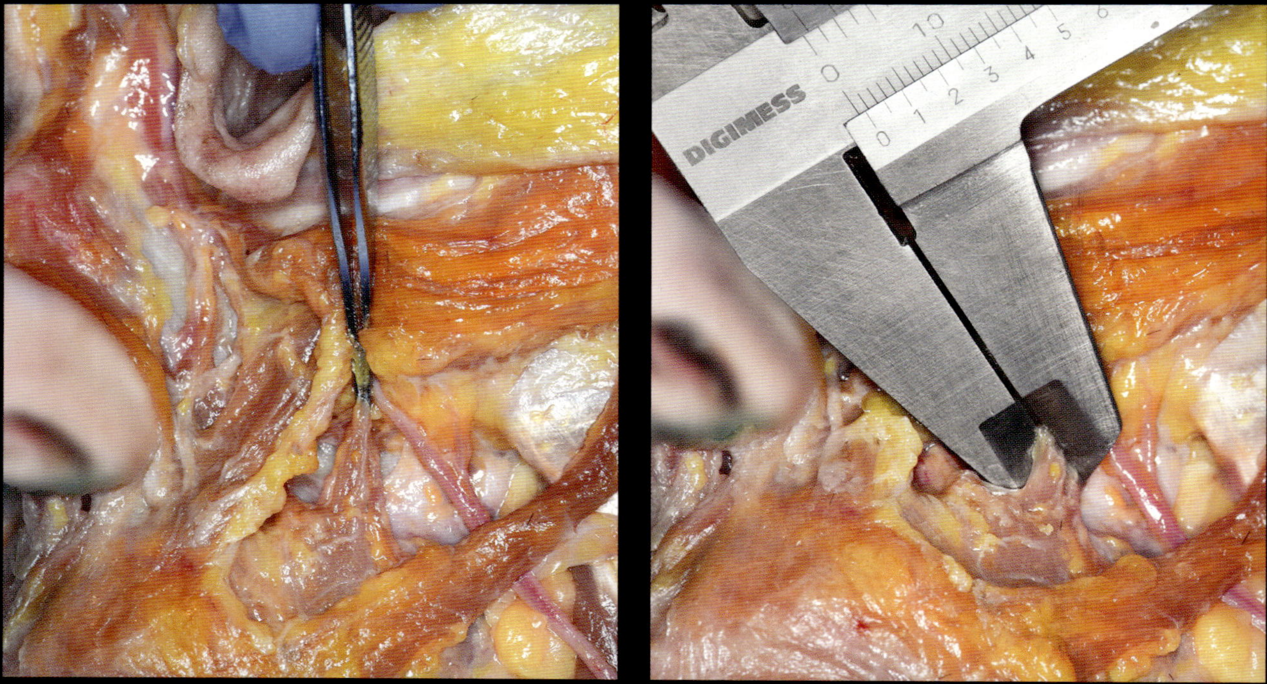

Levator anguli oris thickness = 0.8 mm

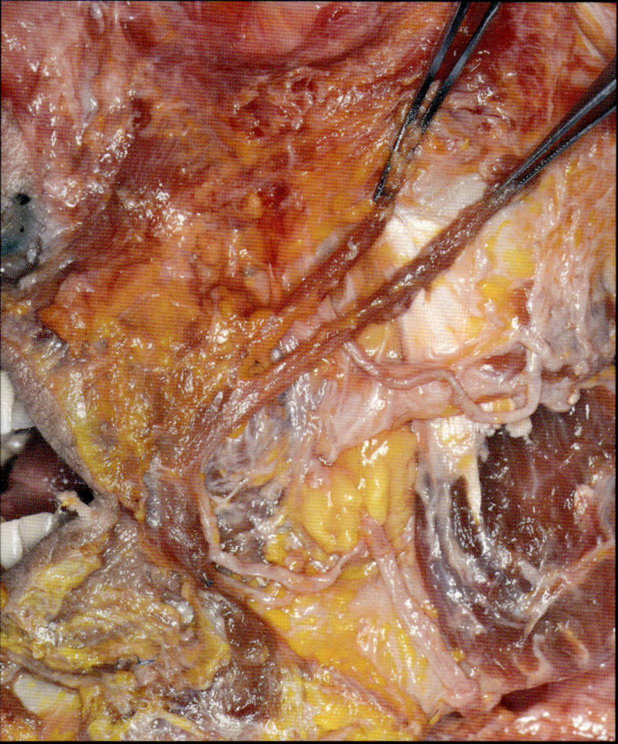

Zygomaticus major and minor

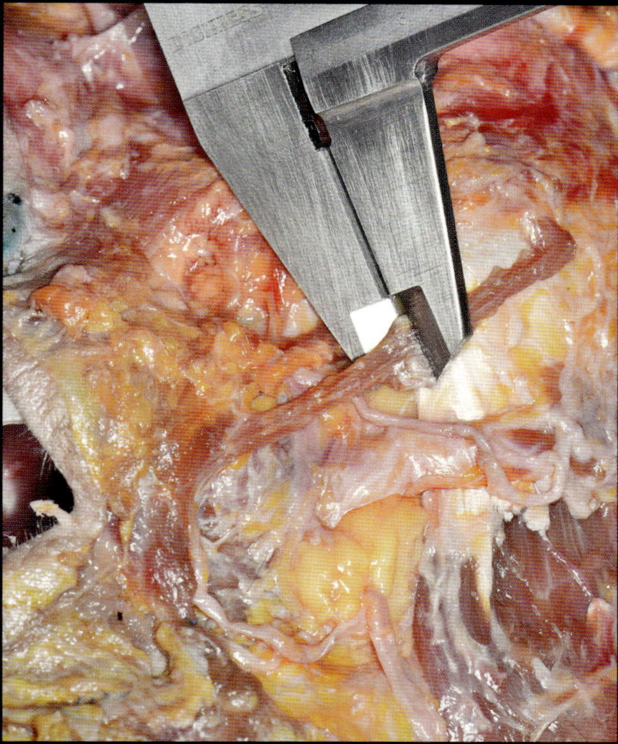

Zygomaticus major thickness = 1.1 mm

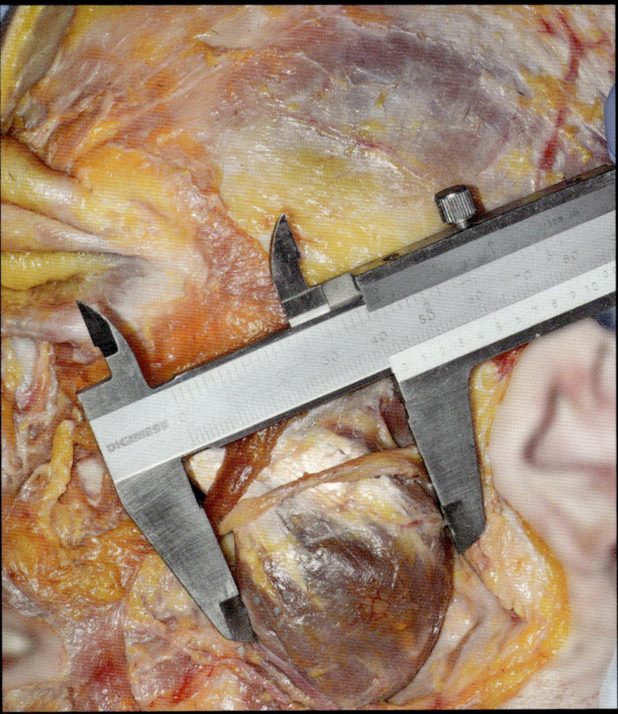

Masseter width = 42.4 mm

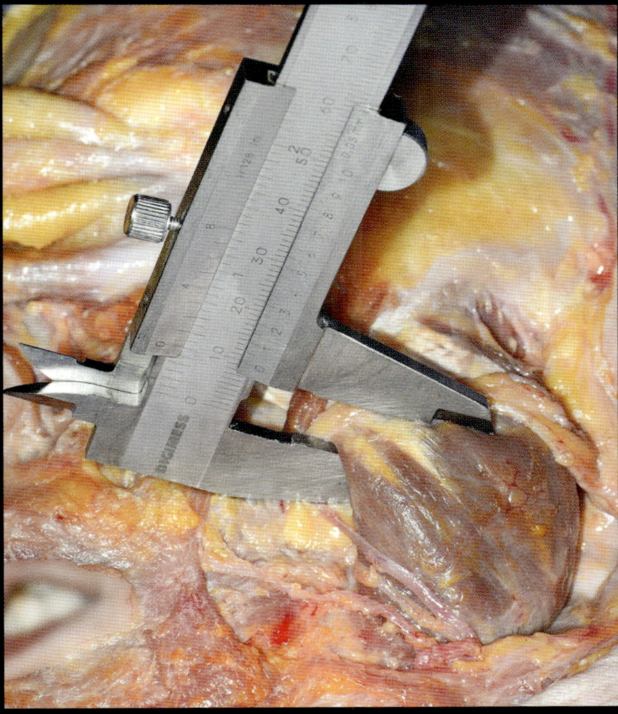

Masseter thickness = 10.0 mm

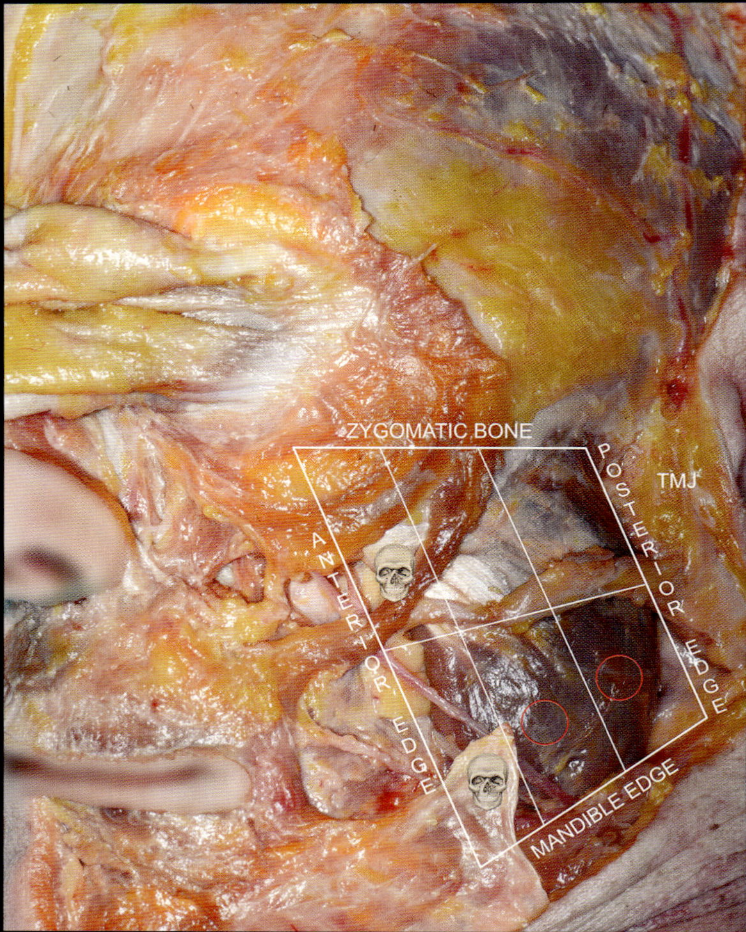

Points to avoid *(skulls)* and to target *(red circles)*

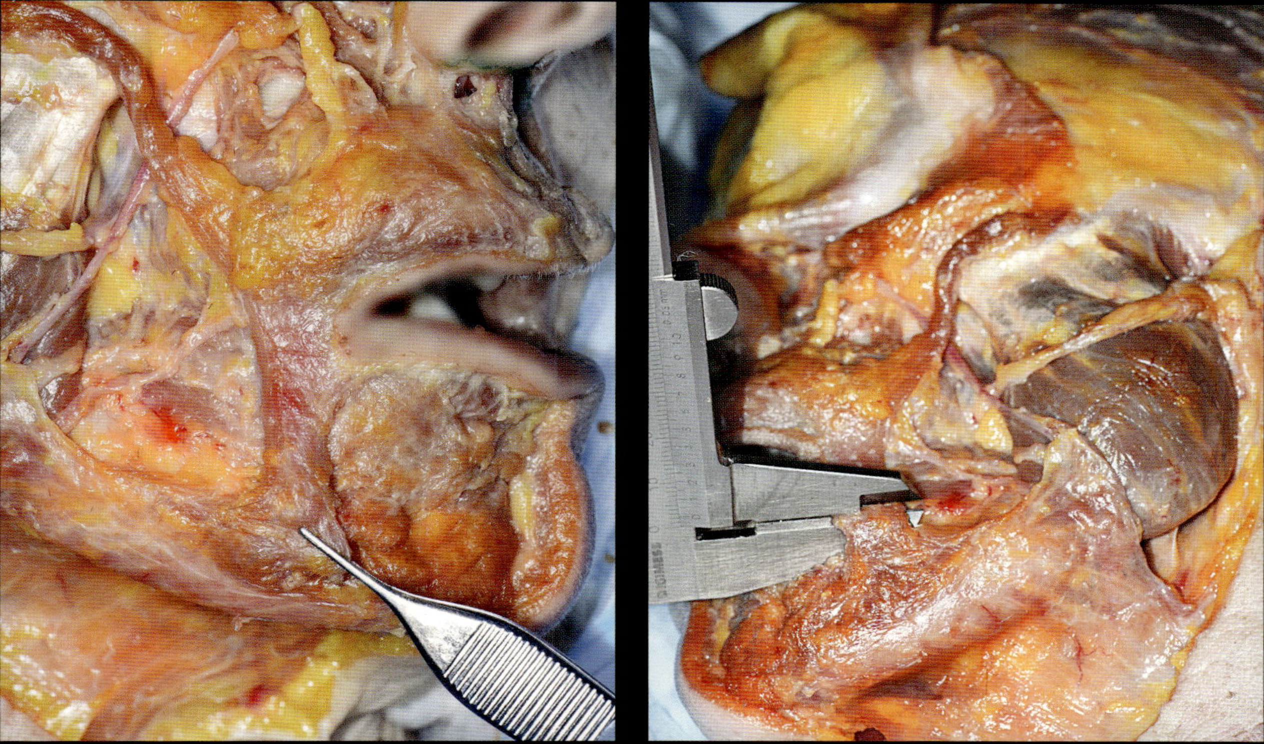

Depressor anguli oris thickness = 2.4 mm

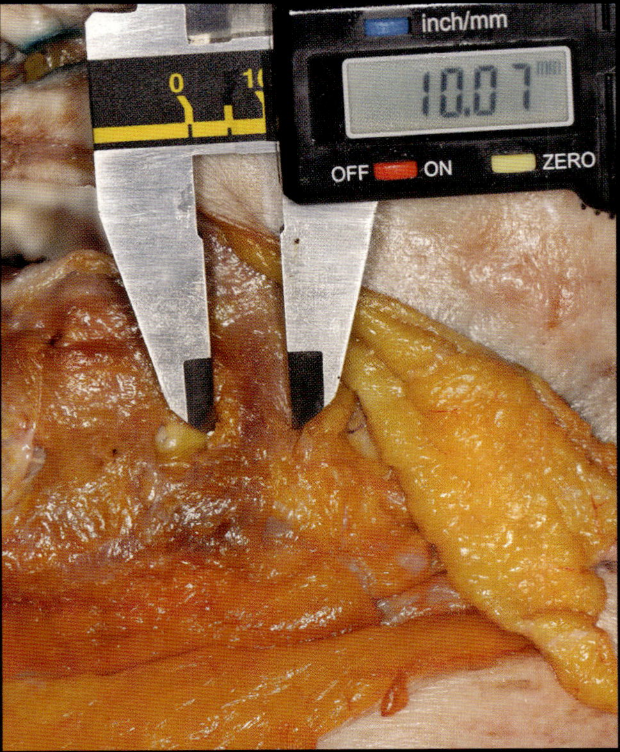

Depressor anguli oris width

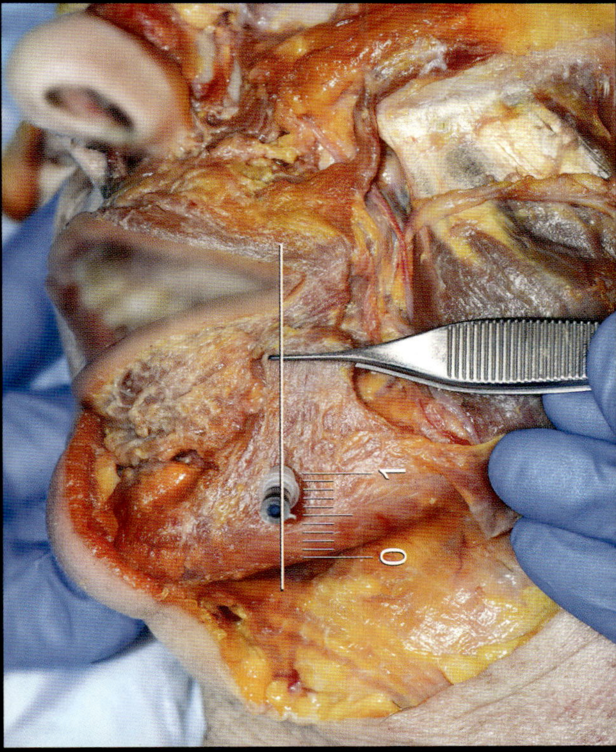

Injection point for the depressor anguli oris

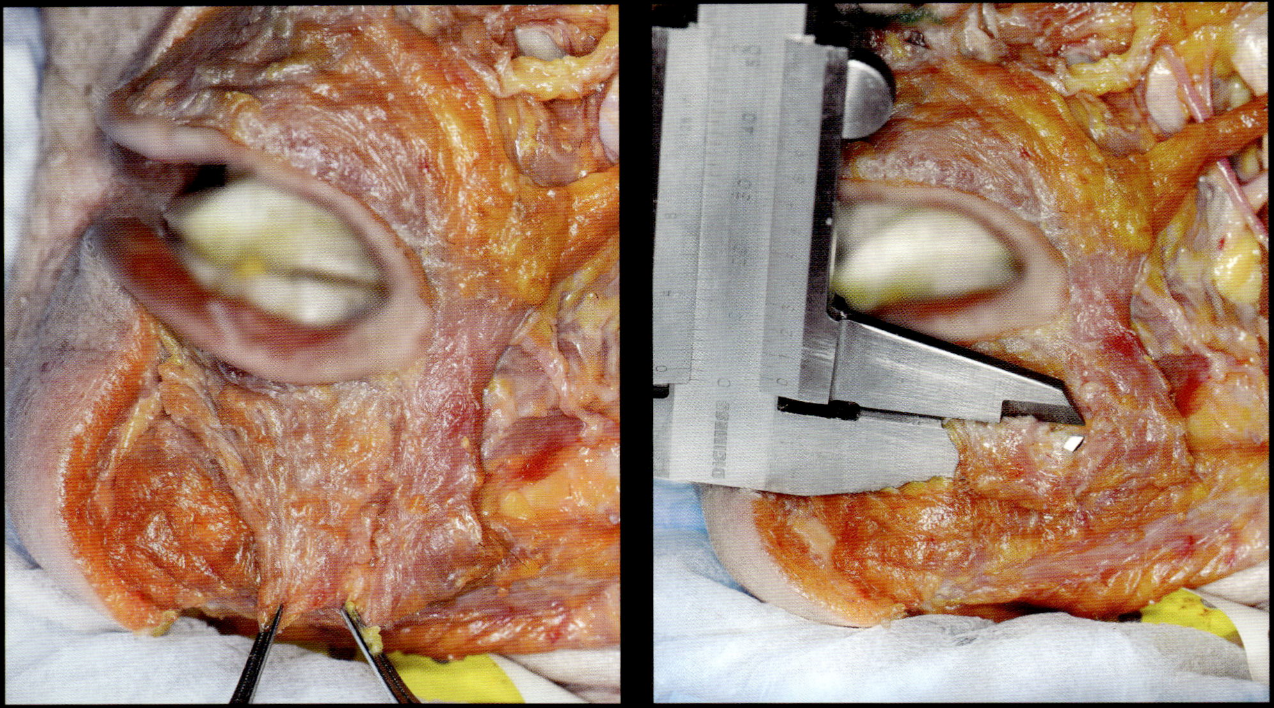

Depressor labii inferioris thickness = 1.5 mm

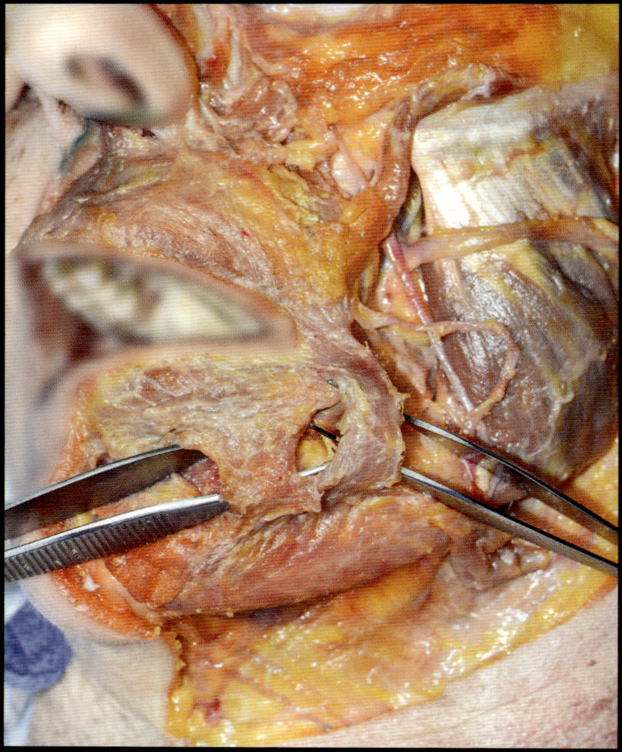

Tweezers on the depressor labii inferioris and depressor anguli oris

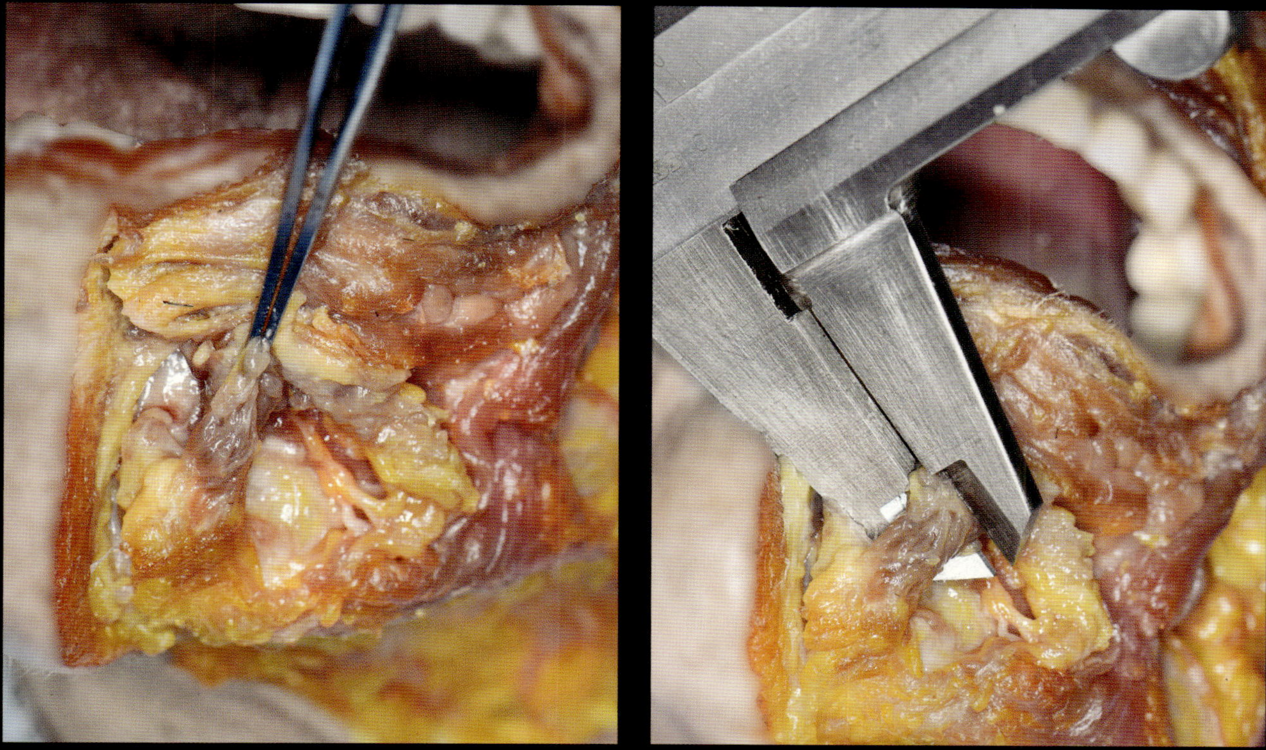

Mentalis thickness = 2.0 mm

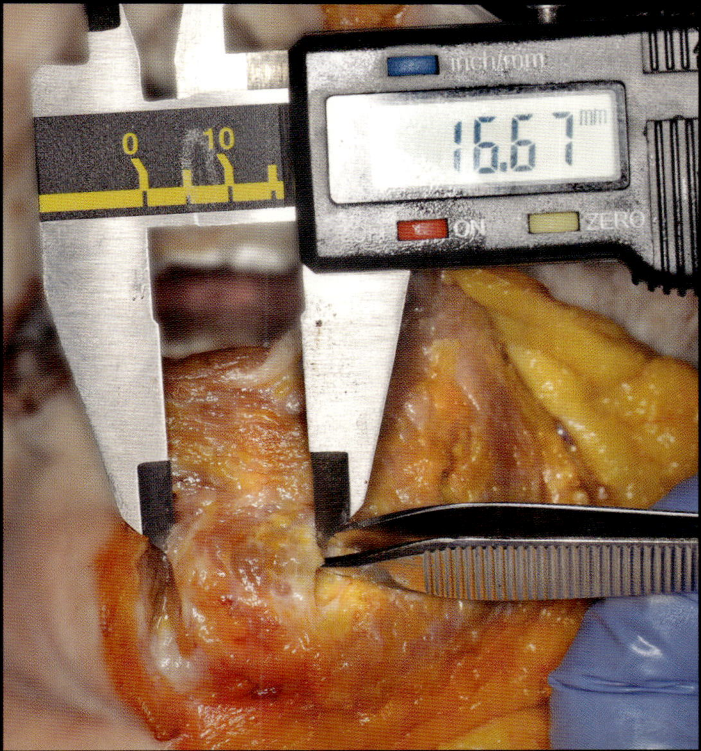

Mentalis width

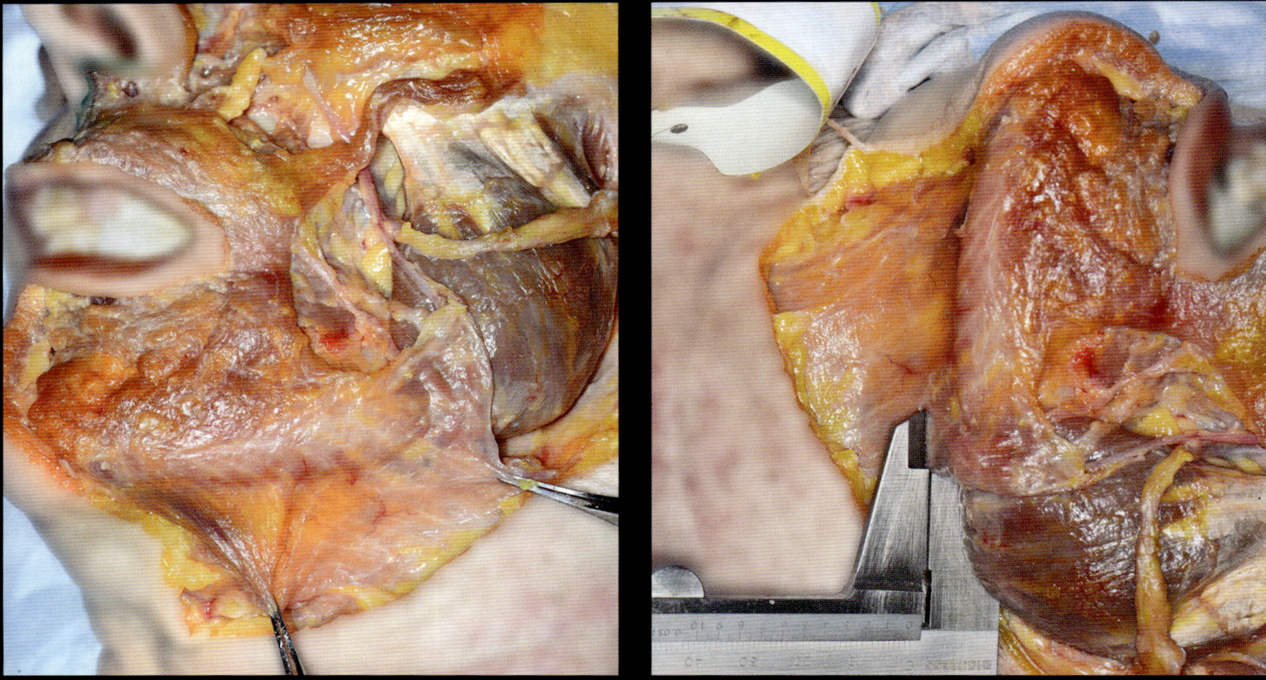

Platysma thickness = 0.5 mm

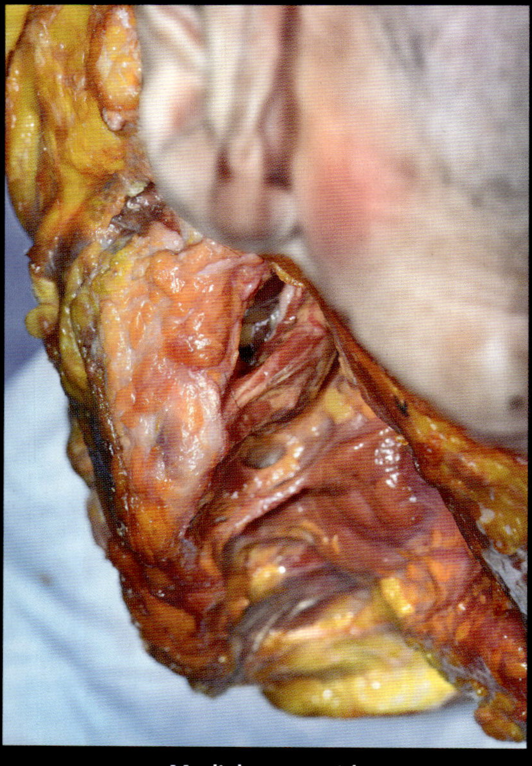

Medial pterygoid

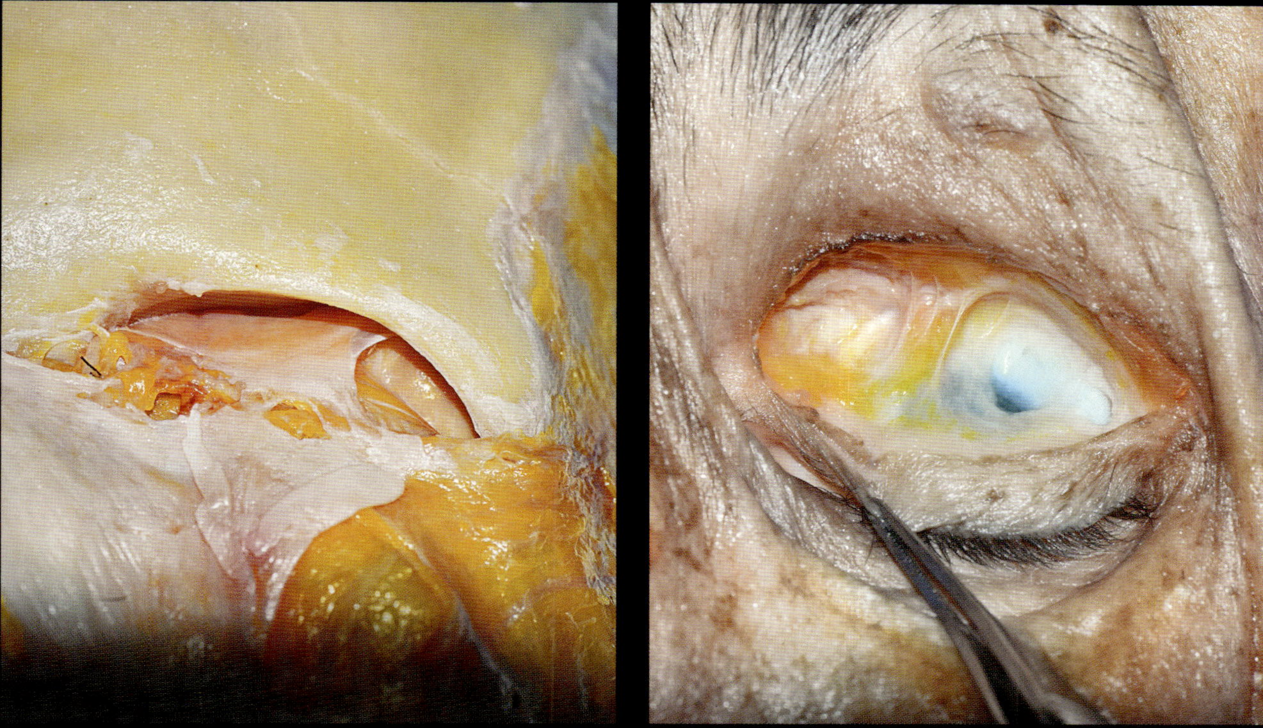

Levator palpebrae superioris

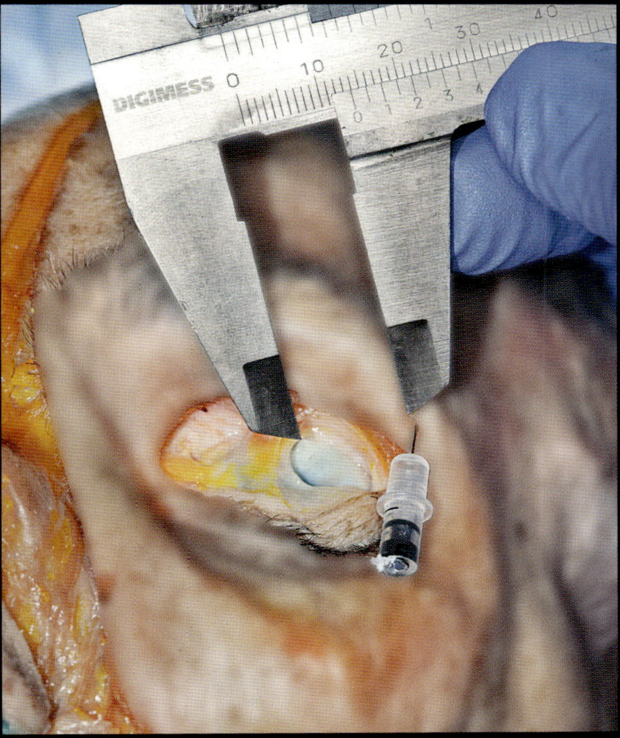

Distance from the eyebrow tail to the levator palpebrae superioris

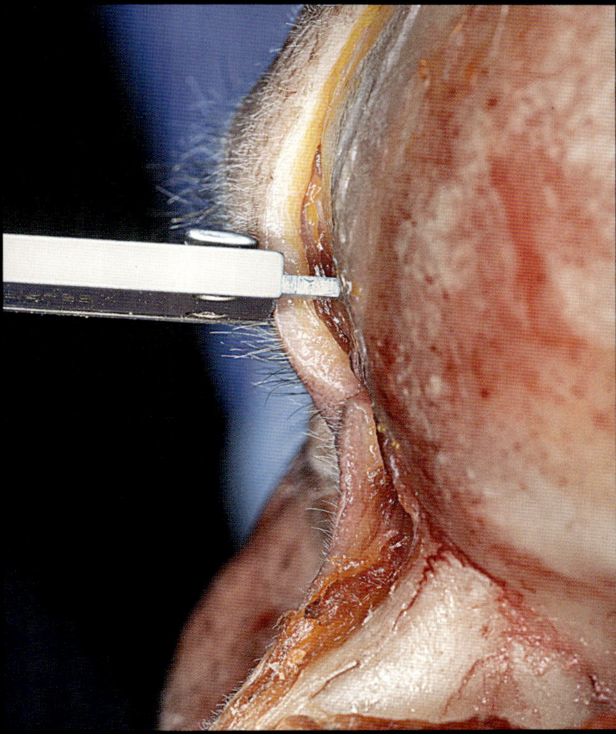

Distance to the procerus = 4 mm

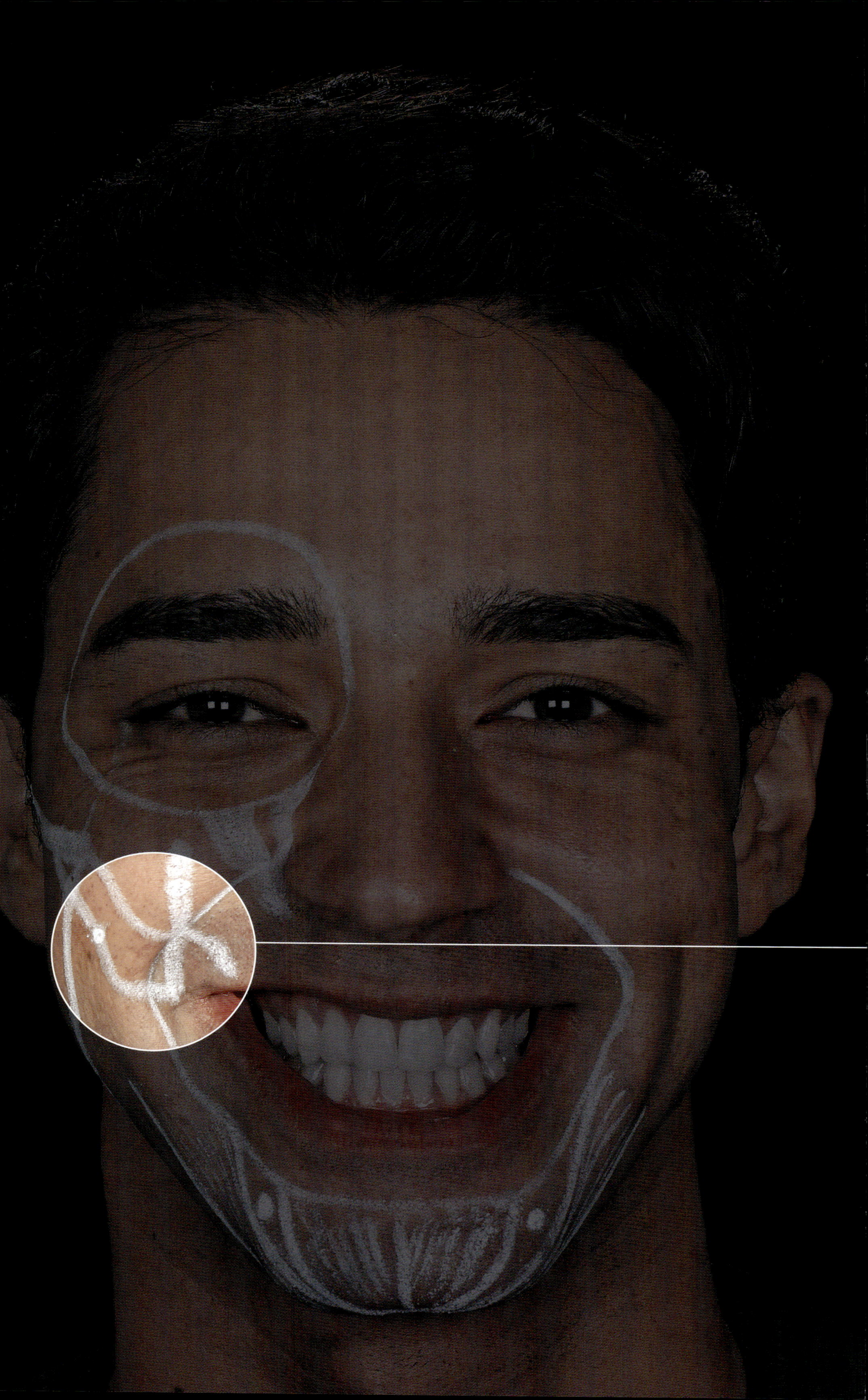

CHAPTER

04

Clinical Cases

Eyebrow Management

Case 1: Eyebrow maintenance

MAIN COMPLAINT: Esthetic deficiency in a 45-year-old woman.

HISTORY OF PRESENT CONDITION: Patient complains about wrinkles in the forehead.

SIGNS AND SYMPTOMS: At rest, the muscle tonus is increased, enabling the visualization of several horizontal volumes in the forehead (Fig 4-1a).

DIAGNOSIS: The occipitofrontalis muscle is hyperkinetic.

FACIAL READING: The skin in the forehead is irregular and wrinkled, making the patient look old.

PROCEDURE PRIORITY LIST: To inject botulinum toxin A (BTX-A) to decrease the tonus of the occipitofrontalis muscle at rest in all muscle width.

THERAPEUTICS: Chemical denervation of the muscles of the forehead was performed to decrease the muscular tonus of the occipitofrontalis muscle. The injections were continuous across the full width of the forehead (Table 4-1 and Fig 4-1b). Figure 4-1c shows the final result.

CAUTION: There is a risk of eyelid ptosis when injecting BTX-A in the occipitofrontalis muscle. A minimum vertical distance of 15 mm from the upper orbital ridge, following the pupil line, should be observed. This approach is necessary to prevent the BTX-A from reaching the levator palpabrae superioris via diffusion and causing eyelid ptosis. This muscle width is similar to the human iris. Carruthers and Carruthers[1] suggested that eyelid ptosis due to intraorbital diffusion can be avoided by applying a high-concentration, low-volume BTX injection 1 cm from the edge of the orbital bone.

Table 4-1 Case 1 Botox injection sites and doses

MUSCLE	DEPTH OF NEEDLE	POINTS PER MUSCLE	UNITS PER POINT	TOTAL UNITS PER MUSCLE
Occipitofrontalis (left)	3 mm	11	2U	22U
Occipitofrontalis (right)	3 mm	11	2U	22U
Procerus	4 mm	1	4U	4U
Corrugator supercilii (left)	4 mm	1	3U	3U
Corrugator supercilii (right)	4 mm	1	3U	3U
Orbicularis oculi (left)	3 mm	3	2U	6U
Orbicularis oculi (right)	3 mm	3	2U	6U
Platysma	3 mm	11	2U	22U

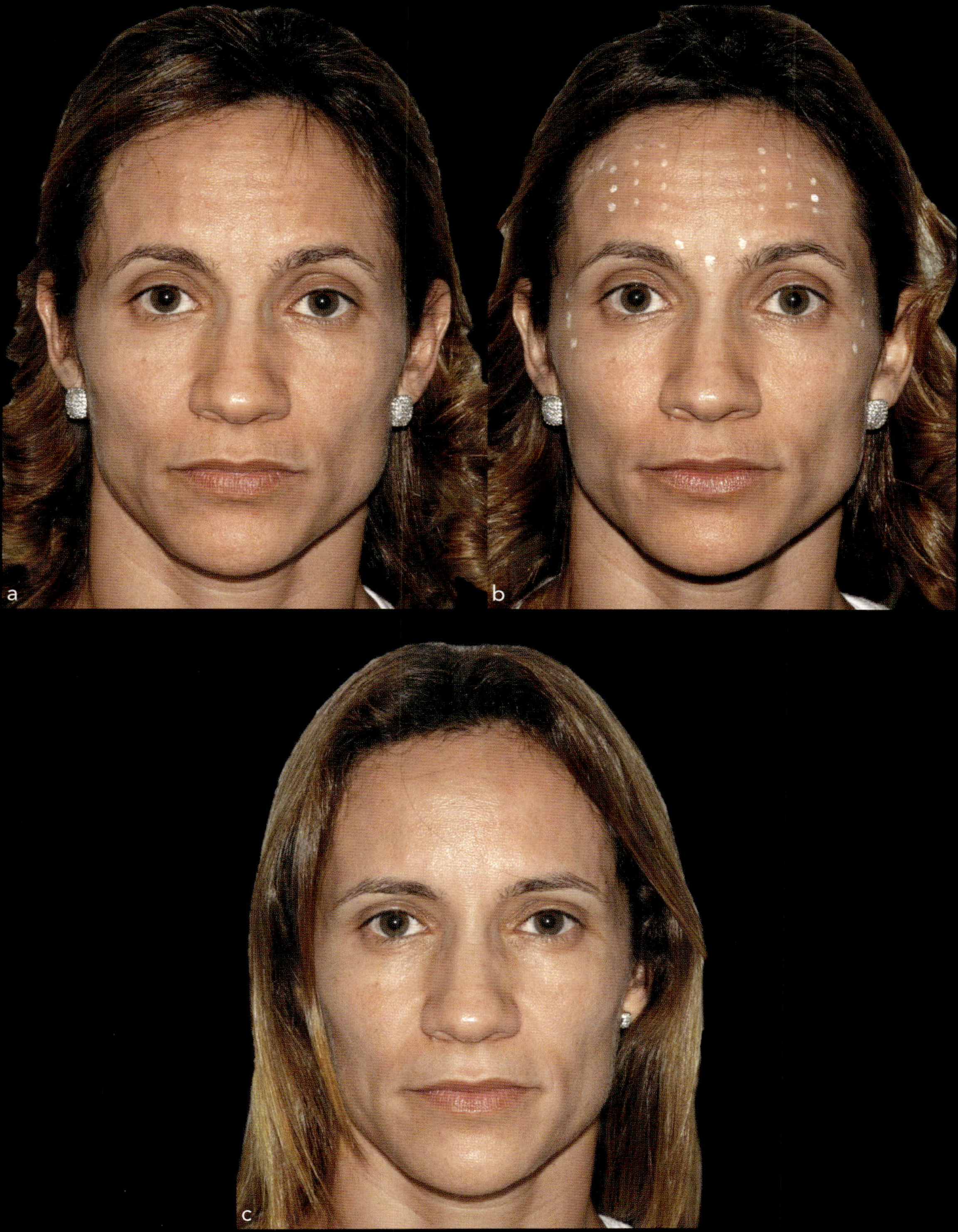

Fig 4-1 Case 1. *(a)* Even at rest, the increased and involuntary tonus of the hyperkinetic occipitofrontalis muscle leads to undulated, irregular-looking skin. *(b)* The occipitofrontalis muscle was marked in all extensions. *(c)* The final result shows a forehead free of irregularities and eyebrows that are not arched, as the patient requested.

Case 2: Eyebrow lifting

MAIN COMPLAINT: Esthetic deficiency in a 50-year-old woman with persistent wrinkles at the lateral canthus.

HISTORY OF PRESENT CONDITION: Persistent wrinkles at the lateral canthus even after BTX injection in this region.

SIGNS AND SYMPTOMS: Slight eyelid ptosis that contributes to the production of wrinkles at the lateral canthus (Fig 4-2a).

DIAGNOSIS: The beginning of an eyelid ptosis is observed, which, along with the sphincter action of the orbicularis oculi muscle, will result in wrinkled skin in the lateral canthus.

FACIAL READING: Wrinkles located at the lateral canthus make the patient look old.

PROCEDURE PRIORITY LIST: To inject BTX-A to decrease the tonus of the occipitofrontalis muscle at rest, not injecting the lateral portion so that this active part can lift the eyebrow tail, stretching the skin in the lateral canthus. To inject BTX-A in the orbicularis oculi muscle to decrease its contraction and consequently reduce the wrinkles at the lateral canthus.

THERAPEUTICS: The muscular tonus of the occipitofrontalis muscle was decreased with injections to the medial and central portions; the lateral portion was not included so that this active part could elevate the eyebrow tail, stretching the skin at the lateral canthus (Fig 4-2b). BTX-A was also injected in the orbicularis oculi muscle to decrease its contraction and consequently reduce the wrinkles at the lateral canthus (Table 4-2). Figure 4-2c shows the final result.

Table 4-2 Case 2 Botox injection sites and doses

MUSCLE	DEPTH OF NEEDLE	POINTS PER MUSCLE	UNITS PER POINT	TOTAL UNITS PER MUSCLE
Occipitofrontalis (left)	3 mm	6	2U	12U
Occipitofrontalis (right)	3 mm	6	2U	12U
Procerus	4 mm	1	4U	4U
Corrugator supercilii (left)	4 mm	1	3U	3U
Corrugator supercilii (right)	4 mm	1	3U	3U
Orbicularis oculi (left)	3 mm	4	3U	12U
Orbicularis oculi (right)	3 mm	4	3U	12U
Platysma	13 mm	4	3U	12U

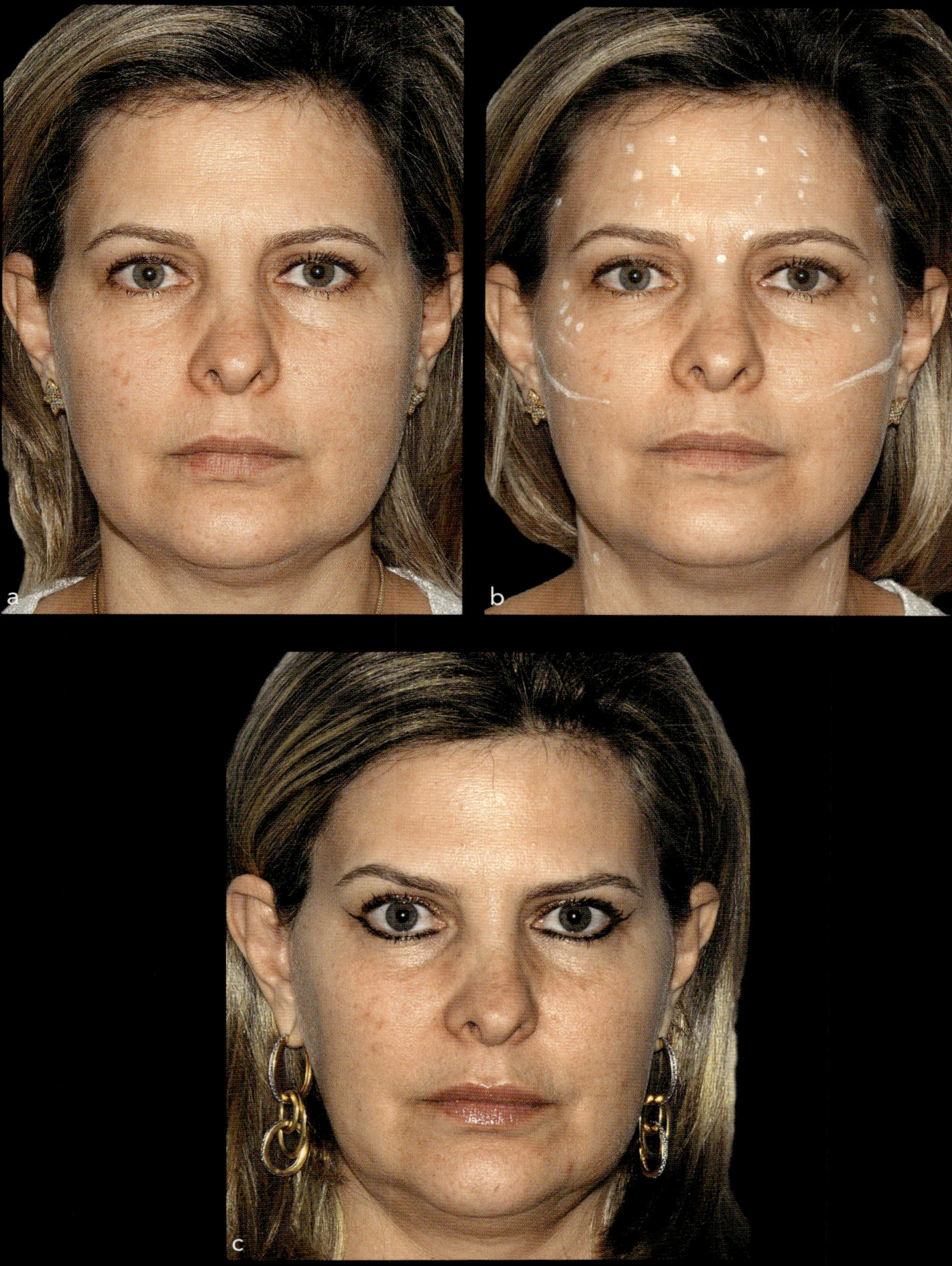

Fig 4-2 **Case 2**. *(a)* Pretreatment view showing discreet static wrinkles in the skin of the left lateral canthus. *(b)* The medial portion of the occipitofrontalis muscle was marked without including the lateral portion. *(c)* The final result shows an eyebrow with an arched lateral third; the skin of the lateral canthus is smoother and more stretched.

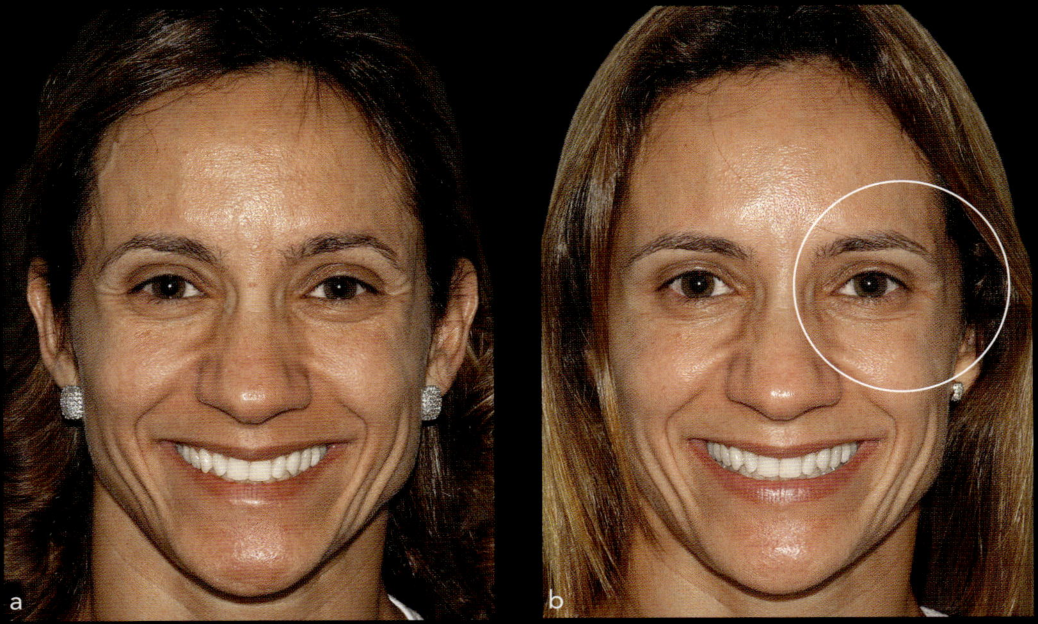

Fig 4-3 *(a)* Pretreatment smile of the patient in case 1. *(b)* Smile 30 days after treatment. The forehead is smooth, and the original shape of the eyebrow has been maintained, as requested by the patient. The periorbital wrinkles have been smoothed.

CAUTION: There is a risk of smile limitation when injecting BTX-A in the orbicularis oculi muscle. A minimum vertical distance of 15 mm from the lower ridge of the zygomatic bone should be observed. This approach is necessary to avoid BTX-A from reaching the zygomaticus major muscle via diffusion and affecting the modiolus position during the smile, thereby leading to asymmetries or limitations in the amplitude of the smile. There is also a risk of strabismus when injecting BTX-A in the orbicularis oculi; a lateral distance of 10 mm from the edge of the orbital bone should be observed. This approach is necessary to avoid BTX-A from reaching the lateral rectus muscle via diffusion and affecting the position of the eyes, thereby leading to strabismus and diplopia. Numerous authors in different studies[1–19] have described these complications as well as how to avoid them.

HINT:

UNDESIRED DIFFUSION: In general to decrease the risk of undesired diffusion, the following should be avoided:

- High doses of BTX-A
- Compressing or massaging the injection site
- Dilutions made with a high amount of saline, which result in a greater volume injected and greater diffusion. The muscles of facial expression do not have a fascia that separates them from one another, hence the easy diffusion. Therefore, more dehydrated dilutions are recommended.

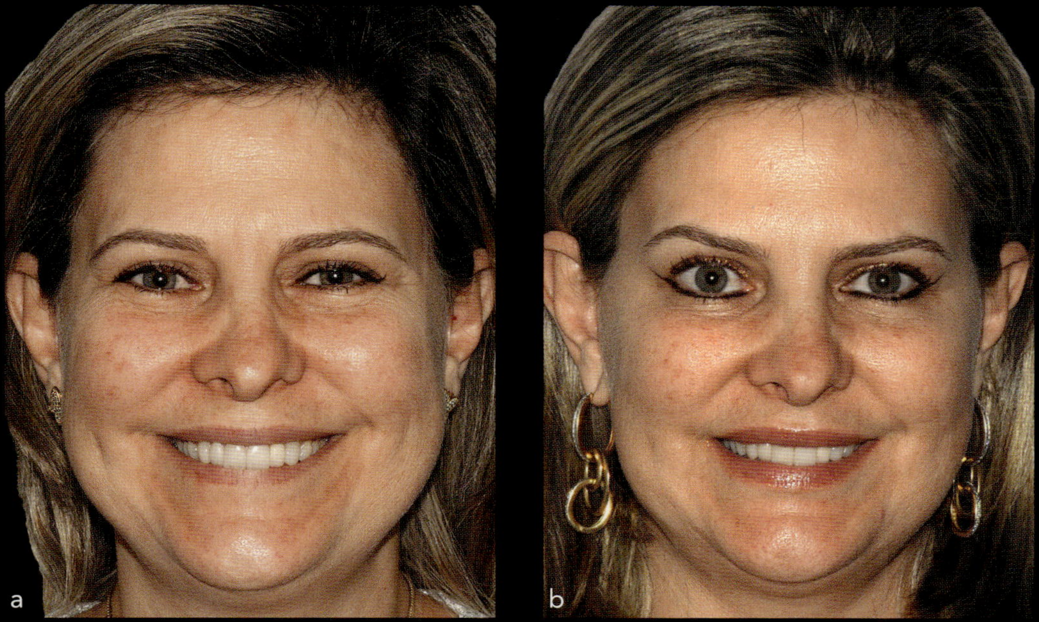

Fig 4-4 *(a)* Pretreatment smile of the patient in case 2. *(b)* Smile 30 days after treatment. Note the lack of dynamic wrinkles in the forehead. The shape of the eyebrow has been altered based on the patient's wishes, and this eyebrow lift has resulted in a more dolichofacial (elongated) face, Consequently, the skin in the lateral canthus has been stretched, eliminating wrinkles in this region. Periorbital wrinkles have also been eliminated.

Marking injection points

Occipitofrontalis muscle: Ask the patient to make a surprised facial expression and mark the top of each defined belly, following a vertical line tangent to the medial palpebral commissure. Another mark should be drawn following the center of the pupil and the third tangent to the lateral palpebral commissure.

When the treatment goal is to lift the eyebrow, toxin should not be injected at the portion of muscle corresponding to the line tangent to the lateral palpebral commissure. If the treatment goal is to extensively lift the eyebrow, BTX-A should also be injected at the eyebrow tail to decrease the strength of the orbicularis oculi muscle, which acts as an antagonist to the occipitofrontalis muscle. This will cause more elevation of the lateral part of the eyebrow.

Orbicularis oculi muscle: Ask the patient to smile and mark the top part of each defined belly, keeping a distance of 10 mm between each site.

Discussion

Both patients were treated by smoothing the upper third of the face, but the therapeutics had one fundamental difference: In case 1, the eyebrow was not lifted as in case 2. This leads to two major differences in the outcome: *(1)* The skin in the lateral canthus is more stretched when lifting the eyebrow, thus effectively eliminating wrinkles in the lateral canthus. *(2)* After the eyebrow lifting, the face looks longer, thinner, and therefore more elegant. Figures 4-3 and 4-4 compare the pretreatment and posttreatment smiles of both patients.

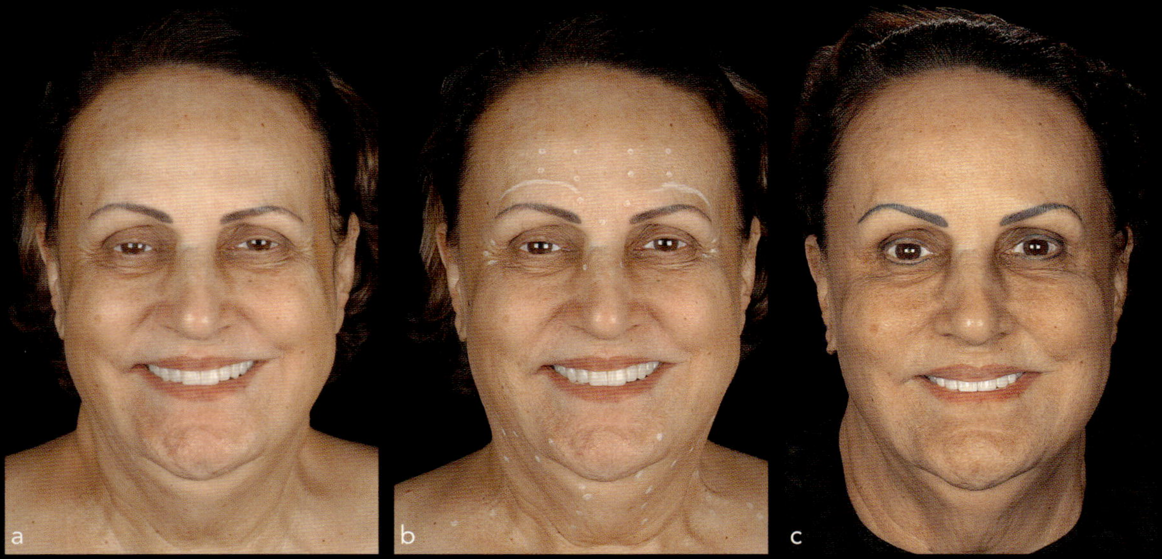

Fig 4-5 **Case 3**. *(a)* Pretreatment photograph of a 72-year-old patient with upper eyelid ptosis. *(b)* Injection points. *(c)* Results 30 days after injecting BTX-A. A great improvement in eye opening was observed. Besides this therapeutic effect, a good cosmeceutical effect was also noticed, as there was a great attenuation of periorbital wrinkles resulting from the eyebrow lift that stretched the skin at the lateral canthus.

Case 3: Eyebrow lifting for eyelid ptosis

Figure 4-5 shows the case of a 72-year-old woman. Similar doses of the toxin to those shown in Table 4-2 were injected, but in this case, the main purpose was therapeutic, with a focus on the upper eyelid ptosis.

Case 4: Eyebrow lifting for a "pity face"

When the lateral portion of the eyebrow is lower than the medial portion, the result is a look of pity the author calls a "pity face." In these cases, maximum arching of the lateral third of the eyebrow is required. This can be accomplished with the following steps:

- Administer one more injection at the eyebrow tail to decrease the force of the orbicularis oculi muscle, which antagonizes the action of the occipitofrontalis muscle responsible for elevating the eyebrow.
- Do not inject BTX-A in the procerus muscle, so that it will keep depressing the medial portion of the eyebrow, thereby increasing the arching.

Figure 4-6 and Table 4-3 illustrate the use of BTX-A in the case of a 52-year-old woman with a "pity face."

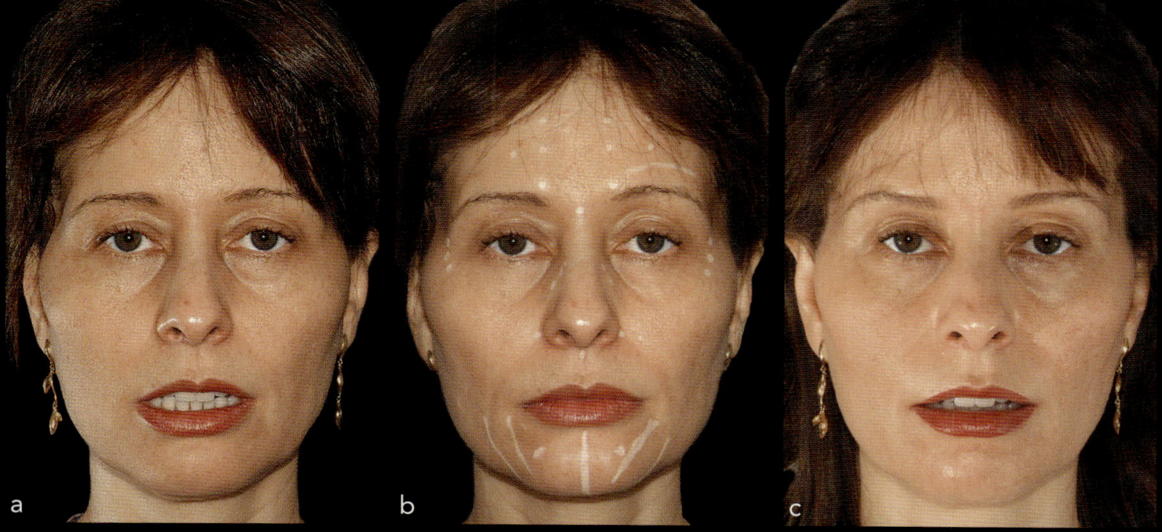

Fig 4-6 **Case 4**. *(a)* Pretreatment photograph of a 52-year-old woman with a "pity face." *(b)* Besides marking injection points to correct the shape of the eyebrow, bilateral applications were made to attenuate wrinkles in the corrugator supercilii and orbicularis oculi muscles. Because there was an excessive exposure of mandibular teeth at rest and during the smile (see Fig 4-9), BTX-A was injected in the right and left depressor labii inferioris muscles to lift the horizontal level of the lower lip. Injections in the depressor septi nasi and right and left levator superioris alaeque nasi muscles were administered to treat the gummy smile (see Fig 4-9). *(c)* Result 30 days after BTX-A injection.

Table 4-3 **Case 4 Botox injection sites and doses for treatment of the "pity face"**

MUSCLE	DEPTH OF NEEDLE	POINTS PER MUSCLE	UNITS PER POINT	TOTAL UNITS PER MUSCLE
Occipitofrontalis (left)	3 mm	4	2U	8U
Occipitofrontalis (right)	3 mm	4	2U	8U
Corrugator supercilii (left)	4 mm	1	3U	3U
Corrugator supercilii (right)	4 mm	1	3U	3U
Orbicularis oculi (left)	3 mm	3	3U	9U
Orbicularis oculi (right)	3 mm	3	3U	9U
Depressor septi nasi	8 mm	1	3U	3U
Levator labii superioris alaeque nasi (left)	4 mm	1	2U	2U
Levator labii superioris alaeque nasi (right)	4 mm	1	2U	2U
Depressor labii inferioris (left)	4 mm	1	2U	2U
Depressor labii inferioris (right)	4 mm	1	2U	2U

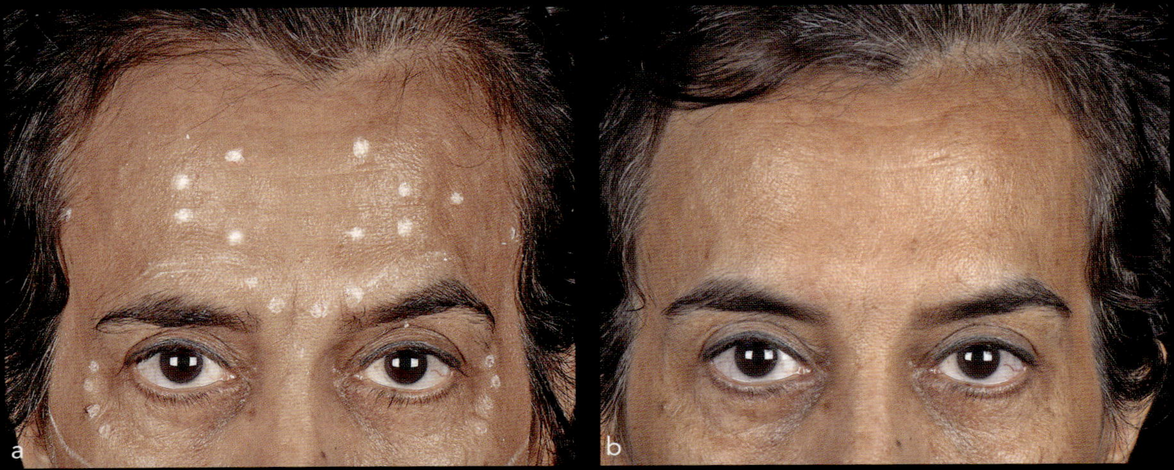

Fig 4-7 Case 5. *(a)* Injection points of BTX in a patient with eyebrow asymmetry. While the injection points vertically aligned with the medial canthus and pupil are symmetric, the points vertically aligned with the lateral canthus are asymmetric. The left eyebrow is higher, so no BTX will be injected on the right side in the site that follows the vertical line of the lateral commissure of the eye, which corresponds to the lateral portion of the occipitofrontalis muscle. BTX-A will only be injected on the left side to reduce the action of this muscle, thereby elevating the eyebrow less and resulting in eyebrow leveling. Each of the points marked received 3U of BTX-A. *(b)* Final result showing the right and left eyebrows at a similar horizontal level.

Case 5: Eyebrow asymmetry

In cases of asymmetric eyebrows, BTX-A injections should also be asymmetric in order to produce distinct effects in each eyebrow aimed at their leveling (Fig 4-7).

Conclusion

- It can be considered as a coadjuvant treatment to smooth periorbital wrinkles when BTX injections in the orbicularis oculi are not enough to smooth and/or eliminate these wrinkles.
- It can be indicated in patients with wider and/or shorter faces because when the eyebrows are higher, the face looks longer and thinner.
- It minimizes eyelid ptosis.
- It can alter the shape of the eyebrow, resulting in arching of its lateral portion.
- In cases of asymmetry, it can be used to level the eyebrows.

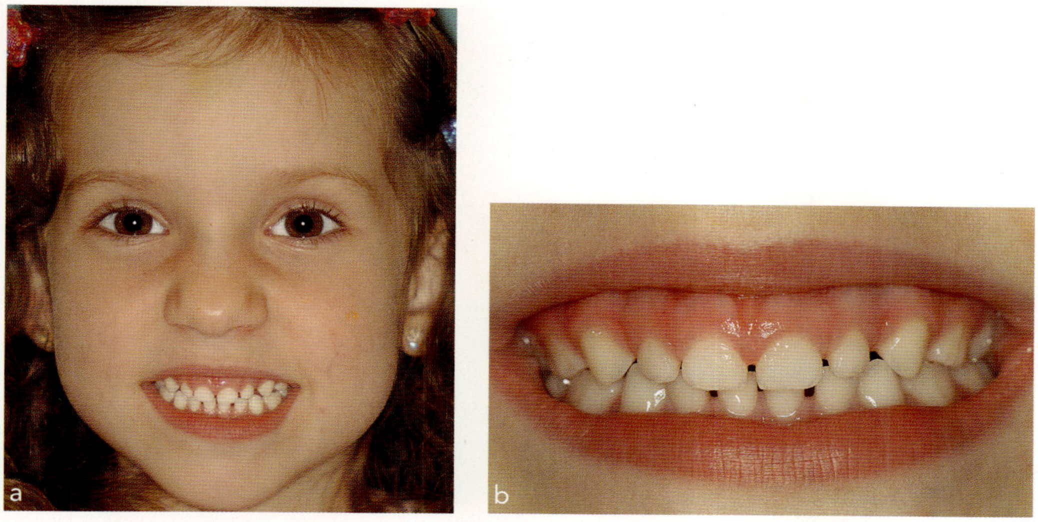

Fig 4-8 *(a and b)* Example of a child's smile.

Gummy Smile

A gummy smile is common in most children, along with diastemas, small teeth, thin lips, and monochromatic teeth (Fig 4-8). However, a gummy smile in an adult gives the face a childlike appearance and is not ideal for esthetics.

Case 4 revisited: Gummy smile

MAIN COMPLAINT: Esthetic deficiency in a 52-year-old woman.

HISTORY OF PRESENT CONDITION: The patient reported discontent in regard to the excessive exposure of gingival tissue during her smile.

SIGNS AND SYMPTOMS: In terms of the muscle dynamics of the smile, excessive exposure of the maxillary gingiva and mandibular papillae were observed, characterizing both an upper and a lower gummy smile (Figs 4-9a and 4-9c).

DIAGNOSIS: In the upper lip, the right and left levator labii superioris alaeque nasi were hyperkinetic, excessively elevating the upper lip. In the lower lip, the right and left depressor labii inferioris were hyperkinetic, excessively depressing the lower lip during the smile.

FACIAL READING: If, when smiling, the patient displays more than 3 mm of gingiva in the region of the maxillary central incisors, the literature[20–24] classifies it as a gummy smile. The lower lip moves less than the upper lip during a smile, ideally descending until it exposes just part of the clinical crowns of the mandibular anterior teeth. However, exposure of mandibular gingival tissue, even if only the papillae, should not occur. In case of mandibular gingival tissue exposure, the smile is characterized as a lower gummy smile. A gummy smile steals the desired dominance of the maxillary teeth and lips during a smile, making it unesthetic.

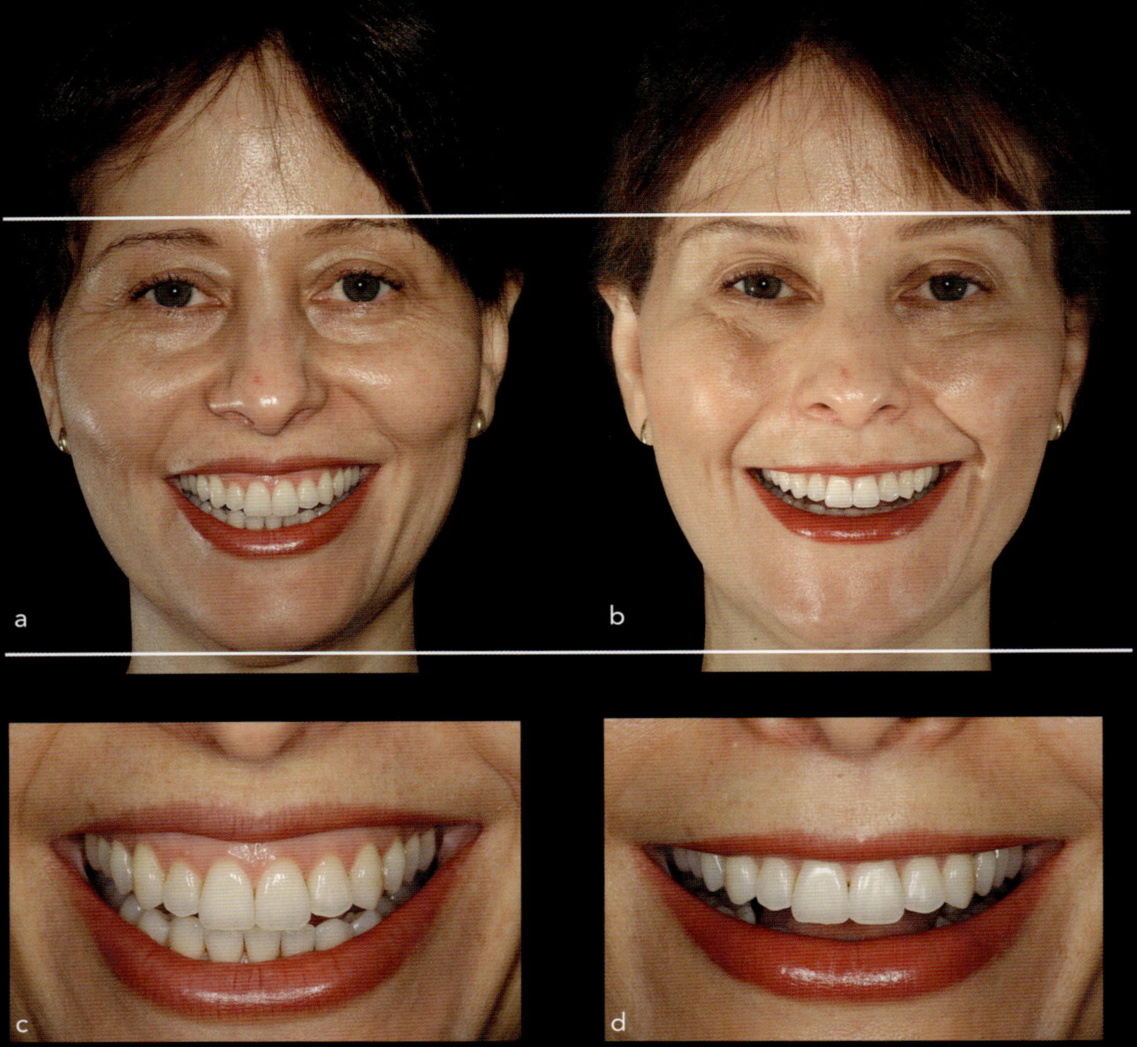

Fig 4-9 **Case 4 revisited**. *(a and c)* Pretreatment views of the gummy smile. *(b and d)* Final views 10 days after the injections.

This patient also has a "pity face" that required eyebrow lifting (see Fig 4-6 and Table 4-3).

PROCEDURE PRIORITY LIST:

1. Use Botox to lower the horizontal level of the upper lip.
2. Use Botox to raise the horizontal level of the lower lip.
3. Use Botox to arch the eyebrows.
4. Use Botox to rejuvenate the upper third of the face.

THERAPEUTICS: The purpose of injecting BTX-A in this case was to promote the chemodenervation of muscles that elevate the upper lip and depress the lower lip during the smile. This would decrease movement of the lips during the smile, leading to less exposure of gingival tissue (Figs 4-9b and 4-9d).

Table 4-4 Case 4 Botox injection sites and doses for treatment of the gummy smile

MUSCLE	DEPTH OF NEEDLE	POINTS PER MUSCLE	UNITS PER POINT	TOTAL UNITS PER MUSCLE
Nasalis (left)	2 mm	2	1U	2U
Nasalis (right)	2 mm	2	1U	2U
Occipitofrontalis	3 mm	8	2U	16U
Corrugator supercilii (right)	4 mm	1	3U	3U
Corrugator supercilii (left)	4 mm	1	3U	3U
Depressor labii inferioris (right)	4 mm	1	1U	1U
Depressor labii inferioris (left)	4 mm	1	1U	1U
Levator labii superioris alaeque nasi (right)	4 mm	1	1U	1U
Levator labii superioris alaeque nasi (left)	4 mm	1	1U	1U
Depressor septi nasi	8 mm	1	3U	3U
Orbicularis oculi (left & right)	3 mm	3	3U	9U

In this specific patient, the gummy smile could not be treated through periodontal plastic surgery (crown lengthening) because the clinical crown ratio was already ideal, harmonic, and esthetically pleasant.

Table 4-4 outlines all of the esthetic applications made in a single treatment appointment.

CAUTION: If, during the initial evaluation of a patient with a gummy smile, the clinician finds that the nasalis muscle is too active during the smile, causing wrinkles in the nose, BTX should be prophylactically injected into this muscle. If not, after injecting the BTX in the levator labii superioris, the nasalis muscle will show an excessive contraction upon smiling, leading to unpleasant esthetics.

HINT:
The needle should be perpendicular to the face so that the toxin effect will be identical on both sides. If the operator uses different inclinations, the effects will also be distinct.

MARKING INJECTION POINTS: Mark an injection point at the levator labii superioris alaeque nasi immediately lateral to the wing of the nose (see Fig 4-6b). Do not mark the point laterally at the end of the nasolabial sulcus; it should always be medial to the sulcus. Only one injection will reach both muscles (levator labii superioris alaeque nasi and levator labii superioris) when done that way.

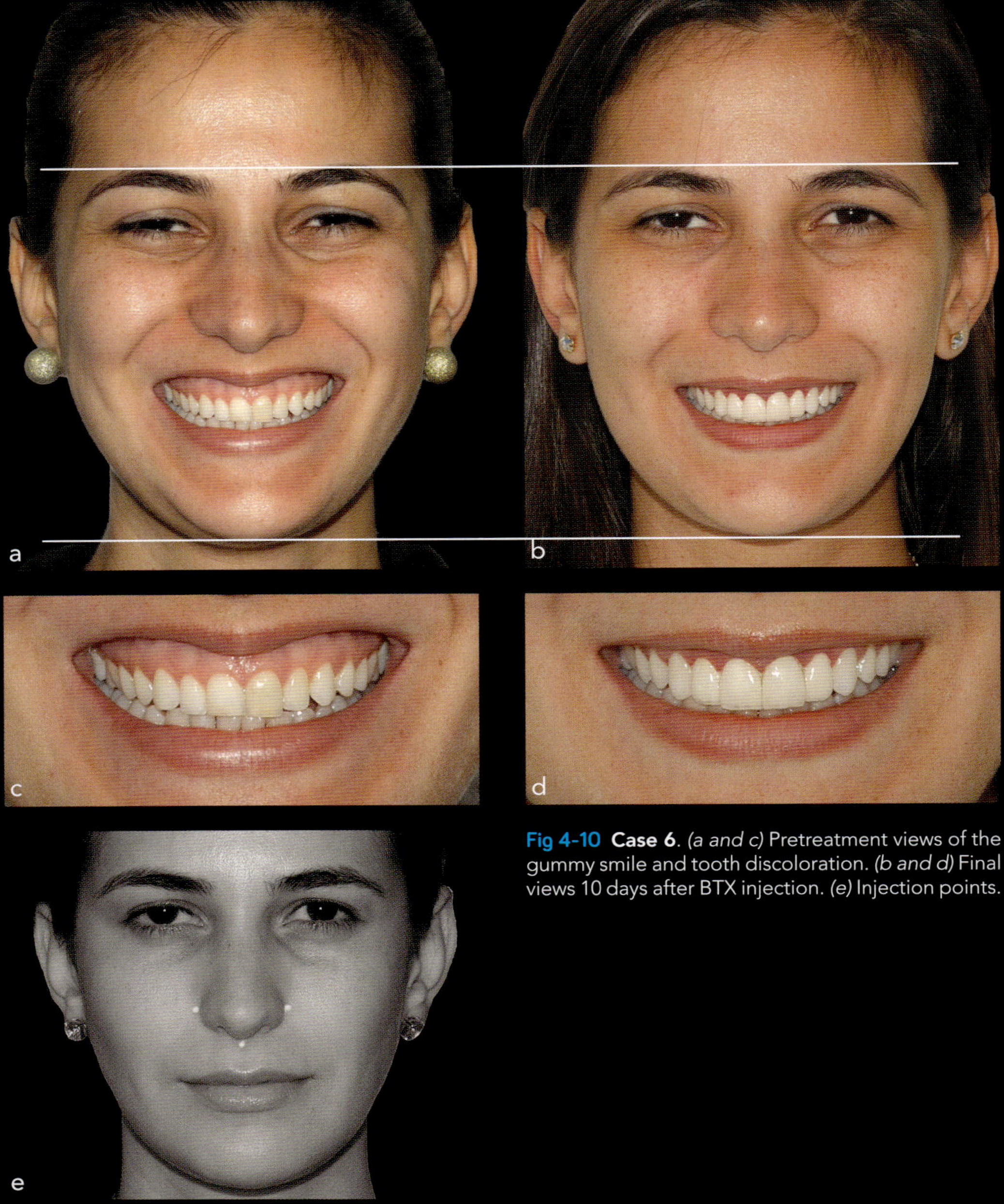

Fig 4-10 Case 6. *(a and c)* Pretreatment views of the gummy smile and tooth discoloration. *(b and d)* Final views 10 days after BTX injection. *(e)* Injection points.

Case 6: Upper gummy smile

MAIN COMPLAINT: Esthetic deficiency in a 34-year-old woman.

HISTORY OF PRESENT CONDITION: The patient reported discontent related to excessive exposure of gingival tissue during the smile and a dark clinical crown of the maxillary left central incisor.

SIGNS AND SYMPTOMS: In terms of the muscle dynamics of the smile, excessive maxillary gingival exposure was observed, characterizing an upper gummy smile. The clinical crown of the maxillary left central incisor was dark due to a trauma that happened when the patient was a teenager (Figs 4-10a and 4-10c).

DIAGNOSIS: In the upper lip, the levator labii superioris alaeque nasi and levator labii superioris were hyperkinetic, excessively elevating the upper lip. The darkened clinical crown could be ex-

Table 4-5 Case 6 Botox injection sites and doses

MUSCLE	DEPTH OF NEEDLE	POINTS PER MUSCLE	UNITS PER POINT	TOTAL UNITS PER MUSCLE
Nasalis (left)	2 mm	2	1U	2U
Nasalis (right)	2 mm	2	1U	2U
Occipitofrontalis	3 mm	8	2U	16U
Corrugator supercilii (right)	4 mm	1	3U	3U
Corrugator supercilii (left)	4 mm	1	3U	3U
Procerus	4 mm	1	5U	5U
Depressor labii inferioris (right)	4 mm	1	1U	1U
Depressor labii inferioris (left)	4 mm	1	1U	1U
Levator labii superioris alaeque nasi (right)	4 mm	1	3U	3U
Levator labii superioris alaeque nasi (left)	4 mm	1	3U	3U
Depressor septi nasi	8 mm	1	3U	3U
Orbicularis oculi (left & right)	3 mm	3	3U	9U

plained by the fact that after the trauma intrapulpal bleeding occurred in the clinical crown, and the iron pigments were not totally removed during the root canal treatment.

FACIAL READING: Besides the gummy smile, another point of concern for the patient was the intense closing of her eyes when she smiled.

PROCEDURE PRIORITY LIST:

1. Use Botox to lower the horizontal level of the upper lip.
2. Make direct resin veneers to restore the natural color of the maxillary left central incisor.
3. Use Botox to rejuvenate the upper third of the face.

THERAPEUTICS: The purpose of injecting Botox was to promote the chemodenervation of muscles that elevate the upper lip and depress the lower lip during the smile. This would reduce movement of the lips during the smile and result in less exposure of the maxillary gingival tissue (Figs 4-10b and 4-10d).

In this specific patient, the gummy smile could not be treated through periodontal plastic surgery (crown lengthening) because the clinical crown ratio was already ideal, harmonious, and esthetically pleasant.

Table 4-5 outlines all of the esthetic applications made in a single treatment session. Figure 4-10e shows the injection sites.

Discussion

The injection of BTX-A to correct a gummy smile has not only an esthetic function but also a functional one, as it helps to eliminate mouth breathing. Mouth breathing can cause negative changes in occlusion, jaw position, tongue position, lip position (flaccidity), tooth position, and facial position and can even adversely affect basal metabolism.[25–27] By decreasing the resting tonus of the target muscles, BTX can help the patient achieve a passive labial seal, which is fundamental for nasal breathing.

A great advantage of using BTX for the treatment of a gummy smile is that it is reversible.[25,26] On the other hand, while surgical resection of the depressor septi nasi muscle certainly reduces its bulk,[28,29] the results of this surgery cannot be quantified by different doses, as is the case with chemical denervation with BTX. This surgery can also lead to a poor result as the patient ages, as it is natural for the upper lip to move downward with age.

Once the BTX is injected in the levator labii superioris alaeque nasi muscle, the nose position will also be affected.

Conclusion

The use of BTX in the depressor septi nasi may change the anatomy of the upper lip, lowering the level of the upper labial tubercle in relation to the lip commissures. Therefore, it should be used in the following cases:

- Cases of excessive gingival display in the anterior maxilla but not the posterior maxilla. In this situation, a single injection only in the depressor septi nasi muscle is recommended.
- Cases of excessive gingival display in the anterior and posterior maxilla where the stomion of the upper lip is lower than the oral commissures. In this situation, injections in the depressor septi nasi muscle as well as in the levator labii superioris alaeque nasi and levator labii superioris muscles are recommended.

Masseter Hypertrophy

Case 7: Masseter pain and clenching

MAIN COMPLAINT: Pain.

HISTORY OF PRESENT CONDITION: The patient complained of preauricular pain when waking up, located at the masseter (right and left), with no tension headache. She also reported diurnal and nocturnal teeth clenching.

SIGNS AND SYMPTOMS: Enamel cracks, dental attrition, limited mouth opening (35 mm), clicking in the right temporomandibular joint with reduction, and maxillary and mandibular bone exostoses.

DIAGNOSIS: Exaggerated, abnormal, and continued tension or contraction of the mandibular elevator muscles peculiar to bruxism.

FACIAL READING: Apparent hypertrophy in the masseter muscles, because the bigonial distance is almost the same as the bizygomatic distance (Figs 4-11a and 4-11b). According to Doncatto and Schwantz,[30] the bigonial width should correspond to 75% of the bizygomatic width. The author observes that the distance between these two measurements must be at least 4%. A smaller number could mean masseter muscle hypertrophy. A difference of 12% is esthetically pleasant. The widening of the lower third of the face reduces the esthetic dominance of the mouth in that region.

PROCEDURE PRIORITY LIST:

1. Use BTX-A to decrease the lower third width.
2. Use fillers to increase the length of the chin and avoid the appearance of a double chin.
3. Use fillers to better sculpt the lips and smooth the nasolabial sulcus.

THERAPEUTICS: The purpose of using Botox was to promote the chemodenervation of the masseter muscles (right and left) and the temporalis muscles (right and left), adjusting their excessive contraction (Figs 4-11c and 4-11d). As a consequence, the pain would be decreased or eliminated, thereby protecting the stomatognathic system from this parafunction. Table 4-6 lists the injection sites and doses.

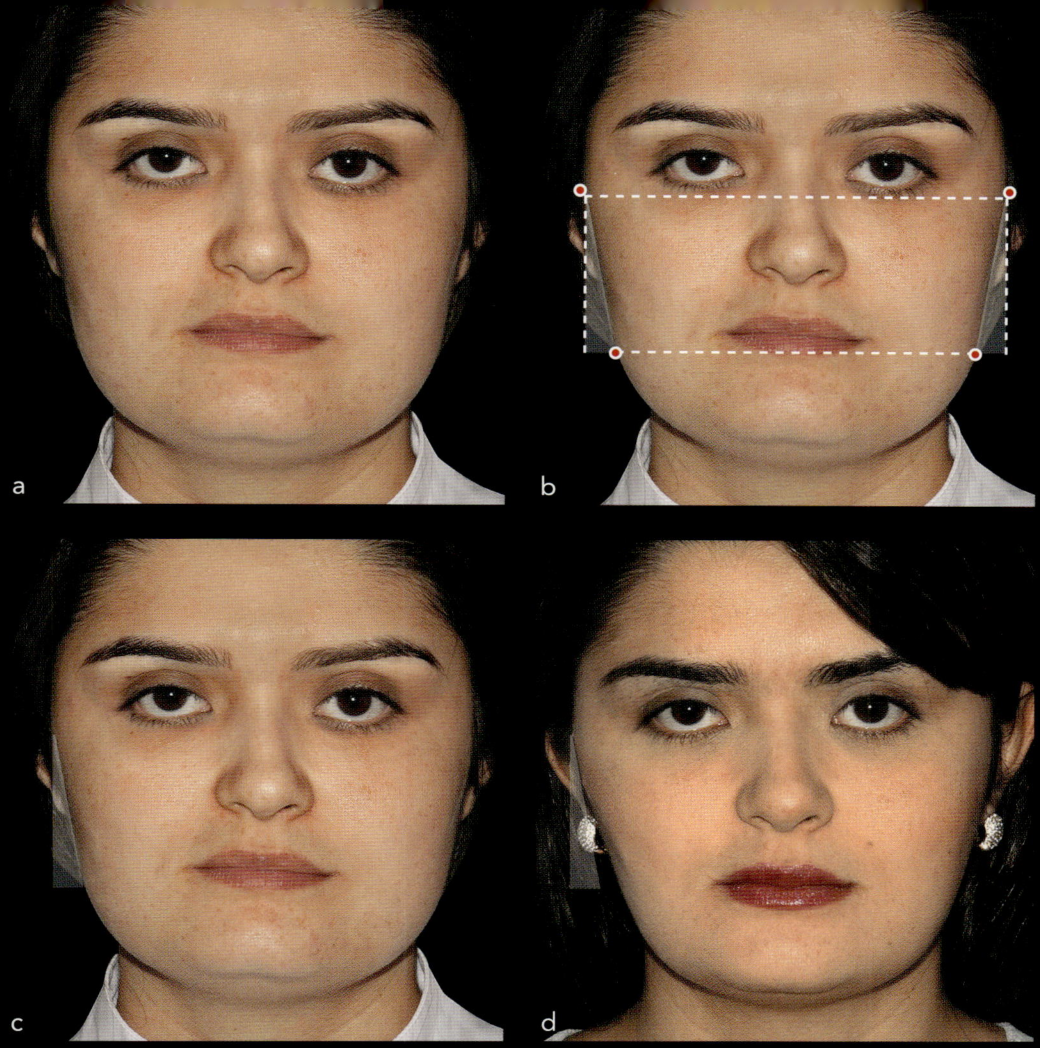

Fig 4-11 Case 7. *(a)* Pretreatment view of the face with a visually wide lower third. *(b)* The top dotted line measures the bizygomatic distance, and the bottom dotted line shows the bigonial distance. The triangle base shows the difference in width between the two measurements. The shorter this distance, the greater the masseter hypertrophy. *(c and d)* Comparison of the pretreatment condition and the result 30 days after the first toxin injection. The triangles in both photographs show the amount of narrowing in the lower third of the face after BTX injection.

Table 4-6 Case 7 Botox injection sites and doses

MUSCLE	DEPTH OF NEEDLE	POINTS PER MUSCLE	UNITS PER POINT	TOTAL UNITS PER MUSCLE
Masseter (left)	13 mm	2	15U	30U
Masseter (right)	13 mm	2	15U	30U
Temporalis (right)	4 mm	1	5U	5U
Temporalis (left)	4 mm	1	5U	5U

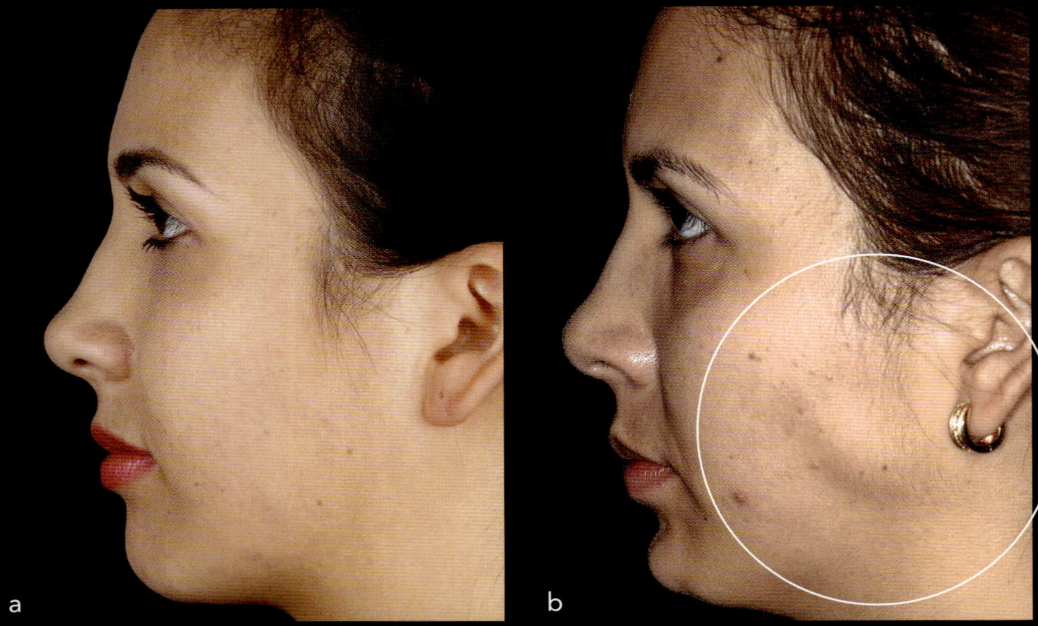

Fig 4-12 *(a)* Preoperative view of a patient with masseter hypertrophy. *(b)* Postoperative view after 5 days showing located hyperkinesia because of BTX injection in the masseter and mentalis muscles. Resolution is spontaneous within 3 weeks, or this hyperkinesia can be addressed by injecting the same dose in the most hyperkinetic points.

CAUTION: Narrowing of the lower third of the face using BTX-A should only be performed in patients with a therapeutic indication, and caution must be used to prevent undesired diffusion (see Fig 4-14). Avoid injecting toxin in the anterior bundle of the masseter muscle because it is too close to the risorius muscle. If accidentally injected, it could cause smile limitations and/or asymmetries. If toxin is injected too close to the zygomatic arch, the diffusion could affect the zygomaticus major muscle, limiting the opening of the buccal corridor during the smile.

In addition, injection of BTX in only one bundle could cause the muscle fibers to be highlighted, resulting in a high volume of the masseter muscle during mastication, which would be painless but unesthetic (Fig 4-12). Furthermore, injecting only one bundle (vertical injection points) would result in decreased contraction in only that bundle, leading to a smaller area of chemodenervation. On the other hand, injection at two horizontal points will affect the posterior and middle third fibers, resulting in more chemodenervation with the same amount of toxin (Fig 4-13).

HINT:
A measurement from the tragus to the injection points marked can be made on one side to accurately reproduce the injection points on the other side.

MARKING INJECTION POINTS: In order to correctly mark the points to be injected, the clinician might mark the area where the masseter muscle is located. Through palpation, mark the following points: *(1)* the lower ridge of the zygomatic bone with the muscle at rest, *(2)* the inferior border of the mandible, and *(3)* the anterior and posterior borders of the masseter during repeated contractions and relaxations. Then divide the masseter muscle into three parts by drawing two inclined vertical lines. The anterior part should not be injected because it is too close to the risorius muscle (lower anterior part of the masseter) and the zygomaticus major and zygomaticus minor muscles (upper anterior part of the masseter) (Fig 4-14).

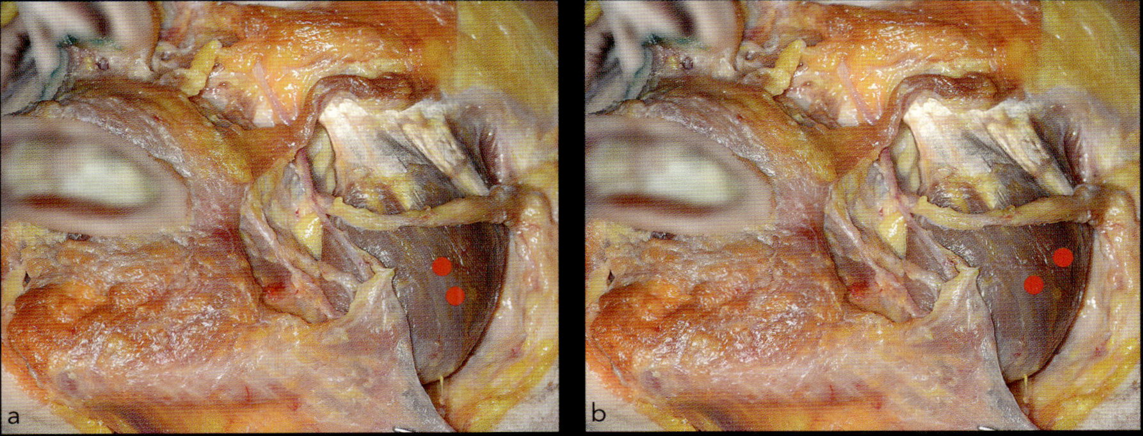

Fig 4-13 Marking injection points in the masseter of a cadaver. *(a)* Marking vertical points that only include the same muscular bundle, which might cause highlighted fibers. *(b)* Marking horizontal points that include middle and posterior fibers of the masseter muscle.

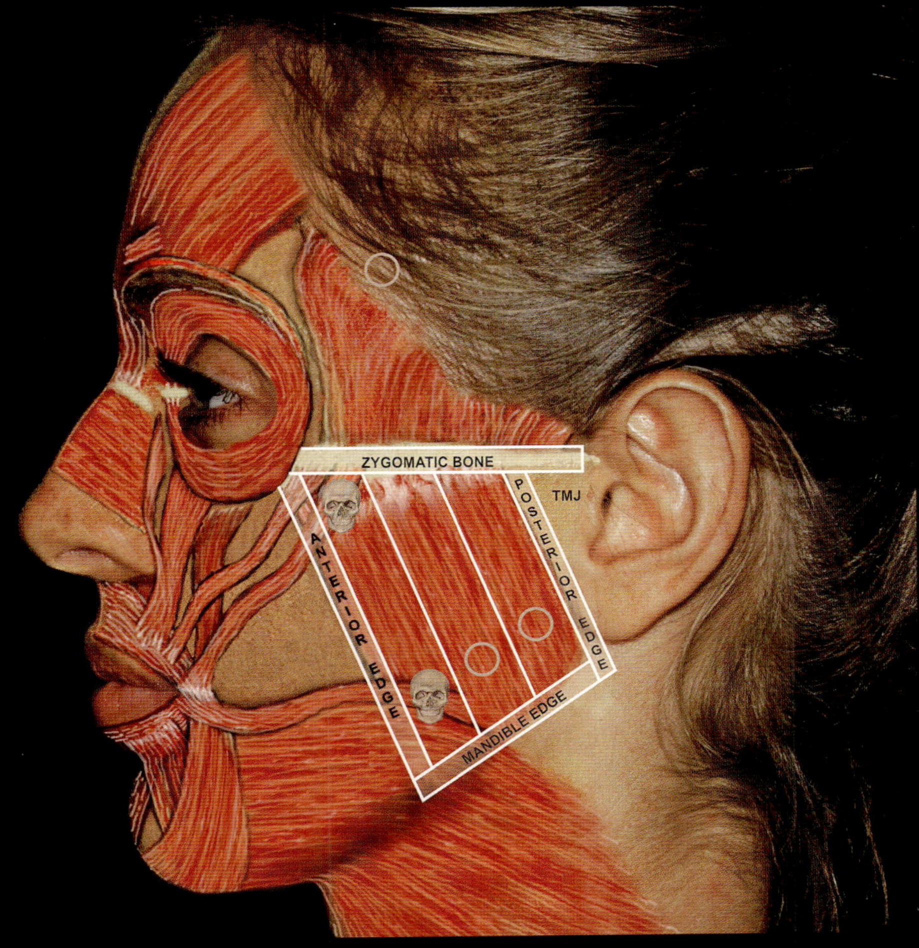

Fig 4-14 Proper marking of BTX-A injections in the masseter and temporalis muscles *(gray circles)*.

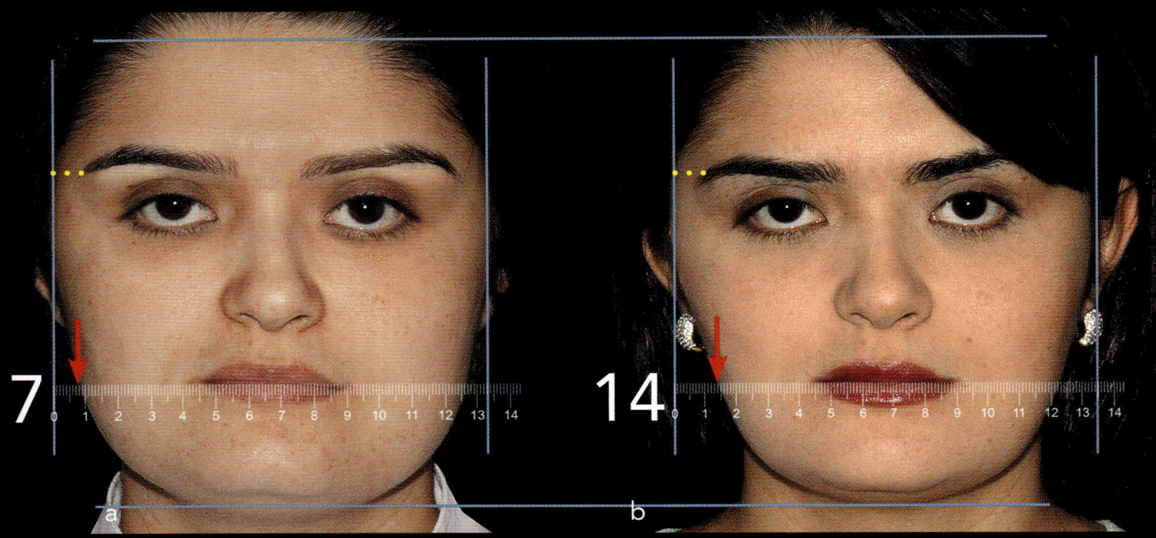

Fig 4-15 *(a and b)* Anthropometrics showing a 14-mm narrowing of the lower third 30 days after the injection.

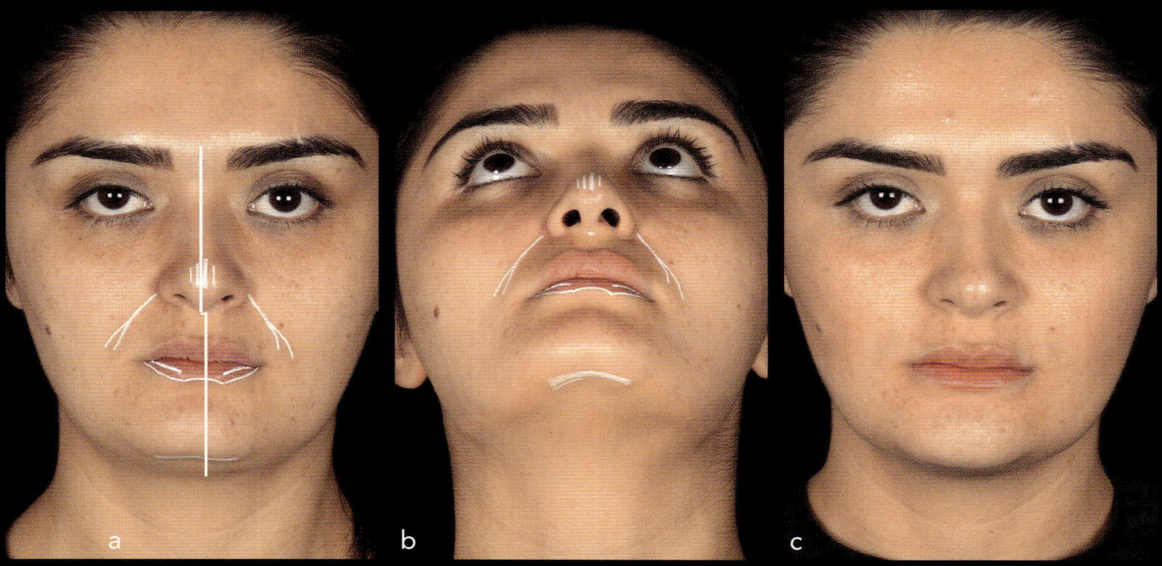

Fig 4-16 *(a)* The vertical line that connects the most anterior part of the glabella to the nasolabial angle should have the same measurement as the vertical line connecting the nasolabial angle to the lower limit of the anterior mandible. This rule suggests that the face should be longer for this patient. *(b)* The horizontal line at the base of the mentalis shows the site where filler will be injected to make the face longer and avoid frontal exposure of the submental region. *(c)* Final result after three toxin injections every 6 months and filler injections at the nasolabial sulcus, lower lip vermilion, and lower limit of the mentalis. Note the drastic change from the pretreatment view (see Fig 4-11a).

DISCUSSION: The patient reported that the pain (chief complaint) decreased 3 days after the injection and disappeared after 8 days. Although the injection was made for therapeutic reasons, a nice cosmeceutical effect was also observed: The lower third of the face was narrowed, making the mouth look bigger. The total narrowing after the first injection was 14 mm (Fig 4-15). The narrowing was even greater after the second injection, and clinical follow-up after repeated injections showed a progressive narrowing of the lower third of the face (Fig 4-16).

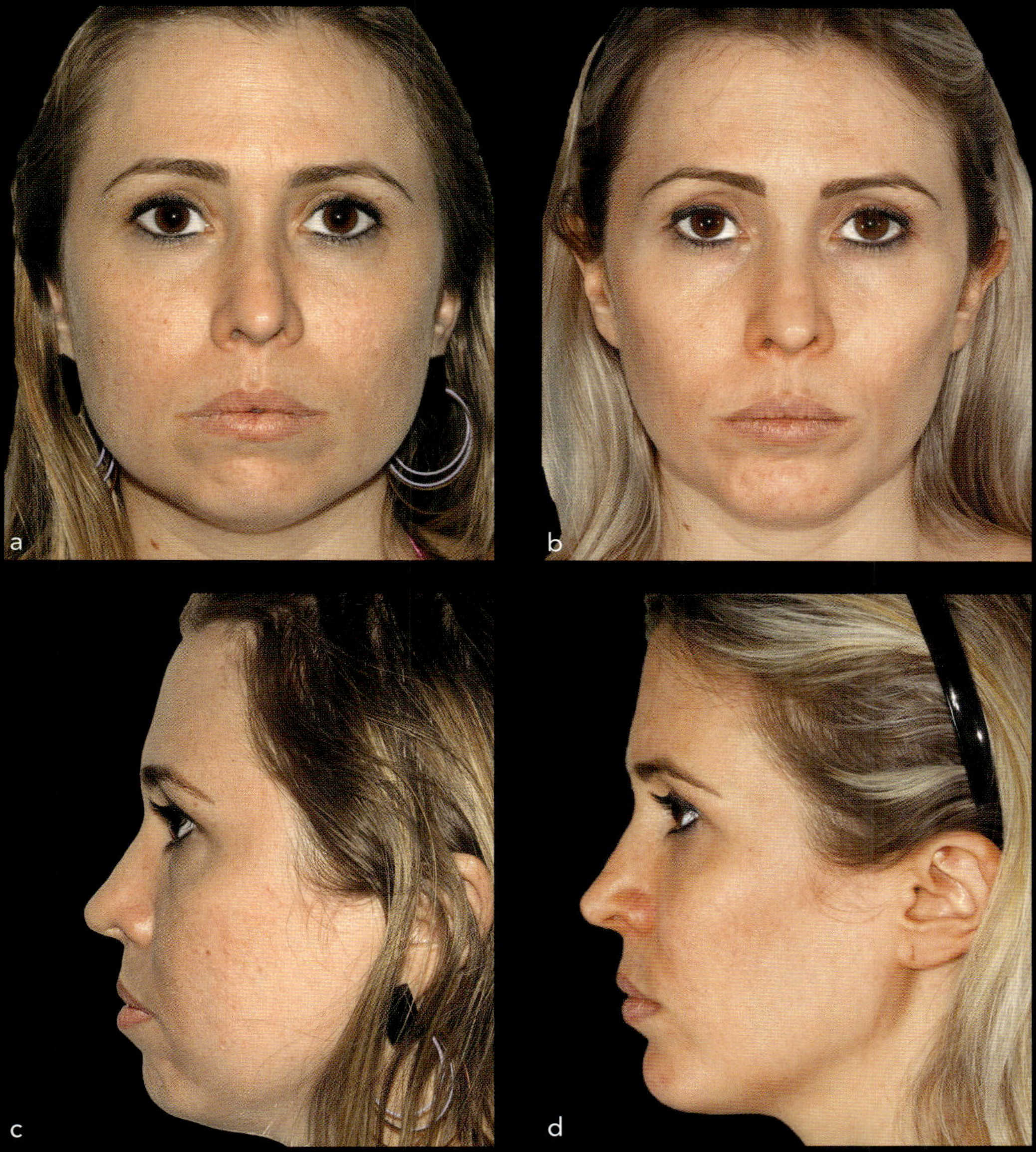

Fig 4-17 **Case 8**. *(a and c)* Pretreatment views of a patient diagnosed with masseter hypertrophy. *(b and d)* Result obtained 30 days after injecting BTX in the masseter muscles and after surgical chin advancement.

Case 8: Masseter hypertrophy

Figure 4-17 illustrates another case of masseter hypertrophy in a 32-year-old woman. The same doses and injection sites as described in Table 4-6 were used for this patient. After the author injected the BTX, the patient was referred to an oral and maxillofacial surgeon, Dr Fernando Saad, who performed her surgical chin advancement.

Conclusion

A systematic review published in 2017 indicated that despite the paucity of works on the topic, BTX-A seems to be a possible management option for sleep bruxism, minimizing symptoms and reducing the intensity of muscle contractions.[31] Of course further studies are necessary, especially as far as the treatment indications for bruxism itself are concerned.

Other possible uses of BTX in the jaw elevator muscles are the following:

- *Unilateral mastication:* Toxin is only injected on the side of the muscle that the individual preferably uses during mastication. By doing so, patients are forced to use the opposite side of their mouth. By the end of the toxin's period of action, some patients have learned bilateral mastication. By then, reinjection is no longer necessary.
- *Severe parafunctional habits in the mixed dentition:* In this case, the resting tonus of the jaw elevator muscles is increased, and the length is decreased. In theory, this could make the lower third of the face shorter. Therefore, the toxin has a preventive effect against this possibility. Besides that, it is important to consider that there is no possibility of using an acrylic nightguard for patients with mixed dentition.

While an acrylic nightguard is a popular and successful intraoral device used for the treatment of bruxism and other parafunctional habits,[32–35] its therapeutic success depends on the patient's cooperation to wear it on a daily basis. On the other hand, the use of BTX is not dependent on the patient's compliance. Furthermore, the toxin has a diurnal and nocturnal effect different from the nightguard. The ideal treatment for a patient with parafunctional habits would be to wear the nightguard and also have BTX injected in the jaw elevator muscles.

Asymmetric Smile

Case 9: Asymmetric oral commissures and buccal corridors

MAIN COMPLAINT: Esthetic deficiency in a 30-year-old man.

HISTORY OF PRESENT CONDITION: The patient complained about his asymmetric smile because he was a fashion model. He stated that he had never had an accident or a disease that could justify the current status. His medical records showed his health status to be very good.

SIGNS AND SYMPTOMS: Oral asymmetry during speech and smile (Figs 4-18a and 4-18b).

DIAGNOSIS: Excessive tension or contraction of the right levator anguli oris and zygomaticus major muscles during the smile.

FACIAL READING: Facial asymmetries are intuitively unesthetic and might adversely affect the judgment of an observer.[36–38] In this patient's case, the right oral commissure is higher than the left, the right buccal corridor is wider than the left, the right wing of the nose is higher than the left, and also the right nasolabial sulcus is more prominent than the left (see Fig 4-18b). This will require multiple treatments for correction.

PROCEDURE PRIORITY LIST FOR FIRST TREATMENT:

1. Use Botox to lower the horizontal level of the right oral commissure.
2. Use Botox to reduce the excessive width of the right buccal corridor.
3. Manufacture and place veneers on the teeth (with Dr Paula Cardoso and Dr Rafael Decurcio).
4. Refer to Dr Márcio Rocha, a plastic surgeon, to correct the protruding ears.

THERAPEUTICS: The purpose of using Botox was to promote the chemodenervation of muscles as follows (Table 4-7):

- To decrease the effect of the right levator anguli oris muscle, which elevates the commissure during the smile. This muscle was chosen instead of the left depressor anguli oris because of the posterior upper gummy smile on this side.
- To adjust the excessive contraction of the right zygomaticus major muscle. As a consequence, this would decrease or eliminate the asymmetric buccal corridor.

Figure 4-18c shows the results after the first treatment.

CAUTION: The ideal treatment for asymmetries is bilateral injections of BTX. Doses on the side with the asymmetry should be higher than the opposite side to avoid a correction that would result in further asymmetry. However, if the operator is experienced and wants to inject only on the asymmetric side, the use of very small doses ranging from 1U to 2U is recommended (see Table 4-7).

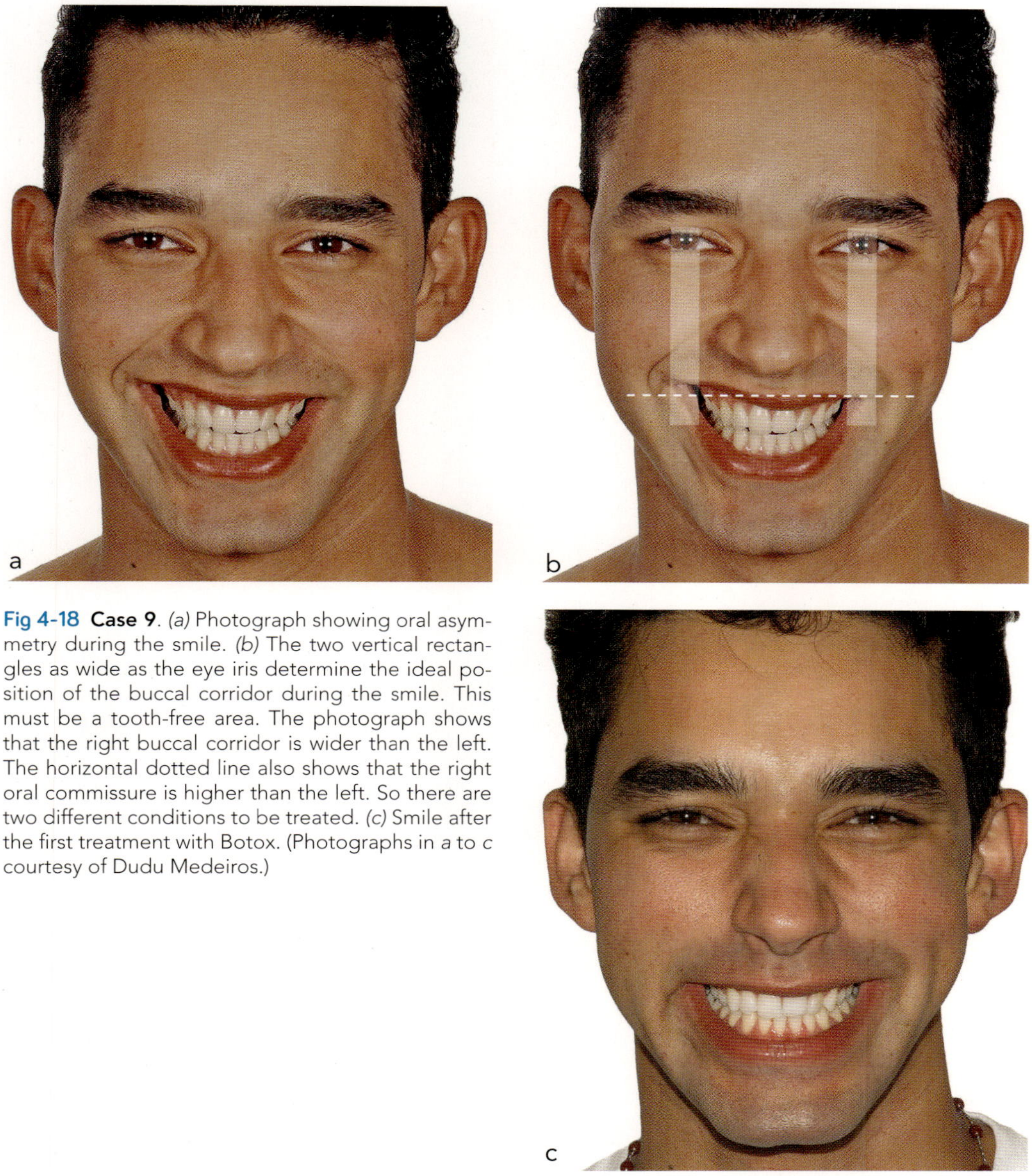

Fig 4-18 **Case 9**. *(a)* Photograph showing oral asymmetry during the smile. *(b)* The two vertical rectangles as wide as the eye iris determine the ideal position of the buccal corridor during the smile. This must be a tooth-free area. The photograph shows that the right buccal corridor is wider than the left. The horizontal dotted line also shows that the right oral commissure is higher than the left. So there are two different conditions to be treated. *(c)* Smile after the first treatment with Botox. (Photographs in *a* to *c* courtesy of Dudu Medeiros.)

→

Table 4-7 Case 9 Botox injection sites and doses

MUSCLE	DEPTH OF NEEDLE	POINTS PER MUSCLE	UNITS PER POINT	TOTAL UNITS PER MUSCLE
First treatment				
Levator anguli oris (right)	8 mm	1	2U	2U
Zygomaticus major (right)	3 mm	1	2U	2U
Second treatment				
Levator anguli oris (right)	8 mm	1	2U	2U
Zygomaticus major (right)	3 mm	1	2U	2U
Depressor labii inferioris (right)	4 mm	1	2U	2U
Depressor labii inferioris (left)	4 mm	1	2U	2U

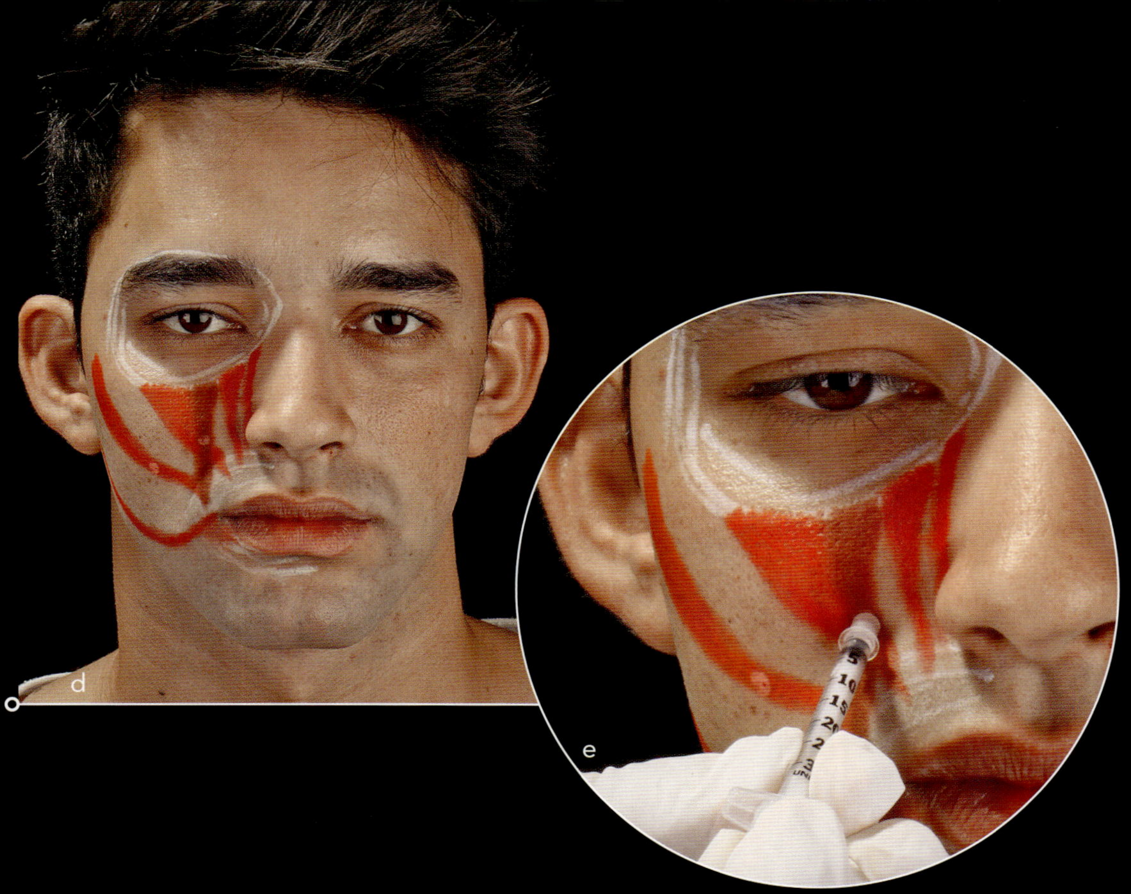

HINT:
There are two options for treatment of asymmetries at the horizontal level of the commissures. The first option is to inject toxin in the levator anguli oris muscle to lower the commissure. The second option is to inject toxin in the depressor anguli oris muscle to elevate the commissure. In order to choose the best option, the clinician should evaluate the amount of clinical crown display of the maxillary premolar. If the lip covers part of the crown during the smile, the latter option should be selected (injection in the depressor anguli oris muscle). The result would be the complete exposure of the first premolars and leveled commissures.

MARKING INJECTION POINTS: The two muscles to be injected are not found via palpation or during facial expressions. To locate the zygomaticus major, draw a line from the anterior lateral aspect of the zygomatic bone to the angle of the mouth (Figs 4-18d and 4-18e). As for the levator anguli oris muscle, the drawing begins in the angle of the mouth and vertically and medially ascends to the maxillary canine fossa (see Fig 4-18d).

PROCEDURE PRIORITY LIST FOR SECOND TREATMENT:
1. Use Botox to lower the horizontal level of the right oral commissure.
2. Use Botox to reduce the excessive width of the right buccal corridor.
3. Use Botox to raise the horizontal level of the lower lip.

Figures 4-18f to 4-18h show the results after the second treatment (see Table 4-7).

PROCEDURE PRIORITY LIST FOR THIRD TREATMENT:
1. Use Botox to lower the horizontal level of the right oral commissure.
2. Use Botox to reduce the excessive width of the right buccal corridor.
3. Use Botox to raise the horizontal level of the lower lip.

Figures 4-18i and 4-18j show the final results of treatment.

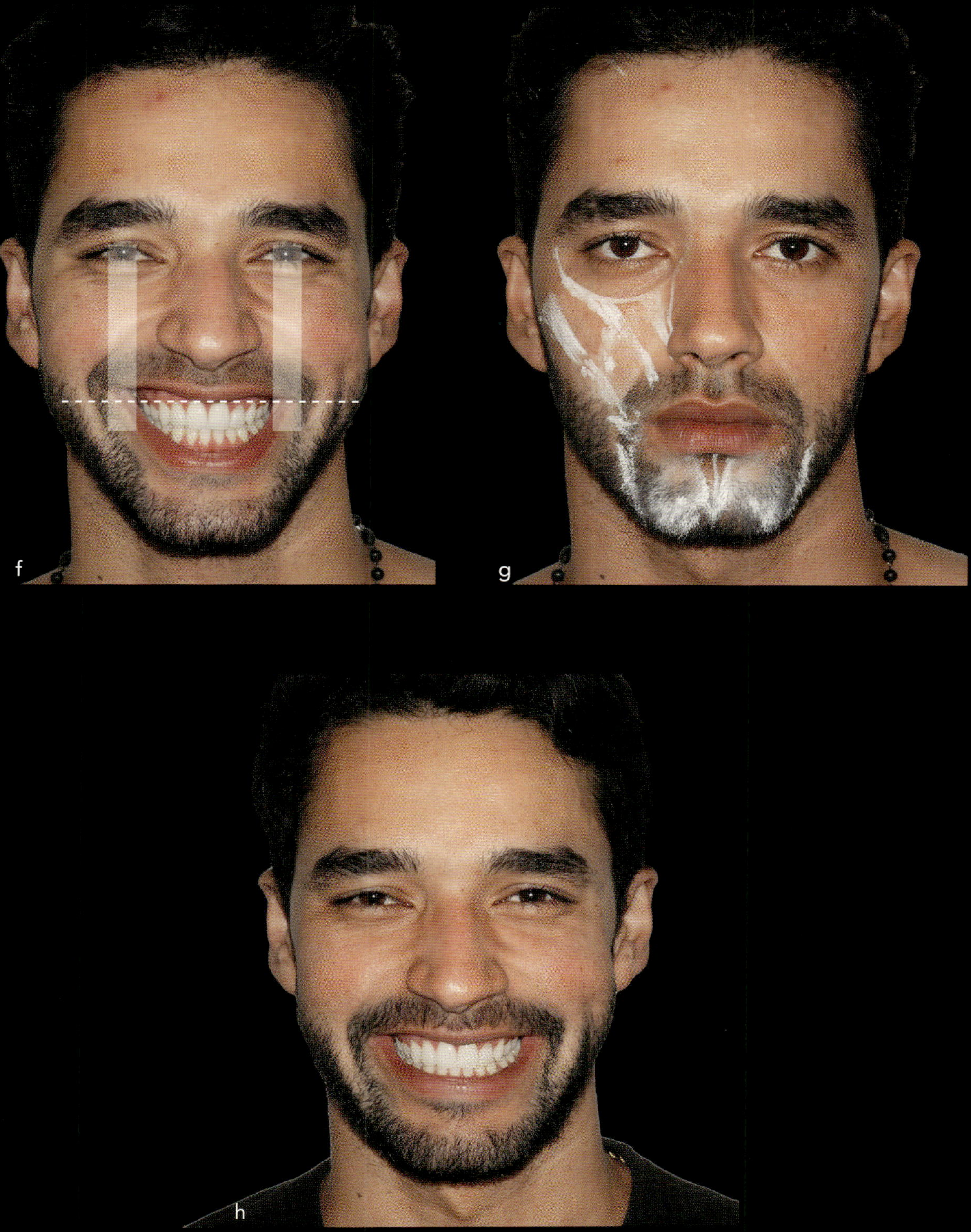

Fig 4-18 *(cont)* *(d)* Marking the injection points (in white) over the drawings of the zygomaticus major muscle (in light red because it is superficial) and the levator anguli oris muscle (dark red because it is deep). *(e)* Because the levator anguli oris muscle is deep, the needle should be inserted the full 8 mm to reach the muscle. On the other hand, because the zygomaticus major muscle is superficial, the needle should be inserted only 3 mm. (Photographs in *d* and *e* courtesy of Dr Marcus Vinícius Perillo.) *(f)* Twelve months after injecting the toxin, its effect was no longer observed. *(g)* A second drawing was made for retreatment but this time included doses to treat a lower gummy smile (see Table 4-7). Veneers were placed on the maxillary anterior teeth after the first treatment, and otoplasty was also performed prior to the second treatment. *(h)* Smile 30 days after the injections. →

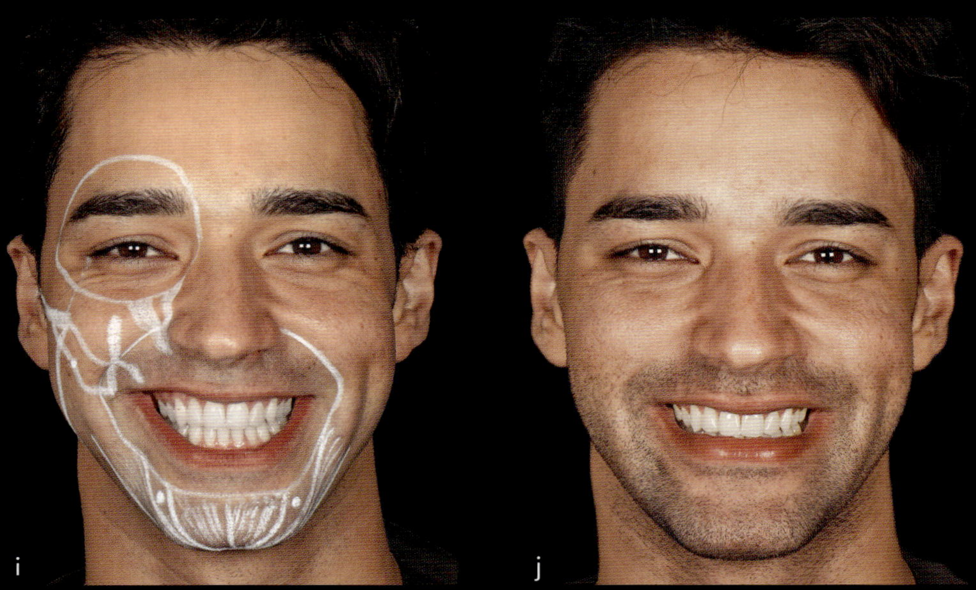

Fig 4-18 *(cont)* *(i)* Six months after the second injection, notice that the toxin effect once again is no longer observed. The muscles were drawn for the third time so injections could be made. *(j)* Results 30 days after the third treatment. Note the difference from the pretreatment smile (see part *a*).

DISCUSSION: The patient described being very happy with the asymmetry correction, as facial esthetics is fundamental in the career of a model. After the first application to correct the asymmetry, the need to also correct a lower gummy smile with bilateral injections of Botox in the depressor labii inferioris muscle was noticed. Later on, the patient was referred to plastic surgeon Dr Márcio Rocha for an otoplasty (see Fig 4-18j).

BTX injections in the upper third of the face are the easiest to perform, whereas injections in the middle third of the face are more difficult, and injections in the lower third are the most difficult. Similarly, injections to smooth wrinkles are considered easy while injections to correct asymmetries are more complex and require more knowledge. The case documented here shows that, although difficult, the technique is effective, as three applications were enough to successfully correct the asymmetry.

Another issue evidenced here is the learning curve required. When the patient first received the toxin, the gummy smile was not treated because it was not diagnosed. During the third treatment, instead of injecting only 1U as in the second visit, the dose was readjusted to 2U, which provided a better final esthetic effect by further elevating the horizontal level of the upper lip.

Case 10: Asymmetric oral commissures

Figure 4-19 shows the case of a 37-year-old man with asymmetric oral commissures but symmetric buccal corridors. Because the buccal corridors were symmetric, the zygomaticus major muscle was not treated as in case 9. However, the horizontal level of the right commissure was higher than the left commissure, displaying an unesthetic gingival band. Treatment included injection of 2U of BTX-A in the right levator anguli oris muscle as well as 2U in the right depressor labii inferioris muscle because the horizontal level of the lower lip was lower on the right side than on the left.

Conclusion

The treatment described in these cases might also be used as part of an approach to smooth unesthetic facial features of patients with facial paralysis and hemifacial spasms where these muscles are involved.

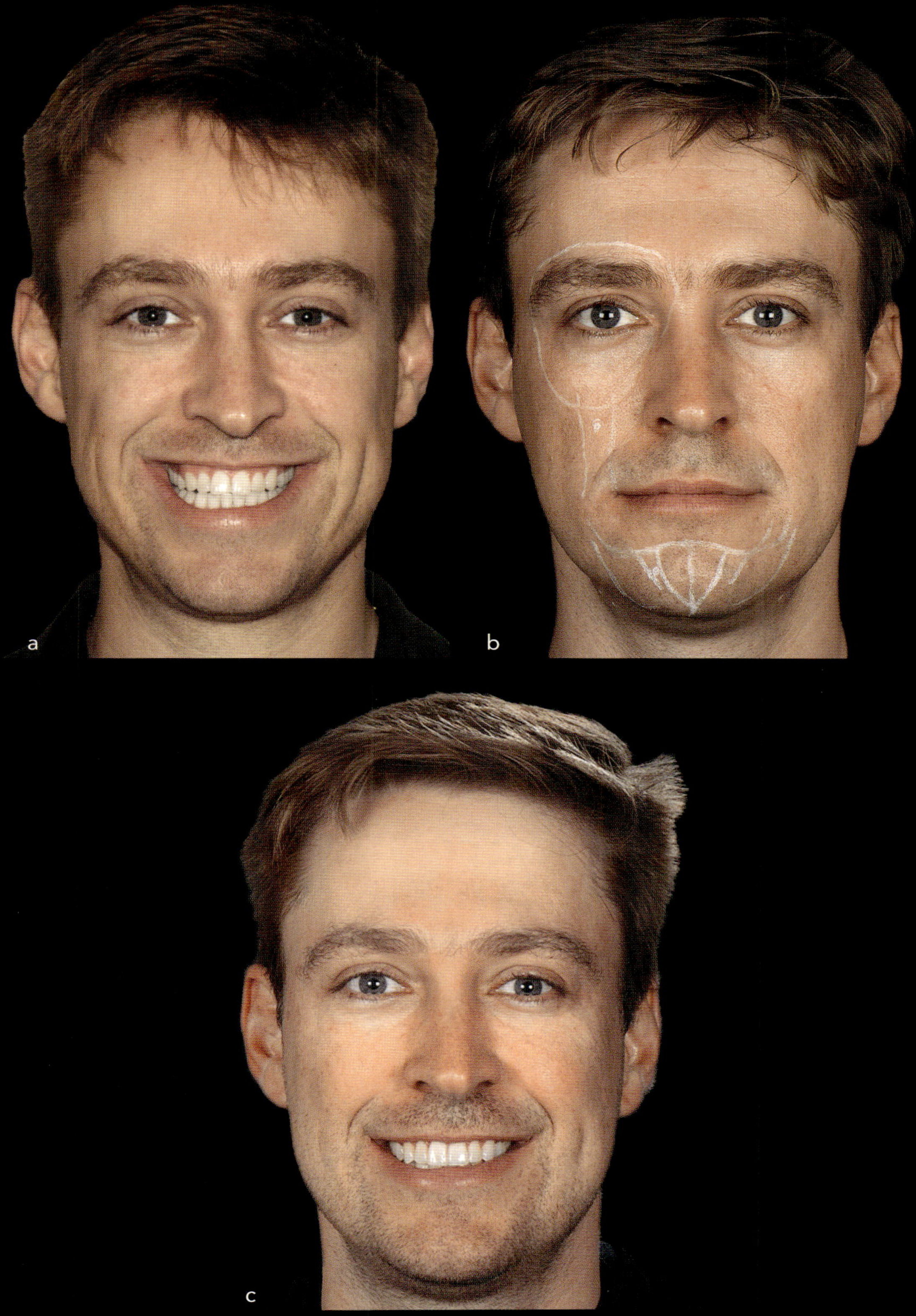

Fig 4-19 **Case 10**. *(a)* Pretreatment photograph of the patient showing an asymmetric smile. *(b)* BTX-A injection points. *(c)* Final result.

Muscle Reduction

Case 11: Unesthetic lower lip at rest

MAIN COMPLAINT: Esthetic deficiency in a 42-year-old woman.

HISTORY OF PRESENT CONDITION: The main complaint in this case was an excessive volume under the skin next to the lower lip vermilion.

SIGNS AND SYMPTOMS: A small amount of skin was visible and palpable when the facial muscles were at rest. During the smile, this unesthetic excess skin disappeared.

DIAGNOSIS: The patient reported the habit of compressing the lips during the day, mainly when she was stressed, which probably led to a hyperkinetic and increased orbicularis oris muscle. This diagnosis was confirmed because the excess was not observed during the smile due to inactivity of the orbicularis oris muscle. This area of skin excess coincided with the region where the fibers blend with the depressor labii inferioris muscle. This muscle was also hyperkinetic during the smile, as evidenced by an excessive display of the mandibular anterior teeth.

Besides the main complaint, the upper third of the face was wrinkled, and the depressor anguli oris muscle was larger than normal. These two issues were included in the treatment planning.

FACIAL READING: One of the parameters to be considered for labial esthetics is the lip eversion. Therefore, it is fundamental that the vermilion of the lips is projected more horizontally than the skin of the lip. In this case, however, the increased volume of the labial skin reduced the perception of the vermilion of the lips, thereby negatively affecting the esthetics of the mouth. Reduction of the lip vermilion is common with aging due to a loss of the collagen responsible for its volume. However, the amount of skin that encircles the lips is maintained because, contrary to the vermilion, the perioral region has muscle fibers. Thus, a patient with an increased volume of skin in relation to the vermilion will look older.

PROCEDURE PRIORITY LIST:

1. Use Botox to decrease the volume of the orbicularis oris muscle.
2. Use Botox to relax the mentalis muscle.
3. Use Botox to relax the depressor anguli oris muscle.
4. Use Botox to rejuvenate the upper third of the face.

Figures 4-20a to 4-20d compare the pretreatment and posttreatment views of the lips both closed and at rest.

THERAPEUTICS: The purpose of injecting the BTX-A was to promote the chemodenervation of the orbicularis oris muscle that presented an excessive volume under the skin of the lower lip. The toxin was injected in the site where the fibers blend with the depressor labii inferioris muscle to decrease its action, resulting in an elevation of the horizontal level of the lower lip (Figs 4-20e to 4-20g). This elevation could be observed both with the muscle at rest and during the smile (Figs 4-20h and 4-20i).

BTX-A was also injected in the depressor anguli oris muscle to decrease its excessive volume perceived during the smile as well as in the facial expression muscles in the upper third of the face to smooth wrinkles. Because the skin in the chin was slightly tensioned, creating the "golf ball" appearance and suggesting hyperactivity of the mentalis muscle, it was also included in the treatment plan. Although the protocol for injection in the mentalis muscle suggests two injection points on each side of the face, in this case only one point on each side was needed because the muscle did not present a lot of hyperactivity.

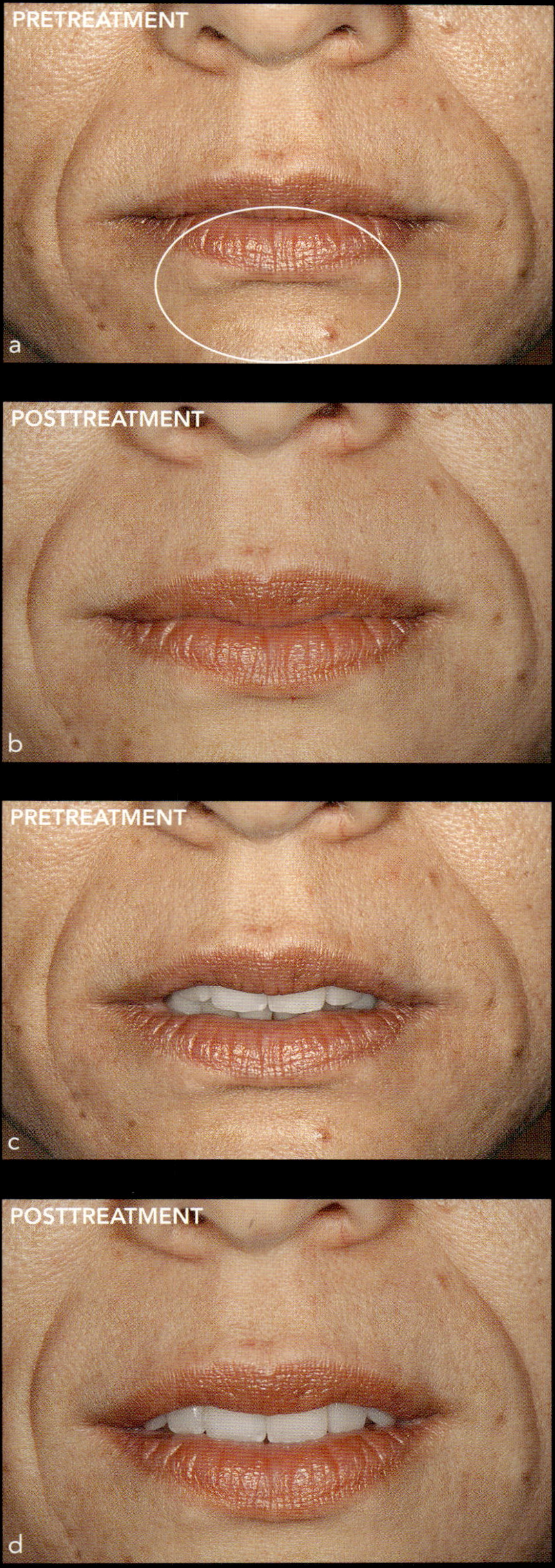

Fig 4-20 Case 11. *(a)* Pretreatment frontal view of the patient with closed lips. There is excessive bilateral volume under the skin of the lower lip. *(b)* Fifteen days after BTX-A injection, the excessive volume is improved. *(c)* Pretreatment frontal view of the patient with lips at rest. The upper border of the lower lip only touches the incisal part of the maxillary left central incisor. *(d)* Fifteen days after BTX-A injection, the upper border of the lower lip now touches the incisal edges of all anterior maxillary teeth, showing that there was an elevation of the horizontal level of the lower lip.

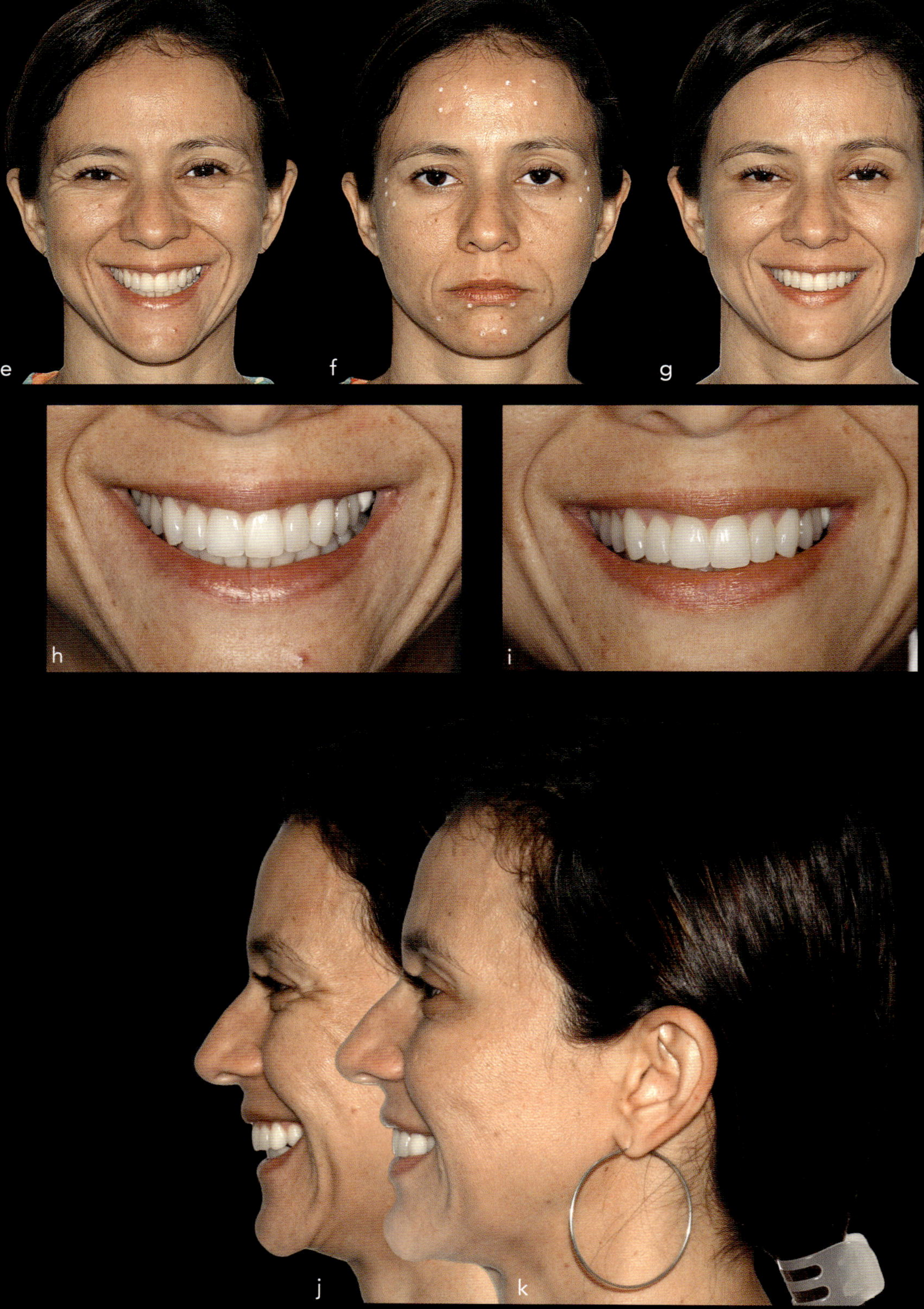

Fig 4-20 *(cont)* *(e)* Pretreatment smile. *(f)* Points marked for BTX-A injections. *(g)* Smile 15 days after BTX-A injection. *(h and i)* Smile views before and after treatment. Before treatment, the definition of the upper edge of the lower lip did not follow the incisal edge of the maxillary anterior teeth. After treatment, the horizontal level of the lower lip was elevated to where its upper edge followed the incisal contour of the maxillary anterior teeth, making the smile more harmonic. *(j and k)* Comparison of pretreatment and posttreatment profiles. The pretreatment view shows a small eversion of the lower lip and several wrinkles in the periorbicular region. The posttreatment view shows an increase in the eversion of the lower lip and accentuated reduction in the number of wrinkles in the periorbicular region.

Table 4-8 **Case 11 Botox injection sites and doses**

MUSCLE	DEPTH OF NEEDLE	POINTS PER MUSCLE	UNITS PER POINT	TOTAL UNITS PER MUSCLE
Occipitofrontalis	3 mm	8	2U	16U
Orbicularis oculi (right)	3 mm	3	2U	6U
Orbicularis oculi (left)	3 mm	3	2U	6U
Depressor labii inferioris and orbicularis oris (right)	3 mm	1	1U	1U
Depressor labii inferioris and orbicularis oris (left)	3 mm	1	1U	1U
Depressor anguli oris (right)	3 mm	1	1U	1U
Depressor anguli oris (left)	3 mm	1	1U	1U
Mentalis (right)	8 mm	1	2U	2U
Mentalis (left)	8 mm	1	2U	2U

Table 4-8 lists all of the esthetic injections performed in the same treatment appointment.

CAUTION: Inform the patient that when injected in the orbicularis oris muscle, BTX-A might temporarily affect the capacity of closing the lips, causing minor side effects such as difficulties in suction. This side effect starts 2 weeks after the injection and lasts for approximately 2 weeks. If the patient agrees to treatment, the use of small doses (0.5U–1U) of BTX-A is recommended just as a precaution.

HINT:
The toxin should be injected in the orbicularis oris muscle before any fillers are used in the vermilion of the lips. BTX-A will relax the perilabial region, making the increase in volume and eversion of the vermilion easier.

MARKING INJECTION POINTS: Inject the toxin in the skin where the volume is higher. Do not inject the toxin at the skin/vermilion limit because it will cause flattening of the labial eversion line. Do not inject toxin close to the modiolus because it will produce saliva accumulation in the commissure. Do not inject toxin close to the upper lip philtrum to avoid flattening this important anatomical structure that gives the person a young look.

DISCUSSION: Fourteen days after injecting BTX-A, the patient was very happy with the results.

By decreasing the muscle volume under the skin, the visual perception of the lip vermilion was increased. Smoothed wrinkles also gave the patient a younger look (Figs 4-20j and 4-20k).

Conclusion

BTX-A can be injected in the orbicularis oris muscle in the following situations:

- When the excessive volume of this muscle decreases the eversion of the vermilion of the lips.
- When the skin of the upper lip is wrinkled due to natural aging or prematurely wrinkled because of the habit of compressing the lips as a response to stress. Smokers also show the same problem from holding the cigarette with their lips.

No other treatment could have shown faster results for this patient, and BTX-A injection has the advantage of not being an invasive approach.

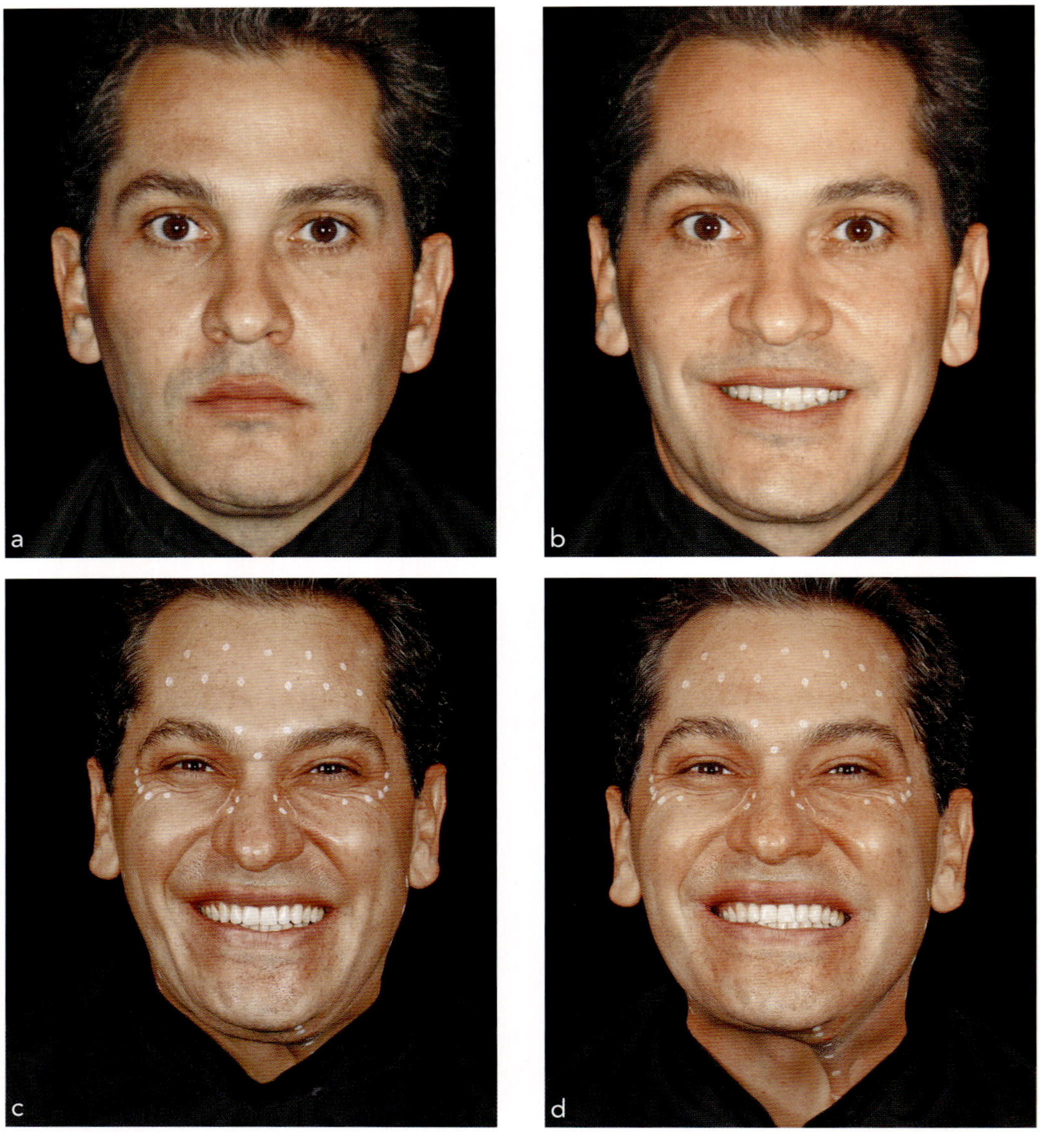

Fig 4-21 **Case 12**. *(a and b)* Pretreatment photographs of the patient. No asymmetry was observed when the lips were closed. But even during a discreet smile, a small asymmetry was noted on the left side of the lower lip, allowing partial exposure of the mandibular left lateral incisor and canine that were not displayed on the right side of the smile. *(c and d)* Injection point markings. During a spontaneous smile *(c)*, an anterior left platysmal band and discreet asymmetry in the lower lip are observed. During a forced smile *(d)*, the same aspects are present but more noticeable.

Platysma Hypertrophy

Case 12: Lip asymmetry and platysma hypertrophy

MAIN COMPLAINT: Esthetic deficiency in a 44-year-old man.

HISTORY OF PRESENT CONDITION: The patient's main complaint was a slight asymmetry of the lower lip while smiling and also an excessive volume below the chin that made shaving difficult.

Table 4-9 Case 12 Botox injection sites and doses

MUSCLE	DEPTH OF NEEDLE	POINTS PER MUSCLE	UNITS PER POINT	TOTAL UNITS PER MUSCLE
Occipitofrontalis	3 mm	11	2U	22U
Orbicularis oculi (right)	3 mm	4	2U	8U
Orbicularis oculi (left)	3 mm	4	2U	8U
Procerus	4 mm	1	4U	4U
Corrugator supercilii (left)	4 mm	1	3U	3U
Corrugator supercilii (right)	4 mm	1	3U	3U
Nasalis	2 mm	4	1U	4U
Platysma (anterior, left)	13 mm	5	2U	10U
Platysma (anterior, right)	13 mm	1	2U	2U

SIGNS AND SYMPTOMS: At rest the lips were symmetric, but when smiling the left side of the lower lip was lower than the right side. At the same time, an anterior platysmal band became more evident.

DIAGNOSIS: The most active muscle involved in the depression of the lower lip is the depressor labii inferioris. However, in this case, when the patient was asked to activate the platysma during the clinical examination, a platysmal band showed hyperkinesia. This band was on the same side as the lip asymmetry, that is, on the left side. Thus, the platysma muscle was diagnosed as responsible for the asymmetry (Figs 4-21a and 4-21b).

FACIAL READING: In the eyes of a layperson, asymmetries might be interpreted as a sign of some type of disease. It is therefore important to resolve asymmetries.

PROCEDURE PRIORITY LIST:

1. Use Botox to decrease the activity of the platysma muscle.
2. Use Botox to decrease the activity of the masseter muscle.
3. Use Botox to decrease the activity of the nasalis muscle.
4. Use Botox to smooth wrinkles in the upper third of the face.

Figures 4-21c and 4-21d show the injection sites.

THERAPEUTICS: The purpose of using BTX-A was to decrease the excessive contraction in one anterior platysmal band on the left side and to minimize the asymmetry in the lower lip (Table 4-9).

CAUTION: It is important to pay attention to the depth of the platysma muscle in relation to the skin. In an individual with an adequate body weight, there is a fat layer approximately 6 mm thick between the skin and the platysma muscle. Thus, to inject BTX-A in the muscle, the whole 13-mm needle should be inserted to cross the skin and fat layers so that the needle bevel in fact penetrates the muscle (Fig 4-22). A 13-mm needle should be inserted but should not depress the skin of the neck (deeply forcing the needle hub) because it would unnecessarily insert the needle deeper.

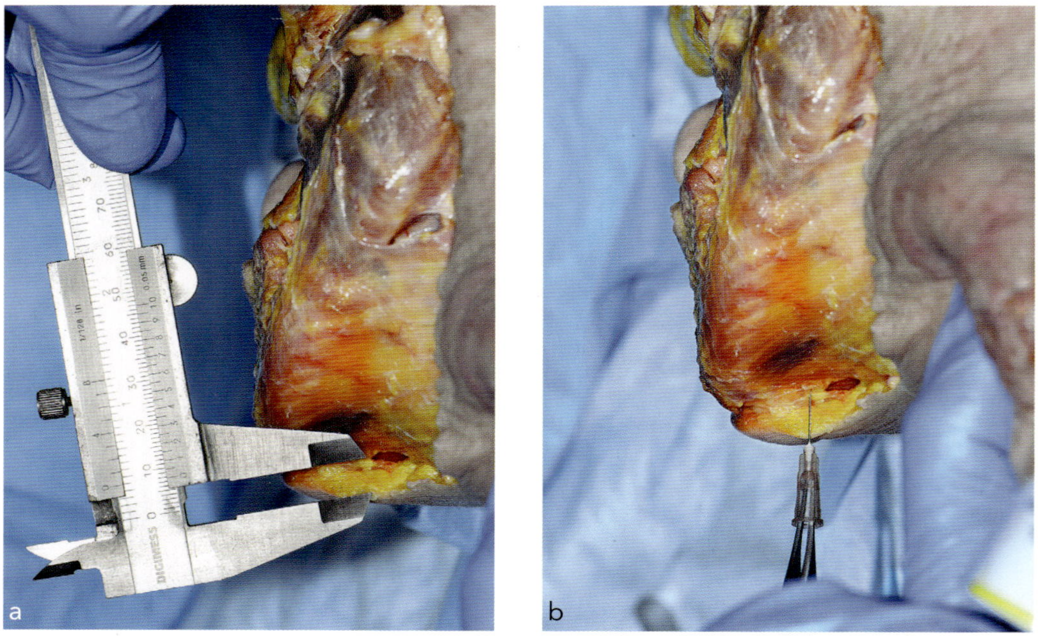

Fig 4-22 Two photos of the same fresh cadaver from the posterior to the anterior direction. The skin of the neck, platysma, and submental fat can be observed in the dissected face. *(a)* Measuring the thickness of the submental fat layer using a mechanical caliper (7.8 mm). *(b)* Simulating an injection with a 13-mm needle.

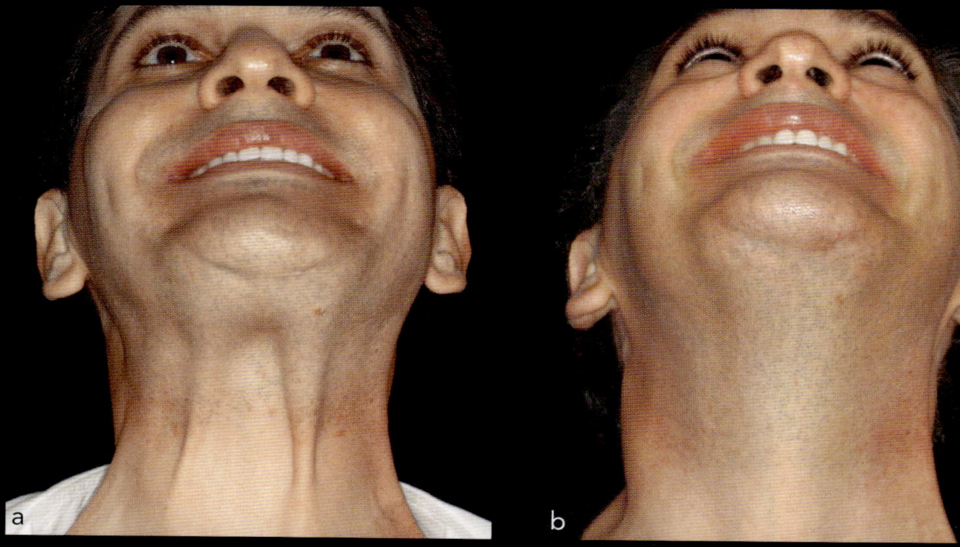

Fig 4-23 *(a and b)* Comparison of the pretreatment and posttreatment views of the neck shows the effect of BTX-A injection on the hyperkinetic platysmal bands. Before treatment, anterior hyperkinetic platysmal bands caused an increased volume in the submental region. The left anterior band presented a higher volume. After treatment, excessive volume is no longer observed in the submental region. The anterior bands are no longer detached from the other parts of the platysma muscle. *(c and d)* Comparison of the pretreatment and posttreatment views at rest. Note the change in the definition of the jawline.

Although the toxin can be used for the treatment of dysphagia and dysphonia, if injected in the platysma, it could lead to difficulty in swallowing and changes in the vocal cords.[39–45] Dysphagia could be manifested by a difficulty in swallowing saliva or, in more severe cases, a difficulty in food deglutition.[41] These adverse effects occur when the suprahyoid muscles are affected. The mylohyoid and geniohyoid muscles facilitate deglutition by pulling the hyoid bone upward and the larynx along with it. In cases of dysphonia, the depth to be injected has to be even greater, going beyond the cricothyroid membrane.[43]

HINT:
BTX-A injections in the platysma muscle should be recommended when this muscle is active during speech and/or while smiling. While asking the patient to force the musculature is standard practice to determine the injection points to be marked, this procedure should not be followed to diagnose the need for BTX-A.

MARKING INJECTION POINTS: Two to three BTX-A injection points can be marked in the hyperkinetic platysmal band (see Fig 4-21d).

DISCUSSION: The decrease in muscular activity of the hyperkinetic platysmal bands allowed for elevation of the horizontal level of the lower lip. This elevation was greater on the left side because a higher dose of BTX-A was injected. This decrease in muscular activity of the hyperkinetic platysmal bands led to a regular and homogenous definition of the neck (Fig 4-23). The patient reported that after treatment, shaving became an easy task.

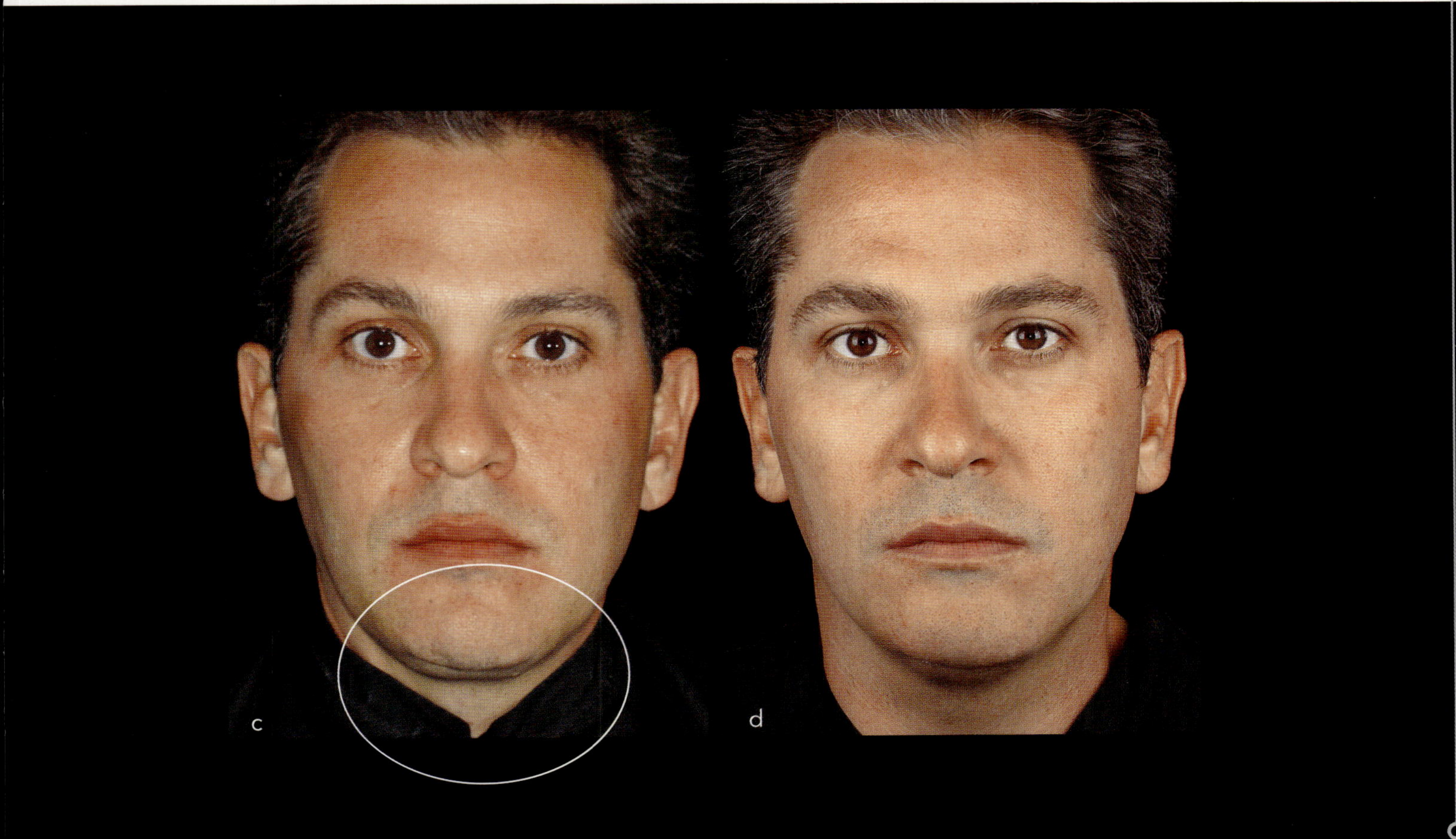

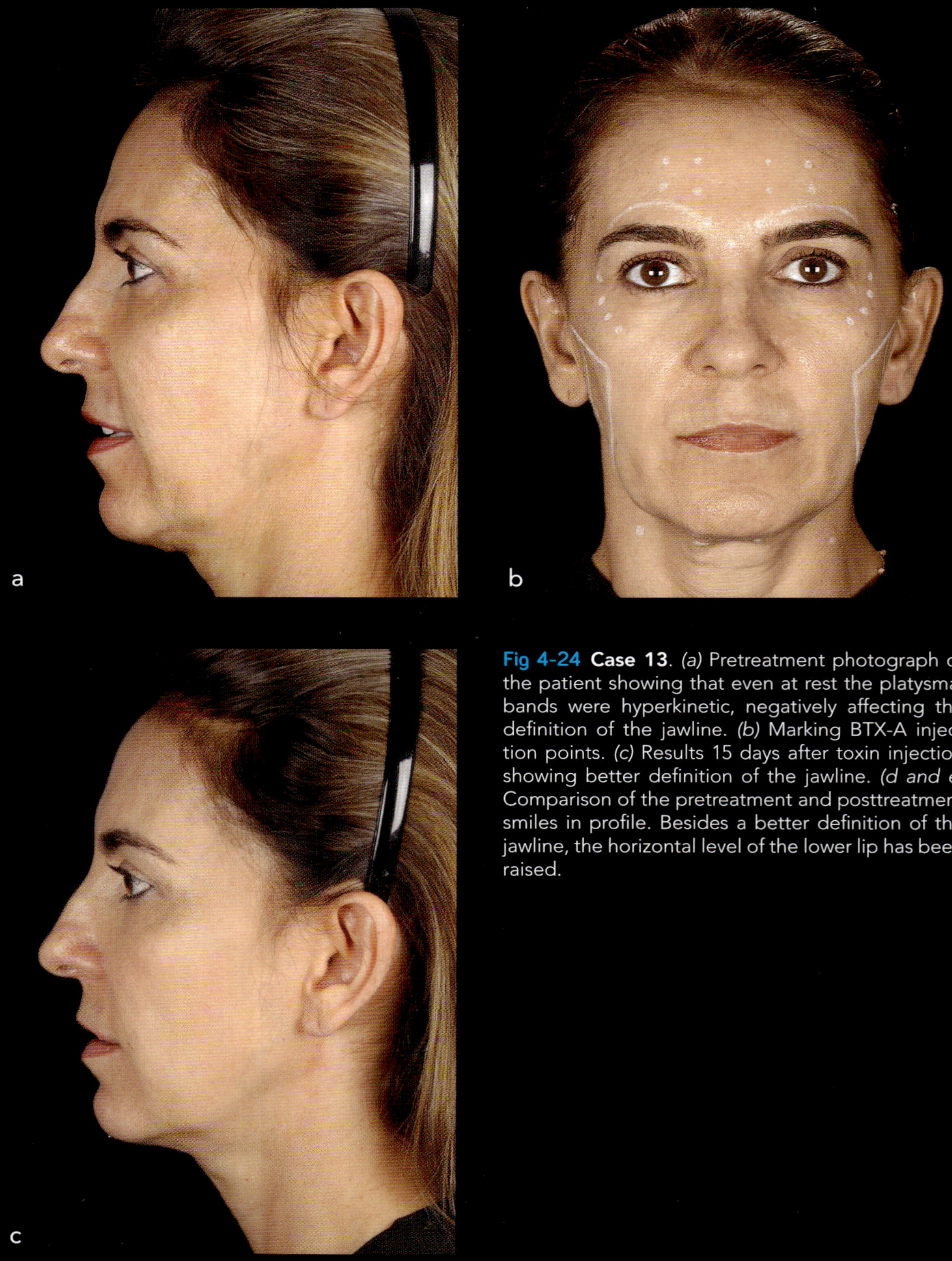

Fig 4-24 **Case 13**. *(a)* Pretreatment photograph of the patient showing that even at rest the platysmal bands were hyperkinetic, negatively affecting the definition of the jawline. *(b)* Marking BTX-A injection points. *(c)* Results 15 days after toxin injection showing better definition of the jawline. *(d and e)* Comparison of the pretreatment and posttreatment smiles in profile. Besides a better definition of the jawline, the horizontal level of the lower lip has been raised.

Case 13: Platysma hypertrophy

Figure 4-24 illustrates the case of a 46-year-old woman diagnosed with hyperkinetic platysmal bands. Besides injections to smooth wrinkles in the upper third of the face, each hyperkinetic platysmal band received only one BTX-A injection. Three units of BTX-A were injected at each point.

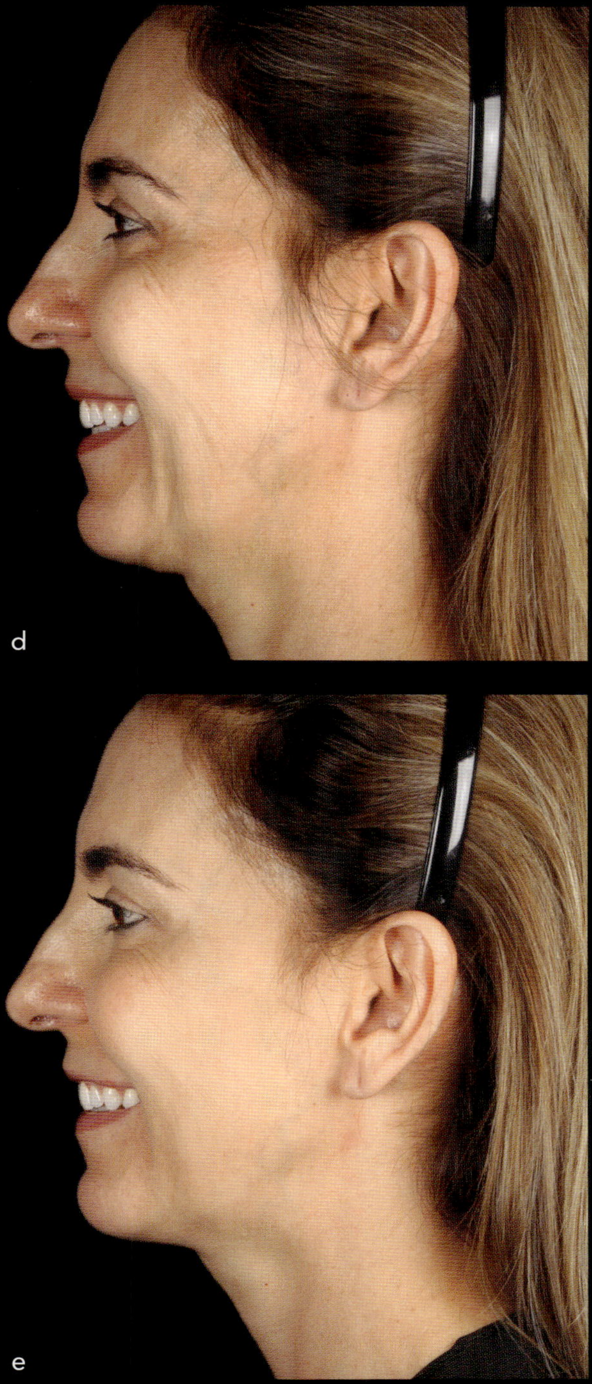

d

e

Conclusion

BTX-A injections in the platysma muscle should be administered as follows:

- When this muscle is hyperkinetic during speech or while smiling
- When the tonus of the muscle is increased even at rest
- To correct minor horizontal level asymmetries between the right and left lower lip
- When the goal is to slightly elevate the lower lip

The expected results are better visual definition of the mandible and neck and slight elevation of the horizontal level of the lower lip.

References

1. Carruthers J, Carruthers A. Complications of botulinum toxin type A. Facial Plast Surg Clin North Am 2007;15:51–54.
2. Başar E, Arici C. Use of botulinum neurotoxin in ophthalmology. Turk J Ophthalmol 2016;46:282–290.
3. Tsui JK. Botulinum toxin as a therapeutic agent. Pharmacol Ther 1996;72:13–24.
4. Kaynak-Hekimhan P. Noncosmetic periocular therapeutic applications of botulinum toxin. Middle East Afr J Ophthalmol 2010;17:113–120.
5. Monheit G, Carruthers A, Brandt F, Rand R. A randomized, double-blind, placebo-controlled study of botulinum toxin type A for the treatment of glabellar lines: Determination of optimal dose. Dermatol Surg 2007;33(special issue):S51–S59.
6. Kane MA, Brandt F, Rohrich RJ, Narins RS, Monheit GD, Huber MB; Reloxin Investigational Group. Evaluation of variable-dose treatment with a new U.S. Botulinum Toxin Type A (Dysport) for correction of moderate to severe glabellar lines: Results from a phase III, randomized, double-blind, placebo controlled study. Plast Reconstr Surg 2009;124:1619–1629.
7. Klein AW. Contraindications and complications with the use of botulinum toxin. Clin Dermatol 2004;22:66–75.
8. Klein AW. Complications and adverse reactions with the use of botulinum toxin. Dis Mon 2002;48:336–356.
9. Zagui RM, Matayoshi S, Moura FC. Efeitos adversos associados à aplicação de toxina botulínica na face: Revisão sistemática com meta-análise. Arq Bras Oftalmol 2008;71:894–901.
10. Carruthers JA, Lowe NJ, Menter MA, et al; BOTOX Glabella Lines I Study Group. A multicenter, double-blind, randomized, placebo-controlled study of the efficacy and safety of botulinum toxin type A in the treatment of glabellar lines. J Am Acad Dermatol 2002;46:840–849.
11. Dutton JJ. Botulinum-A toxin in the treatment of craniocervical muscle spasms: Short- and long-term, local and systemic effects. Surv Ophthalmol 1996;41:51–65.
12. Klein AW. Complications and adverse reactions with the use of botulinum toxin. Semin Cutan Med Surg 2001;20:109–120.
13. Wijemanne S, Vijayakumar D, Jankovic J. Apraclonidine in the treatment of ptosis. J Neurol Sci 2017;376:129–132.
14. Ricci LH, Navajas SV, Carneiro PR, Söderberg SA, Ferraz CA. Ocular adverse effects after facial cosmetic procedures: A review of case reports. J Cosmet Dermatol 2015;14:145–151.
15. Zheng L, Azar D. Angle-closure glaucoma following periorbital botulinum toxin injection. Clin Exp Ophthalmol 2014;42:690–693.
16. Corridan P, Nightingale S, Mashoudi N, Williams AC. Acute angle-closure glaucoma following botulinum toxin injection for blepharospasm. Br J Ophthalmol 1990;74:309–310.
17. Liu M, Lee HC, Hertle RW, Ho AC. Retinal detachment from inadvertent intraocular injection of botulinum toxin A. Am J Ophthalmol 2004;137:201–202.
18. Coté TR, Mohan AK, Polder JA, Walton MK, Braun MM. Botulinum toxin type A injections: Adverse events reported to the US Food and Drug Administration in therapeutic and cosmetic cases. J Am Acad Dermatol 2005;53:407–415.
19. Yamauchi PS. Selection and preference for botulinum toxins in the management of photoaging and facial lines: Patient and physician considerations. Patient Prefer Adherence 2010;4:345–354.
20. Dutra MB, Ritter DE, Borgatto A, Derech CD, Rocha R. Influência da exposição gengival na estética do sorriso. Dental Press J Orthod 2011;16:111–118.
21. Pires CV, Souza CGLG, Menezes SAF. Periodontal plastic procedures in patients with gummy smile: Case report [in Portuguese]. Revista Periodontia 2010;20:48–53.
22. Seixas MR, Costa-Pinto RA, Araújo TM. Checklist dos aspectos estéticos a serem considerados no diagnóstico e tratamento do sorriso gengival. Dental Press J Orthod 2011;16:131–157.
23. Oliveira MT, Molina GO, Molina RO. Sorriso gengival, quando a toxina botulínica pode ser utilizada. Revista Odontol Araçatuba 2011;32:58–61.
24. Al-Fouzan AF, Mokeem LS, Al-Saqat RT, Alfalah MA, Alharbi MA, Al-Samary AE. Botulinum toxin for the treatment of gummy smile. J Contemp Dent Pract 2017;18:474–478.
25. Martins BK. Respiração bucal: Uma abordagem multidisciplinar [thesis]. Florianópolis: Universidade Federal de Santa Catarina, 1999.
26. Guerrer EJ. Respiração bucal: Suas causas e consequências. São Paulo: CEFAC, 2000.
27. Rodrigues SFS. Respiração bucal: Implicações biológicas, fisiológicas e ortopédicas [master thesis]. Porto, Portugal: Universidade Fernando Pessoa, 2014.
28. Freitas RS, Pessoa TJL, Tolazzi ARD, Postai G. Release of the nasal septum depressor muscle for treatment of gingivous smile [in Portuguese]. Rev Soc Bras Cir Craniomaxilofac 2006;9:1–5.
29. Rabelo CC. Libertação do músculo depressor do septo nasal e sorriso gengival. O Jornal Dentistry 2014:26–28.
30. Doncatto L, Schwantz PE. Volumetric analysis of facial proportions in male and female faces. Arquivos Catarinenses de Medicina 2012;41:53–56.
31. De la Torre Canales G, Câmara-Souza MB, do Amaral CF, Garcia RC, Manfredini D. Is there enough evidence to use botulinum toxin injections for bruxism management? A systematic literature review. Clin Oral Investig 2017;21:727–734.
32. Kato T, Thie NM, Montplaisir JY, Lavigne GJ. Bruxism and orofacial movements during sleep. Dent Clin North Am 2001;45:657–684.
33. Tanaka EE, Arita, ES, Shibayama B. Occlusal stabilization appliance: Evaluation of its efficacy in the treatment of temporomandibular disorders. J Appl Oral Sci 2004;12:238–243.
34. Fernandes Neto AJ, Barbosa GAS. Placas oclusais. Federal University of Uberlândia, Brazil, 2006.
35. de Lima DG, Douglas de Oliveira DW, de Oliveira ES, Gonçalves PF, Flecha OD. Placas estabilizadoras em pacientes portadores de DTM: Relato de dois casos. Rev Bras Odontol 2016;73:261–264.

36. Nagi R, Patil DJ, Sahu S, Jain S, Naidu GS. Botulinum toxin in the management of head and neck disorders. Oral Surg Oral Med Oral Pathol Oral Radiol 2017;23:419–428.
37. Cooper L, Lui M, Nduka C. Botulinum toxin treatment for facial palsy: A systematic review. J Plast Reconstr Aesthet Surg 2017;70:833–841.
38. Sahan A, Tamer F. Restoring facial symmetry through non-surgical cosmetic procedures after permanent facial paralysis: A case report. Acta Dermatovenerol Alp Pannonica Adriat 2017;26:41–42.
39. Abramowicz M, Zuccotti G. Botulinum toxin (Botox® cosmetic) for frown lines. Med Lett Drugs Therapeutics 2002;44:47–48.
40. Larrosa F, Idígora A, Aguilar F, Riera L, Martí MJ, Valls J. Resultados de la aplicación de toxina botulínica en el tratamiento de la disfonía espasmódica. Acta Otorrinolaringol Esp 2002;53:27–31.
41. Moguel-Ancheita S, Dixon-Olvera S, Martínez-Oropeza S, Orozco-Gómez LP. Botulinum toxin as a treatment for strabismus in systemic diseases [in Spanish]. Arch Soc Esp Oftalmol 2003;78:9–14.
42. Persaud R, Garas G, Silva S, Stamatoglou C, Chatrath K, Patel K. An evidence-based review of botulinum toxin (Botox) applications in non-cosmetic head and neck conditions. JRSM Short Rep 2013;4:10.
43. Chhetri DK, Jamal N. Percutaneous injection laryngoplasty. Laryngoscope 2014;124:742–745.
44. Park KS, Lee CH, Lee JW. Use of a botulinum toxin A in dentistry and oral and maxillofacial surgery. J Dent Anesth Pain Med 2016;16:151–157.
45. Awan KH. The therapeutic usage of botulinum toxin (Botox) in non-cosmetic head and neck conditions—An evidence based review. Saudi Pharm J 2017;25:18–24.

Index

Page references followed by "f" denote figures; those followed by "b" denote boxes; and those followed by "t" denote tables.

E

F

G

H

I

J

L

M

N

O

P

R

S

T

U

W

X

Z